P9-DVF-740

ORGANOPHOSPHATES AND HEALTH

ORGANOPHOSPHATES AND HEALTH

Editors

Lakshman Karalliedde
Guy's & St. Thomas' Hospital Trust, UK

Stanley Feldman
John Henry
Imperial College School of Medicine, UK

Timothy Marrs
Food Standards Agency, UK

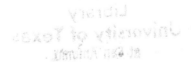

Imperial College Press

Published by

Imperial College Press
57 Shelton Street
Covent Garden
London WC2H 9HE

Distributed by

World Scientific Publishing Co. Pte. Ltd.
P O Box 128, Farrer Road, Singapore 912805
USA office: Suite 1B, 1060 Main Street, River Edge, NJ 07661
UK office: 57 Shelton Street, Covent Garden, London WC2H 9HE

British Library Cataloguing-in-Publication Data
A catalogue record for this book is available from the British Library.

ORGANOPHOSPHATES AND HEALTH

ISBN 1-86094-270-9

Printed in Singapore by World Scientific Printers (S) Pte Ltd

DEDICATION

To our parents, departed and alive, who continue to inspire us.

PREFACE

Without pesticides many millions of the earth's poorest people would be condemned to die from disease and starvation. At present organophosphates are the most effective means of reducing to 30% the proportion of crops that are destroyed by pests and controlling the vectors of diseases such as malaria, filariasis, sleeping sickness, dengue fever and the greatest cause of preventable blindness: trachoma. Unfortunately the price paid in human terms is high. The WHO figures (a gross underestimate in all probability) suggests that each year 3 million people are treated for the effects of OP poisoning of whom 20,000-40,000 die. Unfortunately there is too little co-ordinated research to allow us to know the true extent of the ill health and death rate associated with their use.

Many of the deaths are due to self administration in order to commit suicide. This is especially common in young people in poor rural communities in the Indian subcontinent.

Any agent that kills insects by interfering with its fundamental physiology is going to be lethal, in sufficient dose, in humans. Paracelsus observed that *'all things are poisons and nothing is without poison; the dose alone makes a thing poisonous'*. Indeed oxygen, at high concentrations and water and salt in excessive doses can kill. In the ranking of poisons and substances in our environment the OP pesticides, especially the newer ones, would rank some way down, alongside many domestic products.

OP pesticides are potentially poisonous but whilst Western Nations concern themselves with the possible side-effects of chronic exposure to minute residues of pesticides on the surface of fruits and vegetables, in the Indian subcontinent and Africa they are burying thousands of victims of OP poisoning. This does not diminish the seriousness of the problems of chronic or sub-clinical exposure some of which are real, some probable and others unlikely, nor does it lessen the importance of a possible temporary disturbance to the ecological balance. It does expose the size and nature of the real problem which is less a consequence of the inherent toxicity of the OP pesticides than their misuse. It is a result of those plagues of the developing world - illiteracy, economic deprivation and poverty.

Scientists are producing newer, less toxic agents, however, these are invariably more expensive and therefore unlikely to be readily available in countries with a lack of foreign reserves. As a consequence older and more toxic poisons are used. Whilst committees meet in air-conditioned suites to deliberate on safety criteria, the necessary protective clothing, mixing precautions and safety measures, most of those using these agents live in hot swampy environments where protective clothing, were it available, would be impracticable or add to their discomfort. Even if the safety precautions were printed in many languages it is probable that the peasant farmer would be unable to read them. Instructions to dispose of containers safely are likely to be disregarded when it makes a convenient bucket for someone to whom a water bucket costs a week's wages. When a whole family lives in one room it is impossible to ensure the sack of pesticide is not stored next to the sack of rice.

Without OP pesticides millions would die. The problem with their use is not only due to their inherent toxicity but is also the consequence of illiteracy, hunger and poverty which turns them into a potent cause of death and ill health in the developing world.

It is our intention in this book to present current information associated with OP pesticides with a view to stimulating research and study to narrow the vast gaps in our knowledge.

ACKNOWLEDGEMENTS

We wish to thank Jennifer Butler who spent tedious hours formatting the scripts and Nicola Bates for helping with the Index. We have tried their patience and tolerance to a maximum. To Helaina Checketts our thanks for helping with the literature. Wendy Cox and the staff of the Information Section of the Poison Centre London and the Medical Toxicology Unit for assistance in numerous ways. LK wishes to thank Nimal Senanayake for introducing him to organophosphates and to Professor Tony Adams of Guy's for opening many doors for him. TM thanks Andrew Wadge for encouraging his work. Lastly we wish to thank Geetha Nair of Imperial College Press for co-ordinating all activities associated with this book.

CONTENTS

LIST OF CONTRIBUTORS

Dr Jan L. de Bleecker, MD, PhD. Department of Neurology, University Hospital, B-9000 Gent, Belgium.

Professor Jeffrey Brent, MD, PhD, FACEP, FAACT, Associate Clinical Professor of Medicine, Surgery and paediatrics, University of Colorado Health Sciences Center, Toxicology Associates, 2555 South Downing, Suite 260, Denver, Colorado USA.

Dr Michael Eddleston, PhD. Research Fellow, Centre for Tropical Medicine, University of Oxford, Oxford.

Dr Philippa Edwards, PhD, Department of Health, Skipton House, London SE1 6LW.

Professor Stanley Feldman, BSc, MBBS, FRCA. Emeritus Professor of Anaesthesia, Imperial College School of Medicine, London.

Professor J.A. Henry, FRCP, FFAEM. Academic Department of Accident and Emergency Medicine, Imperial College School of Medicine, St Mary's Hospital, London.

Dr Elwood F. Hill, Wildlife Toxicologist, Adjunct Professor, University Center for Environmental Sciences and Engineering, University of Nevada, Reno, PO Box 1615, Gardnerville, Nevada 89410, USA.

Dr Marcus A. Jackson, MD. Senior Toxicologist, Alpha Gamma Technologies Inc, Raleigh, North Carolina, USA.

Dr Lakshman Karalliedde MBBS, DA, FRCA. Consultant, Medical Toxicology Unit, Guy's and St Thomas' Hospital Trust, London.

Dr Laura Klein, MD. Toxicology Associates, 2555 South Downing, Suite 260, Denver, Colorado USA.

Professor Malcolm Lader, *OBE*, DSc, PhD, MD, FRCPsych, F Med. Sci. Professor of Clinical Psychopharmacology, Institute of Psychiatry, London SE5 8AF.

Professor Marcello Lotti, MD. Dipartimentò di Medicina Ambientale e Sanita Pubblica, Università Degli Studi Di Padova, Via Giustiniani, 2-35128, Padova, Italy.

Dr Timothy C. Marrs, MD, DSc, MRCP, FRCPath, FATS, Senior Medical Officer, Food Standards Agency, Department of Health, Skipton House, London SE1 6LW.

Dr Robert L. Maynard, *CBE*, BSc, MBBCh, FRCPath. Senior Medical Officer Department of Health, Skipton House, London SE1 6LW.

Dr Timothy Meredith, MD FRCP FAACT Coordinator, International Programme on Chemical Safety, UNEP/ILO/WHO, CH-1211, Geneva 27, Switzerland.

Professor Angelo Moretto, MD, Dipartimento di Medicina Ambientale e Sanita Pubblica, Università Degli Studi Di Padova, Via Giustiniani, 2-35128, Padova , Italy.

Dr Virginia Murray, SSStJ: MSc, FFOM, FRCP, FRCPath, FRIPHH. Director, Chemical Incident Response Service, Deputy Medical Director, Medical Toxicology Unit, Consultant, Occupational and Environmental Toxicologist, Medical Toxicology Unit, Guy's and St Thomas' Hospital Trust, Avonley Road, London SE14 5ER.

Professor A.M. Saadeh, MD, FRCPE. Associate Professor of Medicine, Chairman of Internal Medicine, Faculty of Medicine, Jordan University of Science and Technology, PO Box 3030, Irbid, Jordan.

Professor Nimal Senanayake, MD, PhD, DSc, FRCP, FRCPE, FCCP. Senior Professor of Medicine and Head, Department of Medicine, Faculty of Medicine, Peradeniya, Sri Lanka.

Dr H. Frank Stack, MD. Alpha Gamma Technologies Inc, Raleigh, North Carolina, USA.

Professor R. Swaminathan, MBBS, PhD, MSc, MRCPath, FRCPA, FRCPath. Professor and Chairman, Department of Chemical Pathology, United Medical and Dental Schools of Guy's and St Thomas Hospitals, London.

Professor Dr Ladislaus Szinicz, MD. Institute of Pharmacology and Toxicology, FAF Medical Academy, Inglolstaedter Lanolstr 100, Dn 85748, Garching, Germany.

Dr Brian Widdop, PhD, SRCS, CChem, FRSC, FRCPath. Laboratory Director, Medical Toxicology Unit, Guy's and St Thomas' Hospital Trust, Avonley Road, London SE14 5ER.

Professor Michael D. Waters, PhD. US Environmental Protection Agency, Research Triangle Park, North Carolina 27711, USA.

ABBREVIATIONS

2,4-D	2,4-Dichlorophenoxyacetic acid
AAAAI	American Academy of Allergy, Asthma and Immunology
ACD	Acid-citrate dextrose
ACGIH	American Conference of Government Industrial Hygienists
ACh	Acetylcholine
AChE	Acetylcholinesterase
ACOEM	American College of Occupational and Environmental Medicine
ACTH	Adrenocorticotrophic hormone
ADI	Acceptable daily intake
AIDS	Acquired immune deficiency syndrome
ATP	Adenosine triphosphate
BBB	Blood brain barrier
Beta-G	Beta-glucoronidase
Bt H-14	*Bacillus thuringiensis* strain H-14
BTI	*Bacillus thuringiensis israelensis*
BuChE	Butyrylcholinesterase
CA	Chromosome aberration
CaE	Carboxylesterase
CCEP	Comprehensive Clinical Evaluation Program
CD	Communicable disease
CGRP	Calcitonin gene related peptide
ChAT	Choline acetyltransferase
ChE	Cholinesterase
CMAP	Compound muscle action potential
CNS	Central nervous system
COPIND	Chronic OP-induced neurological damage
COSHH	Control of Substances Hazardous to Health (UK)
CPA	N6-Cyclopentyl adenosine
CT	Computer tomography
DALY	Disability-adjusted life year
DEDTP	Diethyldithiophosphate

DEP	Diethylphosphate
DETP	Diethylthiophosphate
DFP	Diisopropyl phosphorofluoridate
DGW	Danish Gulf War
DMDTP	Dimethyldithiophosphate
DMP	Dimethylphosphate
DMTP	Dimethylthiophosphate
DNOC	Dinitro-o-cresol
DTNB	5,5'-Dithiobis (2-nitrobenzoic) acid
ECG	Electrocardiogram
ECPS	Extracorporeal cardiopulmonary support
EEG	Electroencephalogram
EMG	Electromyography
EPA	Environmental Protection Agency (US)
EPN	ISO *(qv)* name for an insecticide: the chemical name is *O*-ethyl *O*-4-nitrophenyl phenylphosphonothioate.
ESCAP	Economic and Social Commission of Asia and the Pacific
ETEC	Enterotoxic *Escherichia coli*
EU	European Union
EUROPOEM	European predictive operator exposure model
E-W nucleus	Edinger-Westphal nucleus
FAO	Food and Agricultural Organization
FSH	Follicle stimulating hormone
FSU	Former Soviet Union
GABA	Gamma aminobutyric acid
GAP	Genetic activity profile
GBS	Guillain Barré syndrome
GC-MS	Gas chromatography-mass spectrometry
GLC	Gas-liquid chromatography
GM	Genetic mutation
HMO	Hepatic mono oxygenase
HMPA	Hexamethylphosphoramide
HPLC	High performance liquid chromatography
HPTLC	High performance thin layer chromatography

HSE	Health and Safety Executive
IARC	International Agency for Research on Cancer
IEI	Idiopathic environmental intolerance
IGR	Insect growth regulator
IMPA	Isopropyl methylphosphonic acid
INN	International non-proprietary name
IOM	Institute of Occupational Medicine
IPCS	International Programme on Chemical Safety
IPM	Integrated pest management
ISO	International Organisation for Standardisation
LC-MS	Liquid chromatography-mass spectrometry
LEAF	Linking environment and farming
LH	Luteinizing hormone
MCS	Multiple chemical sensitivity
ME	Myasthenic encephalitis
MEPC	Miniature end-plate current
MEPP	Miniature end-plate potential
MMPI	Minnesota Multiphasic Personality Inventory
MN	Micronucleus
MRL	Maximum residue limit
NBP	4-(4-Nitrobenzyl)pyridine
NCD	Non-communicable disease
NCI	National Cancer Institute
NECA	5'-N-Ethylcarboxamido adenosine
NIOSH	National Institute for Occupational Safety and Health (USA)
NMDA	N-Methyl-D-aspartate
NMJ	Neuromuscular junction
NTE	Neuropathy target esterase
NTP	National Toxicology Programme
OCP	Onchocerciasis Control Programme
OP	Organophosphate, organophosphorus ester

OPIDP	Organophosphate induced delayed polyneuropathy
OSHA	Occupational Safety and Health Administration (USA)
PEG-ES	Polyethylene glycol electrolyte solution
PET	Positron emission tomography
PON1	Paraoxonase
PPE	Personal protection equipment
PSS	Poison Severity Score
PTSD	Post-traumatic stress disorder
RBC	Red blood cell
RfD	Reference dose
RLN	Recurrent laryngeal nerve
RPTLC	Reversed phase thin layer chromatography
SCE	Sister chromatid exchange
STLC	Sequential thin layer chromatography
TCP	Tricresyl phosphate
TEPP	ISO *(qv)* name for an insecticide: the chemical name is tetraethyl pyrophosphate
TLC	Thin layer chromatography
TOCP	Tri-orthocresyl phosphate
TOF	Train of four
Tris-CP	Tris(2-chloroethyl) phosphate
Tris-DBP	Tris(2,3-dibromopropyl) phosphate
ULV	Ultra low volume
UV	Ultraviolet
WAIS	Wechsler Adult Intelligence Scale
WBI	Whole bowel irrigation

INTRODUCTION

In 1669 in a small laboratory in Hamburg, the alchemist Hennig Brandt was - like many before him - seeking the philosopher's stone that would turn base metals into gold by heating the residues of urine he had boiled down to a dry solid.

"He stoked the small furnace with more charcoal and pumped the bellows until his retort glowed red hot. Suddenly something strange began to happen. Glowing fumes filled the vessel and from the end of the retort dripped a shining liquid that burst into flames. When he caught the liquid in a glass vessel and stopped it, he saw it solidified but continued to gleam with an eery pale-green light and waves of flame seemed to lick its surface. Fascinated, he watched it more closely, expecting this curious cold fire to go out, but it continued to shine undimmed hour after hour. Here was magic indeed. Here was phosphorus." (1)

Phosphorus was the thirteenth chemical element to be discovered and proved to be one of the most remarkable and dangerous. It occurs naturally tightly guarded by a protective cage of four oxygen molecules which, if stripped away - by heating to one thousand degrees centigrade - seek to recombine and in doing so generate the same amount of energy that was originally required to separate them. Naked phosphorus is a tiger which over the subsequent three hundred years has had a profound effect for both good and evil - in each of its three major applications to human affairs.

Its spontaneous flammability gave rise to the phosphorus match that ended thousands of years of struggling with flint and tinder to light fires, oil lamps and candles. But it also led to the phosphorus bombs which when they rained down on the German city of Hamburg in the second World War created a fire storm that killed 37,000 people. Phosphorus as a chemical fertiliser transformed agricultural production, increasing crop yields sixfold but also had devastating environmental effects clogging up lakes and rivers with algae. The collection of essays in this book deals with its third major application as a pesticide. Here, too, its potential for good must be balanced against its potential for harm as the widespread benefits of organophosphates (OPs) in protecting humans and animals against infestation must be set against an estimate by the WHO (not, admittedly, the most reliable of sources) of three million severe poisonings and two hundred thousands deaths every year. (2)

The organophosphates were first synthesised by reacting alcohol and phosphoric acid, thus replacing one of the cage of four oxygen molecules with carbon and attaching chemical groups to the others. In this form they damaged the nervous system, making them powerful poisons. Accordingly, in 1936, Gerhard Schrader, a chemist working for the massive German chemical company, 1 G Farbenindustrie set out to synthesise as many OPs as possible in the hope that they might prove to be useful insecticides. Compounds that can damage the nervous system of mites and lice will, at much higher doses, have the same effect on humans and, with the prospect of a European war imminent, the German military authorities promptly classified Schrader's research as top secret and redirected it towards the manufacture of chemical warfare agents.

In 1942, the most potent of these, tabun, a phosphorus-cyanide compound, entered large scale production and by the end of the second war the Nazis had manufactured sufficient quantities to kill 12 trillion people.

"There is still a mystery why Hitler did not authorise the use of tabun against the Allied forces following the Normandy invasion. The likely explanation must be that the Office of Strategic Services had successfully generated the rumour amongst the German high command that the Allies were prepared to retaliate in kind." (3)

It was not until after the war - in 1946 - that the precise mode of action of the OPs was clarified when two scientists, Koelle and Gilman, showed they deactivated acetyl cholinesterase (AChE) which neutralises the neurotransmitter acetyl choline (ACh).

The persistence of ACh at the neural junction means the muscles, glands and nerves remain in a state of constant stimulation producing a wide range of acute symptoms. They affect the CNS to cause giddiness, anxiety, headaches, confusion and respiratory difficulties. They disrupt the regulation of the various glands of the body leading to excess salivation, copious phlegm and profuse sweating. Finally they interfere with muscle action leading to miosis - those affected have the impression that everything has suddenly gone very dark - stomach cramps, diarrhoea, breathlessness and dysrythmias. This constellation of signs and symptoms is known by the mnemonic SLUDGE (salivation, lacrimation, urination, defaecation, gastroenteritis and emesis).

Following the declassification of Gerhard Schrader's research at IG Farbenindustrie at the end of the war, chemical companies around the world realised the potential of his original intentional use for OPs - as insecticides. They proved to be wonderfully toxic against the army of mites, lice, ticks and blowfly that afflict humans and animals. They are certainly much superior to the many other compounds that have been used in the past - lime, lead oxide, mercury, arsenic and most recently the organochlorines that notoriously persist in the environment.

Their potency against infestation is of almost inestimable benefit but as the essays of this book point out, their use remains controversial because of the hazards they pose to humans from acute and chronic exposure.

The main burden of toxicity remains in developing countries where 99% of pesticide poisonings occur with 25 million episodes annually especially amongst agricultural workers. (5) These include the acute neurological effects from the suppression of AChE already described that usually occur within 24 hours of exposure. They have also been associated with the development of a peripheral neuropathy two to three weeks later. The most contentious issue, however, centres around the question of whether they are responsible for long term neuropsychological problems. These were first reported back in 1961 in the form of sixteen case reports described by S Gershon and F H Shaw of the University of Melbourne. (6). In one incident a 43 year old greenhouse technician who had been exposed to OPs for ten years consulted a psychiatrist complaining of depression, irritability and insomnia. His memory was impaired and he could no longer recall the number and names of plants under his care and had 'difficulty in understanding anything he read'.

More recently the role of OPs in causing such neuropsychological problems have been extensively investigated in the West in two major groups - sheep farmers and the veterans of the Gulf War. There are more than 42 million sheep in Britain alone all of which in time had to be dipped twice a year to control blowflies and 'scab' - a horrible disease caused by mites that drive sheep to distraction by its persistent itchiness. Soon after the introduction of OP pesticides some farmers claimed they made them ill. Their most formidable spokesperson is the Countess of Mar who was accidentally poisoned by an OP sheep dip back in 1989. She now attributes her fluctuating symptoms of mood swings, difficulty in concentration, speech and writing difficulties and respiratory problems to OPs.

Most shepherds and sheep dip contractors, however, claim no ill effects. As one 'dipper' puts it: "I have had massive exposure, and I am not alone. I can get pretty depressed at times but I don't think it's OPs. We use dips sensibly. If you wear protective clothing I think it's OK." (7)

The 700,000 troops sent to the Gulf War in 1981 were exposed to OPs when their quarters and tents were sprayed as a precautionary measure against malaria causing mosquitoes. It has been suggested that some may also have been exposed to the OP chemical warfare agent sarin deployed by the Iraqis, eight tonnes of which were subsequently captured by the Allied forces. Many soldiers consequently developed what has become known as Gulf War Syndrome, which features many of the neuropsychological problems associated with OPs - including fatigue, depression and weakness.

The Gulf War Syndrome and the effects of OP sheep dip have been the subject of numerous reports but the protean nature of symptoms reported and the lack of hard clinical signs of neurological damage has made it difficult to reach a definitive verdict about the scale - or indeed the reality - of OP poisoning. This collection of essays is an important contribution to the ongoing and important debate on this issue.

James Le Fanu

Medical Journalist

References

1. John Emsley, The Shocking History of Phosphorus, Macmillan 2000.
2. World Health Organisation. Public Health Impact of Pesticides used in Agriculture. Geneva *WHO* 1990.
3. Dherage Khurana, Organophosphorus Intoxication. *Archives of Neurology* 2000; **57**: 600-2.
4. Koelle G B, Gilman A. The relationship between cholinesterase inhibition and the pharmacological action of DFP. *Journal of Pharmacology* 1946; **87**: 421-47.
5.Rosenstock, L. et al. Chronic and Central Nervous System Effects of Acute Organophosphate pesticide intoxication, *Lancet* 1991; **338**: 223-7.
6.Gershon, S., Shaw, F.H. Psychiatric Sequelae of Chronic Exposure to Organophosphorus Insecticides. *Lancet* 1961; **ii** :1371-5
7. Richard D North, Personal Communication.

CHAPTER 1

Organophosphates: History, Chemistry, Pharmacology

Timothy C Marrs

1.1. INTRODUCTION

Organophosphorus (OP) compounds are widely used in agriculture, horticulture and veterinary medicine. They also include the nerve gases and poisons which are amongst the most feared and toxic group of chemical warfare agents. Exposure to these poisons has been mercifully infrequent, comprising a few instances of exposure during study, mostly within the confines of research establishments. They have been used at Halabja in Iraqi Kurdistan and by terrorists in Japan. By contrast, residues of anticholinesterase (antiChE) OPs, used as insecticides in agriculture and as pesticides in animals, are found in crops, fruits and vegetables, and meat. Moreover, OP insecticides are frequently used around the house, in public hygiene and in tropical countries to control vectors of disease. Additionally, certain OP agents have been used in human medicine. Thus the pharmacology and toxicology of OPs are of importance to many different groups of health professionals.

1.2. HISTORY

Holmstedt (1963) has reviewed the history of OPs. Particular reference to chemical warfare agents is found in the work of SIPRI (1963), Maynard and Beswick (1992) and Marrs et al (1996). Organic compounds of phosphorus were first made in the 19th century. Philippe de Clermont synthesised tetraethyl pyrophosphate in 1854, tasting it without harming himself. However, little was known of the toxicity of OP compounds until the 1930s. At that time, the chemistry and toxicity of certain such compounds was investigated as part of a programme to develop synthetic insecticides undertaken by the German company IG Farbenindustrie. Gerhard Schrader led this project. In the latter half of the 1930s, the Hitler government required that information on toxic compounds be reported to the War Ministry.

Amongst the compounds reported were tetraethyl pyrophosphate (TEPP) and tabun and sarin (GA and GB), two of the earliest G-type chemical warfare poisons. A pilot manufacturing plant was established at Münster-lager and a larger one at Dühernfurt near the upper River Oder, north of Breslau in Prussian Silesia (now Dyhernfurth and Wrocław in Poland).

Both the German military and industry carried out studies into the toxicology of these compounds. These revealed the cholinesterase inhibiting effects of these compounds which explained the parasympathomimetic effects of the OP intoxication. During World War II work in Germany produced soman (GD), another G agent. During the same period, studies were carried out in Cambridge on the OPs with particular emphasis on fluorine-containing organic phosphates. Development of insecticide OPs was directed at producing greater specificity by increasing their toxicity to insects whilst minimising their effect on non-target species, such as humans. The history of the second main group of OP chemical warfare agents, the V agents such as VX is more complicated than that of the G agents. Amiton, an ICI compound, [O,O-diethyl (S-2-diethylaminoethyl phosphorothioate)], was found to be an effective experimental insecticide but of high mammalian toxicity. Similar compounds were synthesised in a number of laboratories, largely S-dialkylaminoethyl O-alkyl alkylphosphonothioates. These compounds have a much lower vapour pressure than the G agents but many were found to be even more toxic than G agents, especially by the percutaneous route. By contrast, the objective of the development work on the insecticides has been directed at seeking greater toxicity to the pest whilst minimising toxicity to non-target species. One major advancement in that direction was the introduction of =S phosphorothioates. These agents require desulfuration before they acquire antiChE activity (see below).

1.2.1 THERAPY

The development of treatments for OP poisoning started with the recognition of the efficacy of atropine as an antidote for their parasympathomimetic effects. The usefulness of oximes, such as pralidoxime salts, in reactivating inhibited esterases was discovered in the 1950s (Wilson and Ginsberg, 1955). A further landmark in treatment was the addition of anticonvulsants to the combination of oximes and atropine. It was noticed that soman-inhibited antiChE enzyme was refractory to reactivation by oximes, a phenomenon now known as ageing.

This observation led to the development of carbamate prophylaxis for nerve agent poisoning (see Inns and Marrs, 1992). Much of the work on the treatment of OP poisoning by the use of antidotes was undertaken at defence research establishments such as that at Edgewood Arsenal in Maryland, USA, Porton Down near Salisbury in England, Suffield in Canada and at various laboratories in Germany and the former USSR.

Table 1.1. Outline history of OPs

Event	Date
Philippe de Clermont tastes tetraethyl pyrophosphate	1854
Pure tetraethyl pyrophosphate synthesised by Nylén	1930
Ginger jake paralysis	1930s
Lange and von Krueger synthesise alkyl esters of fluorophosphoric acid	1932
Schrader starts to work on organophosphates as insecticides for IG Farbenindustrie	1936
Tabun and sarin synthesised	1937
Construction of a chemical warfare agent factory in Dyhernfurth near Wrocław (then Dühernfurt)	1940-2
Diisopropyl phosphorofluoridate synthesised	1941
Soman synthesised	1944
Paraoxon and parathion synthesised	1944
Malathion introduced as an insecticide	1950
Accidental poisoning of two subjects with mipafox, an insecticide under development, produces organophosphate-induced delayed polyneuropathy	1951
Amiton described	1955

1.2.2. Organophosphate Induced Delayed Polyneuropathy (OPIDP)

Some OP antiChEs have effects other than those explained by cholinesterase inhibition. This was first clearly shown when mipafox, a candidate insecticide, was undergoing development. Two human subjects were accidentally poisoned. They initially developed the acute cholinergic syndrome (see below) but some time after recovering from its effects they developed a neuropathy, now recognised to be organophosphate-induced delayed polyneuropathy (OPIDP).

This had previously been described with compounds with weak or absent antiChE effects, such as phosphocreosote, when used as an antituberculous medication. More notorious was ginger jake paralysis which occurred during the era of prohibition in the USA in the 1930s when OPIDP was caused by the adulteration of beverages with tri-o-cresyl phosphate (see review by Davies, 1963).

1.2.3. Intermediate Syndrome

A third syndrome, in addition to the acute cholinergic syndrome and OPIDP, has been described: this consists of a proximal and reversible paralysis, including the muscles of respiration (Senanayake and Karalliedde, 1992; see Chapter 6). This syndrome occurring 24 hours to 4 days after exposure to OP poisoning has been termed the 'intermediate syndrome'.

1.2.4. Long Term Effects on the Central Nervous System

More recently, it has been recognised that apparent recovery from acute OP poisoning may be followed by long term neurological sequelae. Some authorities have speculated this may also result from long term low dose exposure to OPs (see Chapter 8).

1.3. STRUCTURE AND NOMENCLATURE OF ORGANOPHOSPHATE ANTI ChEs

Literally the term organophosphorus (OP) compound means any organic compound containing phosphorus. However, the term has come to be used as shorthand for a group of compounds that are esters of phosphoric acid, phophorothioic acid, phosphonic acid, phosphonothioic acid and the corresponding dithioic acids, which have antiChE activity. The term organophosphate is best restricted to esters of phosphoric acid. Phosphoric acid esters have all three substituents linked to the phosphorus atom through an oxygen atom whereas phosphonic acid derivatives have one substituent linked directly to the phosphorus atom. Phosphinic acid derivatives, such as glufosinate, which have two substituents linked directly to the phosphorus atom generally lack antiChE activity.

In many OPs, used as insecticides, the oxygen that is attached to the phosphorus atom by a double bond is replaced by sulfur, giving one type of phosphorothioate. OPs with a P=S structure are sometimes known as phophorothionates, but will be referred to in this chapter as P=S phosphorothioates. There are also phosphorothioates in which one of the substituents is attached to phosphorus via a sulfur atom: these are sometimes called phosphorothiolates, but will be referred to below as S-substituted phosphorothioates. Dithioates and trithioates are also used as agrochemicals. It will be apparent that both of these may exist as one or other of two types, depending on whether or not one of the sulfur atoms is attached to the phosphorus by a double bond. Phosphorotetrathioates are also theoretically possible. Analogous phosphonothioates are also possible as well as dithioates and trithioates (Table 1.2. See also WHO [1986]).   OPs, other than those exploited for their antiChE properties, are discussed briefly at the end of this chapter.

The typical general structure of organophosphate antiChEs is:

$$R \diagdown \underset{\diagup}{\overset{\displaystyle O \atop \displaystyle \parallel}{P}} - X$$

where the R groups are similar or dissimilar alkoxy groups. The X group which is linked directly to the phosphorus atom is more labile than the alkoxy groups and is known as the leaving group. In the nomenclature and structures illustrated in Table 1.2. the leaving group is not distinguished from the alkoxy groups. The leaving group is usually not a simple alkyl or alkoxy group like the other two substituents. It can be one of a large number of moieties. In many G-type nerve agents the leaving group is fluorine, as it is with the laboratory chemical, diisopropyl phosphorofluoridate (DFP). The structure of the leaving group provides one way in which OPs can be classified (see Table 1.3.) (Gallo and Lawryk, 1991). This classification is of little use to the pesticide toxicologist as the overwhelming majority of pesticides belong to a single group (IV). The classification is useful in that it is predictive of biological properties: compounds of group I, which have a choline-like structure, are highly toxic as are most of the phosphorofluoridates (group II).

This group includes the G chemical warfare agents, sarin and soman. In the classical OP antiChE structure, given above, the nature of the alkoxy groups is important in determining reactivity and especially reactivation rates as discussed below. In the case of most insecticides both alkoxy groups are methoxy or ethoxy groups: notable exceptions are EPN, leptophos and cyanofenphos which have one alkoxy and one phenyl group and methamidophos which is a methoxy S-methyl compound. Trichloronat, which is a phosphonate has one ethoxy substituent and one ethyl group attached direct to the phosphorus atom.

Table 1.2. Main groups of organophosphates

Type	Structure	Examples
Phosphate	O ‖ R^1O–P–OR^3 | OR^2	Dichlorvos[a] Chlorfenvinphos[a] Heptenophos[a] Tri-o-cresyl phosphate[b]
Phosphonate	O ‖ R^1O–P–OR^3 | R^2	Trichlorfon[a]/metrifonate[c] Glyphosate[d]
Phosphinate	O ‖ R^1O–P–R^3 | R^2	Glufosinate[d]
Phosphorothioate = S type	S ‖ R^1O–P–OR^3 | OR^2	Diazinon[a] Parathion[a] Bromophos[a] Pyrazophos[e] Fenitrothion[a]

Type	Structure	Examples
Phosphorothioate S-substituted	$$\begin{array}{c} O \\ \| \\ R^1O-P-SR^3 \\ \| \\ OR^2 \end{array}$$	Demeton-S-methyl VG [f]
Phosphorodithioate	$$\begin{array}{c} S \\ \| \\ R^1O-P-SR^3 \\ \| \\ OR^2 \end{array}$$	Malathion[a] Dimethoate[a] Disulfoton[a]
Phosphorotrithioate	$$\begin{array}{c} O \\ \| \\ R^1S-P-SR^3 \\ \| \\ SR^2 \end{array}$$	S,S,S–Tributyl phosphorotrithioate (DEF)[g]
Phosphonothioate =S type	$$\begin{array}{c} S \\ \| \\ R^1O-P-OR^3 \\ \| \\ R^2 \end{array}$$	Leptophos[a] EPN[a]
Phosphonothioate S-substituted	$$\begin{array}{c} O \\ \| \\ R^1O-P-SR^3 \\ \| \\ R^2 \end{array}$$	VX[f]
Phosphoramidate	$$\begin{array}{c} O \qquad R' \\ \| \quad / \\ R^1O-P-N \\ \| \quad \backslash \\ OR^2 \quad R'' \end{array}$$	Fenamiphos[a] Tabun[f]
Phosphorothioamidate =S type	$$\begin{array}{c} S \qquad R' \\ \| \quad / \\ R^1O-P-N \\ \| \quad \backslash \\ OR^2 \quad R'' \end{array}$$	Isofenphos[a] Propetamphos[a]

Type	Structure	Examples
Phosphorothioamidate S – substituted	$\begin{array}{c} O \\ \parallel \quad\nearrow R' \\ R^1O-P-N \\ \mid \quad\searrow R'' \\ SR^2 \end{array}$	Methamidophos[a]
Phosphorofluoridate	$\begin{array}{c} O \\ \parallel \\ R^1O-P-F \\ \mid \\ OR^2 \end{array}$	DFP[h]
Phosphonofluoridate	$\begin{array}{c} O \\ \parallel \\ R^1O-P-F \\ \mid \\ R^2 \end{array}$	Sarin[f] Soman[f] GE[f]

Key to Table 1.2.

   a   insecticide

   b   Industrial chemical

   c   INN name; used as human pharmaceutical

   d   herbicide

   e   fungicide

   f   chemical warfare agent

   g   defoliant

   h   laboratory chemical

Note trichlorfon and metrifonate are the same substance

Certain other structures are consistent with antiChE effects, thus TEPP, sulfotep and schradan, all pesticides, are derivatives of pyrophosphoric acid. Some OPs have no clearly defined leaving group, for example the cotton defoliant S,S,S-tributyl phosphorotrithioate, a weak cholinesterase inhibitor, and the industrial chemical tri-o-cresyl phosphate.

Table 1.3. OPs classified by the nature of their leaving group

Group	Structure of Leaving Group	Examples
I	Quaternary nitrogen	Ecothiopate
II	Fluorine atom	Sarin, soman, DFP, mipafox
III	Cyanide, cyanate, thiocyanate, halogen atom other than fluorine	Tabun
IV	Other moieties	Many insecticides

1.3.1. Nomenclature of Special Groups of Substances

Pesticides and drugs have systematic chemical names, trade names and generic names (see below). The usual practice is to capitalise the initial letter of the trade name; tabun, sarin and soman (chemical warfare agents) are of course not trade names.

1.3.1.1. Pesticides

In addition to their chemical names pesticides have national (for example British Standards Institute [BSI]) common names as well as ISO (International Organisation for Standardisation) common names (ISO, 1965, 1981). Furthermore, there are both English language and French language ISO names and rules for translating ISO names into other languages, such as Dutch. The English language ISO name is not always the same as the British or US common name. The agent with an ISO name jodfenphos has a British common name, iodofenphos. Pesticides will have one or more trade names in addition.

1.3.1.2. Nerve Agents

Some OP chemical warfare agents have, in addition to their chemical names, common names as well as codes (see above); others such as GE and VX have no common name.

1.3.1.3. Drugs

A few OPs are used as drugs either in human or veterinary medicine. Drugs used in human medicine include ecothiopate used in the treatment of glaucoma, whilst in veterinary medicine OPs are used as anthelmintics and in the treatment of infestation by ectoparasites especially in hairy animals. Phosmet is used to combat warble fly infestation in cattle, diazinon, chlorfenvinphos and propetamphos are used to treat scab and fly-strike in sheep and tetrachlorvinphos is commonly used to combat fleas in pet cats. When used as pharmaceuticals, OPs have international non-proprietary (INN) names. In some cases these differ from the ISO pesticide names, thus trichlorfon, a pesticide, is the same as metrifonate, a pharmaceutical used in human medicine.

1.4. EFFECTS OF OPs

The fundamental toxicological activity of OPs in humans is due to the inhibition of esterases. This results in three or possibly four syndromes. The acute cholinergic syndrome and the intermediate syndrome are the result of inhibition of the enzyme, AChE. The syndrome of organophosphate induced delayed polyneuropathy (OPIDP) is associated with inhibition of another enzyme, neuropathy target esterase (NTE).

Table 1.4. Syndromes associated with OPs

Syndrome	Time in Association with Exposure
Acute cholinergic syndrome	Immediate; lasting a few days
Intermediate syndrome	Commencing a few days after poisoning and lasting a few days further
Organophosphate—induced delayed polyneuropathy (OPIDP)	Starting a week or two after poisoning and, at least to some extent, persistent
Chronic OP-induced neurological damage (COPIND)	Persistent

1.4.1. Cholinesterases

Two main classes of cholinesterases are recognised, those whose preferential substrate is acetylcholine (ACh), named acetylcholinesterases (AChE), and those whose preferential substrate is butyrylcholine, named butyrylcholinesterases (BuChE) or pseudocholinesterases. The structure of both of esterases has been extensively studied (Massoulié and Bon, 1982). There is a high degree of homology in the amino acid sequences of the active sites in all cholinesterases, even those of distantly related organisms (La Du and Lockridge, 1986). Because it is found in red blood cells, AChE is sometimes called red cell or erythrocytic cholinesterase (RBC AChE). BuChE similarly has the appellation of plasma cholinesterase because it occurs in the plasma. This nomenclature has its drawbacks in that this distribution, while true of man, does not hold for all species.

As well as differing in preferred substrate, the two enzymes, AChE and BuChE also have different inhibition characteristics, which can be exploited in biochemical assays, and histochemical staining techniques.

1.4.1.1. Acetylcholinesterases (AChEs)

AChE is found in many tissues in human beings. It is found in erythrocytes where its role is not understood. It is present at many sites in the nervous system where ACh is the neurotransmitter. It is found at the neuromuscular junction (NMJ), in the autonomic ganglia and at parasympathetic effector organs.

The role of the enzyme at these sites is to hydrolyse ACh so terminating its action. ACh binds to and acetylates AChE at a serine group at its esteratic site resulting in hydrolysis of the ACh. The enzyme also binds the quaternary nitrogen of the choline group, at the so-called anionic site, by weak electrostatic forces. All the evidence suggests that AChE is a single gene product in any individual human or vertebrate animal although the catalytic domain can be associated with different C-terminal peptides. This gives rise to distinct subunits and different molecular forms. These can be divided into asymmetric and globular forms (Massoulié and Bon, 1982; Massoulié et al., 1999). The asymmetric forms (also termed long tailed cholinesterase) tend to be concentrated at synapses and in the synaptic cleft of the motor endplates. Because erythrocyte AChE inhibition is similar to that in nervous tissue the level of its activity is frequently used as a marker of the severity of OP poisoning.

However, the correspondence is not perfect because of the relative accessibility of poison in the plasma to the enzyme in the red cell compared to the CNS and to a lesser extent, the NMJ (see also Chapter 9). Moreover, the rate of resynthesis of AChE varies with tissue and species. The red cell in mammals lacks the ability to synthesise protein. Therefore, after irreversible inhibition, reappearance of erythrocyte cholinesterase is a function of the life of that erythrocyte in that species. After irreversible inhibition in humans recovery of red cell AChE activity is thus usually slower than recovery of BuChE in the plasma.

After irreversible inhibition, brain esterase activity reappears surprisingly quickly in animals. Twenty-four hours after poisoning mice with DFP, Wehner *et al.* (1985), observed approximately 30% recovery in cholinesterase activity in CNS reaggregates. Recovery of brain AChE is generally faster than recovery of activity in the erythrocyte but may be slower than recovery in BuChE in plasma (Lim *et al.*, 1989). See below for a discussion of the interaction of inhibition, synthesis, reactivation and ageing on interpretation of ChE activity.

1.4.1.2. Butyrylcholinesterase (BuChE)

As well as being present in the plasma, BuChE is found in the CNS, liver and other organs, but the physiological role of plasma and brain BuChE is unknown. The plasma enzyme is a tetramer in most mammalian species although the monomer and dimer are present to some extent (see, Masson *et al.*, 1982). Plasma BuChE activity is controlled by a number of allelic genes. Families are known with atypical or absent plasma cholinesterase activity; the main importance of this phenomenon is that such individuals react to the muscle relaxant, suxamethonium, by developing prolonged apnoea (Kalow and Gunn, 1957; Østergaard *et al.*, 1992). Some of these variant plasma cholinesterases are abnormally resistant to inhibitors of cholinesterase activity such as dibucaine or fluoride, while an "absent" gene also occurs. The affected families appear normal, despite atypical, low or even absent plasma BuChE. Hence, the role of the BuChE in the plasma is obscure. However, it seems unlikely that this enzyme evolved millions of years ago in order that, many years later, an anaesthetic adjunct could be used safely.

It has been hypothesised that plasma or BuChE might act as a sink in antiChE poisoning, preventing inhibitors reacting with the more physiologically important AChE in nervous tissue particularly with OP nerve agents which are active at extremely low molar concentrations. BuChE is also of importance in OP poisoning for two reasons. Firstly, inhibition of the enzyme tends to be more long lasting and less rapidly reversed by reactivation (see below) than that of erythrocyte AChE, especially in humans (Reiner, 1971; Škrinjaric-Špoljar et al., 1973; Worek et al., 1999), although there are exceptions (Hinz et al., 1998). As a result the degree of inhibition of plasma BuChE activity can be a useful marker of exposure. Secondly, in the event of a subject undergoing a surgical procedure in the aftermath of substantial OP exposure, suxamethonium apnoea may occur. This has only been reported with any frequency in animals (e.g. Keller and Müller, 1978) when hairy animals have been exposed to OPs, used as ectoparasiticides, regularly and at high doses. In humans this is rarely the case and more typical sources of human exposure result in a much lower dose of OP.

When BuChE is used to monitor exposure to antiChEs it should be remembered that plasma BuChE is synthesised in the liver and low levels can also result from liver disease. Because of this and the wide normal range for plasma cholinesterase activity (Brock, 1991; Brock and Brock, 1993), levels can be difficult to interpret unless the subject has had the enzyme assayed in the recent past. (See also Chapters 5 and 15)

1.4.1.3. Interaction of OPs with Cholinesterases

The interaction of AChEs with OPs is a complex set of reactions of which two are closely analogous to the reaction of the natural substrate ACh with the enzyme. The interaction with BuChE is mechanistically similar although the kinetics are not the same. The severity of the clinical effects at any time depends on the totality of these reactions of OPs with AChE.

1.4.1.4. Mechanism of Inhibition and Reactivation

In normal circumstances, ACh binds to cholinesterases at two sites, the anionic site, where the quaternary nitrogen of choline forms an electrostatic link and at the esteratic site where the carbonyl group binds to a serine residue.

The binding of ACh to the enzyme, which results in acetylation of the serine at the active site of the enzyme, causes loss of the choline moiety. The reaction for ACh can be envisaged as shown, E being the enzyme, AX ACh, EAX is a reversible Michaelis–Menten complex and A is acetate:

$$
E + AX \underset{k_{-1}}{\overset{k_{+1}}{\longleftrightarrow}} EAX \overset{k_2}{\rightarrow} \underset{+X}{EA} \overset{k_3}{\rightarrow} E + A \tag{1.1}
$$

k_{+1}, k_{-1}, k_2, k_3 are rate constants. Inhibition with OPs, takes place by a process analogous to the reaction of ACh with the enzyme, by a non-reversible reaction in which the leaving group is lost and the esterase is phosphorylated at the hydroxyl group of the serine residue. One major difference is that the OPs' interaction with the anionic site of the enzyme occurs only with ecothiopate-like OPs. The key to the powerful antiChE effects of OPs is what happens after inhibition. When the enzyme is acetylated, as occurs when it interacts with its normal substrate ACh, reactivation by hydrolysis of the acetylated enzyme (EA → E + A) occurs very quickly. In the case of OPs, hydrolysis is much slower. In a process that is independent of the nature of the leaving group, reactivation by hydrolysis of the dialkoxyphosphorylated enzyme occurs at a clinically significant rate with nearly all important OPs but this is always much slower than when the enzyme is acetylated by its natural substrate. The enzyme deacetylates in microseconds, but dephosphorylates in a matter of hours to days. While the active site of the enzyme is phosphorylated it is unavailable for the hydrolysis of ACh. Hence it results in an accumulation of ACh at the receptor sites in the body.

Most pesticides produce either dimethoxyphosphorylated enzyme or diethoxyphosphorylated enzyme. Reactivation is much more rapid in the case of the former than the latter (Vale, 1998). Furthermore, reactivation is more rapid if one of the alkyl groups is linked to phosphorus through a sulfur atom. In the case of large substituent groups such as isopropyl and sec-butyl groups, for example DFP, spontaneous reactivation is so slow as to be clinically insignificant (see Marrs and Dewhurst, 1999), and recovery depends upon the resynthesis of the enzyme. It should be noted that, as discussed above, resynthesis rates for AChE in the central nervous system are not negligible and that resynthesis may contribute substantially to the recovery of activity that is observed with OPs that form complexes that reactivate slowly.

The difference in reactivation rates may be clinically important in the treatment of pesticide poisoning. As a result of these differences it can be expected that poisoning with dimethoxy compounds will be more short-lived than with diethoxy compounds (see Table 1.5).

The affinity with which ACh or an inhibitor such as an OP binds to AChE is described by the dissociation constant for the complex EAX, K_D. This is equal to k_{-1}/k_{+1}.

For inhibitors whose complexes with AChE reactivate slowly, such as OPs, k_3 can be ignored and the reaction with AChE can be described by a bimolecular rate constant, k_i as follows:

$$E + AX \quad \rightarrow \quad X + EA$$
$$k_i \tag{1.2}$$

Further $k_i = k_2/K_D$ (Main and Iverson, 1966). The relationship $k_i = \ln 2/I_{50}t$ allows an easy estimation of k_i (Aldridge, 1950). I_{50}, the concentration of inhibitor which inhibits 50% of the ChE in a given time (t), is another expression of inhibitor potency. These constants have been measured for many OPs, especially OP chemical warfare agents (e.g. Gray and Dawson, 1987).

It should be noted that some OPs have a chiral structure and enantiomers exist that may have a major difference in antiChE activity.

Table 1.5. Main groups of pesticides grouped by alkoxy group

Dimethoxy pesticides	Diethoxy pesticides
Azinphos-methyl	Chlorfenvinphos
Chlorpyrifos-methyl	Chlorpyrifos
Dichlorvos	Diazinon
Malathion	Disulfoton
Mevinphos	Ethion
Parathion-methyl	Mephosfolan
Pirimiphos-methyl	Parathion
Temephos	Phorate
Trichlorfon	Phosalone

1.4.1.5. Ageing

The development of enzyme reactivators for the treatment of OP poisoning revealed that these substances were ineffective in the case of poisoning with soman unless given very soon after exposure. The reason for this is that the complex that soman forms with AChE rapidly loses its bulky pinacolyl group to leave a monoalkyl phosphonylated complex. This chemical structure is refractory to oxime-induced reactivation and does not reactivate spontaneously. Monodealkylation occurs to some extent with all dialkoxyphosphorylated AChE complexes but it is, in general, only significant in relation to the treatment of poisoning with soman. The $t_{1/2}$ for ageing of soman-inhibited AChE is a matter of a few minutes (Talbot et al., 1988) which is too short for oximes to be effective, except in the most exceptional circumstances. The $t_{1/2}$ for pesticides is much longer, it is 2–9h in the case of dimethoxy OPs and > 36h in the case of diethoxy OPs (see Wilson et al., 1992).

Nevertheless, failure of oximes to be effective in pesticide poisoning has, from time to time, been ascribed to ageing (Glickman et al., 1984; Gyrd-Hansen and Kraul, 1984). There are two circumstances where ageing is likely to be of importance: firstly, where treatment is greatly delayed. Secondly, and possibly more importantly, it might be speculated that recurrent moderate exposure, insufficient to cause serious clinical effects, might result in a gradual increase in the proportion of enzyme in the aged form, in which it would be unable to reactivate either spontaneously or with reactivating oxime antidotes. This might be particularly likely to occur with dimethyl OPs, where both reactivation and ageing occur relatively fast. Furthermore, the phenomenon suggests that to be optimal oxime therapy should be carried out promptly. It should be noted that the failure of certain reactivators to work on tabun-inhibited esterases is not due to ageing but to other factors (Heilbron, 1963).

1.4.1.6. Reactivation, Synthesis *de novo* and the Use of Measurement of Cholinesterase Activity in Diagnosis and Treatment

From the above it will be clear that the degree of enzyme inhibition after OP exposure will at any time be a function of a number of processes occurring concurrently, namely, inhibition, reactivation, ageing and resynthesis.

With dimethoxy OPs, by far the most important process is spontaneous reactivation by hydrolysis of the dimethoxyphosphorylated enzyme unless substantial ageing has occurred. With OPs with larger alkyl groups resynthesis predominates. In measurements, where AChE activity in red cells is being used as surrogate for the enzyme in the nervous system, it should be remembered that red cells cannot synthesise the enzyme. This does not hold for neuronal AChE, so that measurement of erythrocytic AChE may over-estimate the severity of exposure. However, AChE in the red cell is more accessible than that in the CNS, so early in poisoning when inhibition is occurring, erythrocytic activity may also give an over-estimate of effect. With plasma BuChE, often more sensitive than AChE to inhibition, resynthesis can occur, unlike erythrocytic AChE. Therefore generally, where return of esterase activity is by synthesis *de novo* rather than reactivation, BuChE activity will return faster than red blood cell AChE activity. These complex situations can be summarised by saying that the level of red cell cholinesterase is a moderately good surrogate measurement for the vital enzyme in the nervous system, except where resynthesis is the main means whereby enzymatic activity is restored; in those circumstances BuChE can be useful. In other situations, BuChE activity is best treated as a marker of exposure, nothing more.

1.4.2. The Acute Cholinergic Syndrome

The major toxicological effects of OPs result from esterase inhibition rather than any direct effect on receptors. Of these effects, the most important in the acute syndrome, are those that result from the inhibition of AChE. The symptoms and clinical signs of this syndrome result from an excess of ACh resulting from a failure of its hydrolysis. To understand the toxicology of antiChE OPs it is necessary to consider the role of ACh as a neurotransmitter.

1.4.2.1. Acetylcholine (ACh)

ACh is one of a number of neurotransmitters in nervous tissue and is responsible for transmission of nerve impulses in the autonomic nervous system from preganglionic to postganglionic neurones in the parasympathetic and sympathetic nervous system, postganglionic parasympathetic fibres to effector organs and sympathetic fibres to sweat glands.

ACh is also the neurotransmitter at the skeletal muscle neuromuscular junction and some nerve tracts in the CNS.

The essential features in this system are a synthetic enzyme, choline acetyltransferase (ChAT); the neurotransmitter itself; a hydrolytic enzyme, AChE and specialised receptors, with which the ACh interacts. ChAT is synthesized in the perikaryon of cholinergic neurones and transported to nerve terminals, where it exists in soluble and membrane-bound forms.

The action of ChAT is the synthesis of ACh, from choline and acetyl coenzyme A, at sites of cholinergic neurotransmission. The ChAT gene also encodes another protein besides ChAT, vesicular ACh transporter. This protein in responsible for transporting ACh from the neuronal cytoplasm to the synaptic vesicle (Oda, 1999). At ganglia, ACh is released in response to an action potential triggering opening of voltage-gated calcium channels in the presynaptic terminal. The ACh crosses the synaptic cleft and contact of the ACh with specialised receptors (see below) at the proximal end of the post-ganglionic nerve fibre results in localised depolarization of the postsynaptic membrane and generation of the nerve impulse in the postganglionic nerve fibre. Transmission is similar at parasympathetic nerve endings except that the ACh stimulates receptors at parasympathetic effector organs and also at the neuromuscular junction, at which muscle fibre depolarization is initiated at the motor end plate following a similar sequence of events. In the cases of both autonomic ganglia and muscle, it is necessary for the depolarization to exceed a certain threshold to produce postjunctional activity e.g. initiate an action potential in a postsynaptic nerve cell or muscle fibre.

1.4.2.2. Hydrolysis of ACh.

In normal circumstances ACh is hydrolysed almost immediately by AChE at sites of action, as is discussed above. The effect of antiChEs is to block hydrolysis and cause the accumulation of ACh. This causes overstimulation and sometimes depolarization blockade. At the neuromuscular junction, where accumulation of ACh initially causes fasciculation (uncoordinated contraction of muscle fibres), continued accumulation produces flaccid type paralysis due to depolarization blockade.

1.4.2.3. Autonomic Nervous System

The autonomic nervous system consists of both afferent and efferent components, the afferent components being much less well understood than the efferent components. The afferent component is concerned with visceral sensation and its fibres are to be found in both the cranial nerves, such as the vagus and also the pelvic and splanchnic nerves. Afferent fibres also arise from more specialised structures such as pressor receptors and chemoreceptors in the aorta, carotid artery and carotid body. These are part of the system of vasomotor and respiratory reflexes. Less is known about the afferent fibres associated with the chemoreceptors in the aorta and carotid artery. The cell bodies of many afferent visceral fibres lie in the dorsal root ganglia or cranial nerve sensory ganglia. The nature of the neurotransmitters involved in the afferent nerves is mostly unknown, although some afferent fibres make connections with post-ganglionic sympathetic neurones and, at these sites, the transmitter is substance P. The location of CNS autonomic integrative system is thought to be the hypothalamus for regulation of blood pressure, water balance, sexual responses and other autonomic functions, while the medulla oblongata is also involved in the control of respiration and blood pressure but many other CNS structures including the cortex are involved in autonomic modulation. By contrast the nature of the neurotransmitters involved in the efferent system is well understood. The efferent system consists of two major components, the sympathetic system and the parasympathetic system, which act on smooth muscle and glands, often with opposite effects. Both systems differ from somatic nerves by having ganglia that are situated peripherally, moreover most postganglionic autonomic nerve fibres are unmyelinated. Furthermore unlike skeletal striated muscle, smooth and cardiac muscle innervated by the autonomic nervous system has intrinsic activity, which is modified rather than initiated by nervous action.

The sympathetic system is concerned with response to stress ("fight and flight") and is not necessary for life except at times of stress. Although ACh is the neurotransmitter at sympathetic ganglia, at effector organs norepinephrine is released, i.e. the fibres are adrenergic, a major exception being the sweat glands. The cell bodies of the sympathetic preganglionic fibres lie in the spinal cord in the thoracic and upper lumber segments. There are 22 pairs of paravertebral sympathetic ganglia on either side of the vertebral column as well as prevertebral ganglia in the abdomen and pelvis and additionally intermediate ganglia. The adrenal medulla is also part of the sympathetic nervous system but releases epinephrine rather than norepinephrine.

In contrast to the sympathetic nervous system, the parasympathetic nervous system is essential to life. This system utilises ACh as its neurotransmitter both at ganglia and at effector organs. Moreover the ratio of postganglionic to preganglionic neurones is generally considered to be smaller than that prevails in the sympathetic system, although this difference is not universal (Wang *et al.*, 1995). The preganglionic fibres have their origin in the Edinger-Westphal (E-W) nucleus in the mid brain, the superior and inferior salivary nuclei of the medulla oblongata and the sacral part of the spinal cord. The fibres from the E-W nucleus are found in the occulomotor nerve (IIIrd cranial) supplying the ciliary muscle and circular muscle fibres of the iris. Pre-ganglionic fibres arising in the superior salivary nucleus, run in the facial (VIIth cranial) nerve and divide to enter the greater petrosal nerve and the chorda tympani: the former to the sphenopalatine ganglion, the latter to the submandibular ganglion. Post-ganglionic fibres from the sphenopalatine ganglion supply the lachrymal gland and glands of the nasal mucosa and palate. Post-ganglionic fibres from the submandibular ganglion supply the submandibular gland and join the lingual nerve to supply the sublingual gland and the glands of the tongue. Fibres from the inferior salivary nucleus run in the glossopharyngeal (IXth cranial) nerve and supply the parotid gland. The preganglionic fibres in the vagus nerve are notably long extending, for example, to ganglia in the plexuses of Auerbach and Meissner in the gut. Post-ganglionic fibres from these plexuses supply the gut musculature and glands. The vagus also supplies the heart via the deep cardiac plexus. The sacral outflow cells synapse in ganglia around or in the bladder and organs of reproduction.

1.4.2.4. Neuromuscular Junction.

Somatic motor neurones innervate the striated (voluntary) musculature. The axons divide into branches each innervating a single muscle fibre. The muscle fibres supplied by a motor neurone are collectively called a motor unit. The neuromuscular junction (motor endplate) consists of the termination of the motor neurone axon and a specialized part of the muscle fibre membrane, the neurotransmitter at the neuromuscular junction being ACh. An impulse in the motor nerve fibre triggers ACh release and this ACh interacts with the ACh receptor in the post-synaptic membrane giving rise to an endplate potential. Each nerve impulse synchronously releases about 60 ACh-containing vesicles, that is about 10,000 molecules of ACh. This is roughly 10 times the amount needed to trigger a full end-plate potential (EPP). Miniature endplate potentials (MEPPs) are caused by the random release of single vesicles.

1.4.2.5. Central Nervous System.

Cholinergic neurones are found in many areas of the CNS, and interact with many other neurotransmission systems. The neurological control of the cerebral vasculature depends to some extent on cholinergic neurotransmission.

1.4.2.6. Cholinergic Receptors

Cholinergic receptors are divided into muscarinic and nicotinic on the basis of their sensitivity to pharmacological stimulation by muscarine and nicotine, respectively; muscarinic receptors are found in parasympathetic effector organs, whereas nicotinic receptors are found at autonomic ganglia and the neuromuscular junction. More or less specific antagonists are available; thus atropine antagonises muscarinic agonists at muscarinic sites but has little effect at the neuromuscular junction, whereas the reverse is true of tubocurarine. The two types of receptor are fundamentally different, muscarinic receptors using a second-messenger system, whereas nicotinic receptors are ligand-gated ion channels.

1.4.2.7. Muscarinic Receptors.

Five subtypes of muscarinic receptor, designated M_1 to M_5, have been cloned. Each receptor has a serpentine structure that spans the cell membrane seven times. The receptor is coupled via G-proteins (guanosine triphosphate-binding proteins) to the enzymes adenylate cyclase or phospholipase C. M_1 receptors are found in neuronal tissue and activation of M_1 receptors leads to an increase in Ca^{2+} conductance of local ligand-gated Ca^{2+} channels.

These calcium channels are ligand-gated unlike those in the presynaptic or prejunctional terminals which are voltage-gated. Influx of calcium ions via open channels is both electrically driven by the negative intracellular potential and concentration driven: the intracellular free Ca^{2+} concentration being about 100 nmol/l whilst the extracellular concentration is about 1,200,000 nmol/l (Ganong, 1991). Activation of M_2 receptors leads to a decrease in Ca^{2+} conductance. M_2 receptors may play a role at prejunctional sites in modulating the activity at the neuromuscular junction. M_2 receptors are also found in the heart and mediate the depressor effects of parasympathetic activity via the vagus nerve.

The distribution and some functions of the other subtypes have also been characterised (Eglen and Whiting, 1990; Jones, 1993). M_3 receptors are found in glandular tissue, M_4 in the striatum and M_5 in the hippocampus and brainstem.

1.4.2.8. Nicotinic Receptors.

Nicotinic receptors, found at all autonomic system ganglia and at the skeletal neuromuscular junction have been well characterised at a molecular level. The receptors are composed of multiple subunits and a number have been cloned (Boyd, 1997). Each receptor seems to comprise five sub-units arranged around a channel that passes through the cell membrane. Binding of ACh leads to a widening of the channel and an increase in Na^+ conductance. Influx of Na^+ ions leads to depolarization of the cell membrane.

In the CNS both muscarinic (M_1, M_2 and others) and nicotinic receptors are found.

1.4.2.9. Effects of Accumulation of ACh.

Traditionally these effects are divided on the basis of whether the effect in question is mimicked by muscarine or nicotine, which is to say whether muscarinic or nicotinic receptors are involved. Effects in the CNS are considered separately as there is evidence that both types of receptors are involved, and the mechanisms involved have been less well-characterised.

1.4.2.10 Muscarinic Effects

Muscarinic effects mediated by the parasympathetic nervous system include miosis, which causes dimming of vision, spasm of the ciliary muscle, bronchorrhea, bronchoconstriction, rhinorrhea, lacrymation, salivation, sweating, abdominal colic, involuntary micturition and defecation and bradycardia. In very mild oral poisoning with OP antiChEs the only effect may be abdominal cramps, caused by muscarinic effects on the smooth muscle of the small intestine.

1.4.2.11. Nicotinic Effects

Nicotinic effects are those at sympathetic ganglia which may include pallor and tachycardia. Effects at the NMJ include fasciculation and in severe cases muscle paralysis due to depolarization blockade. As the diaphragm may be affected, respiratory failure may occur.

1.4.2.12. Central Effects.

In mild cases of OP exposure ACh accumulation will cause loss of concentration, nightmares, fear, dysarthria and, in more severe cases, convulsions and coma. Broadly speaking the changes that take place in OP poisoning are reversible; as has been described above, reactivation of AChE occurs with most pesticidal OPs and even with soman resynthesis occurs at measurable rates. In general this reversibility seems true of the central effects although where animals or man survive high doses of nerve agents or insecticides pathological changes are sometimes found in the CNS, which would suggest that permanent structural and functional change was likely.

These changes have been best described in experimental animals after dosing with nerve agents such as soman—cellular, particularly astrocytic, edema, perivascular hemorrhages and neuronal degeneration or necrosis, may be seen with occasional infarcts (McLeod, 1985). These changes may be followed by an encephalopathy affecting typically the cortex, hippocampus, and thalamic nuclei (McLeod, 1985; McDonough et al., 1986; McDonough et al., 1989). This distribution may indicate that the cause of the histopathological changes in the brain is anoxia. Quite clearly, at high exposures OP poisoning may cause anoxia through convulsions, effects on the respiratory system or the heart or perhaps through a combination of these. The correlation of the changes with seizure activity (Carpentier et al., 1988; Kadar et al., 1995) and the protective effect of diazepam (Martin et al., 1985; Filliat et al., 1999) suggest that convulsions are a major factor. On the other hand the distribution of the histopathological changes reported in a study by Petras (1981) regions were not typical of the distribution of the lesions after anoxia. Furthermore, Carpentier et al. (1988) observed histopathological changes in rat brains after convulsions during which which hypoxia had not been observed. In a study using rat hippocampal slices in vitro, Labeda et al. (1988) found differences between morphological changes induced by soman in pyramidal nerve cells and those induced by anoxia.

Although the existence of a correlation between histopathological changes in brain cells and anoxia does not prove causation (they might both have a common origin), explanations other than anoxia advanced so far for the distribution of the lesions, need further study: thus the work of Carpentier *et al.* (1990) suggested that soman-induced seizures might produce reversible opening of the blood-brain barrier. The cause of the histopathological changes observed in acute OP poisoning is an important question as the role of anticonvulsants in the prevention of long-term brain damage is underpinned by the possibility that drugs such as benzodiazepines will prevent such effects. There is indeed some experimental evidence that the prevention of convulsions induced by soman not only thwarts the development of histopathological changes induced by soman, but also impedes the development of memory-impairment in the rat (Filliat *et al.*, 1999). The somewhat conflicting data described above may be explicable on the basis of more than one mechanism of toxicity acting at once, and Ray (1998) concluded that the pathogenesis of the changes seen in experimental high dose OP exposure in animals probably involve a combination of hypoxia, cholinergically-mediated excitotoxicity with an element of secondary glutaminergic excitotoxicity.

There is evidence from human studies of patients who have suffered OP poisoning of long term deleterious effects on the CNS (e.g. Savage *et al.*, 1988); although some caution is needed in interpreting such results (it is difficult to obtain an appropriate reference group for epidemiology studies), these results may be the correlate in man of the results in experimental animals discussed above. The effect of long-term low dose exposure has received attention in many countries, in the UK especially because of the exposure of sheep farmers and shepherds to OP sheep dips and also in connection with Gulf War Syndrome, although in the latter case the evidence for exposure was tenuous. The epidemiological evidence for the existence of such effects is a matter of some controversy and some have interpreted the evidence as supporting the existence of a distinct syndrome (chronic OP-induced neuropsychiatric disorder [COPIND]) (Jamal, 1997; Ahmed and Davies, 1997), whereas others have found the evidence for such a discrete syndrome unconvincing (e.g. COT, 1999). At this time any discussion of mechanisms for COPIND is premature, although it is worth considering the possibilities. It is difficult to conceive straightforward antiChE effects that would occur at exposures of the type received during even moderately sensible working practices.

Effects on other enzymes, esterases other than cholinesterases or peptidases, within the CNS would be a possibility especially in view of the generalised antiesterase activity of OPs. One such esterase, neuropathy target esterase is discussed later in this book (Chapter 7) but there are numerous other enzymes in the CNS with esterase activity. This subject was reviewed by Ray (1998), who also pointed out that down-regulation of cholinergic systems occurred with low dose OP exposure, although this is likely to be an adaptive response, and therefore unlikely to interfere with function.

1.4.2.13. Changes in Peripheral Sensory and Motor Nerves

OPIDP is a syndrome that is well recognised and discussed elsewhere in this book. There is some evidence for peripheral nerve damage unrelated to OPIDP. Early studies showed no change or only minor changes in peripheral nerve conduction (e.g. Kimura, 1974; Stålberg et al., 1978).

In a study by Richter (1991), there was weak evidence of changes in peripheral nerve conduction, but confounding factors especially alcohol were present. Other workers have found evidence of decrement in peripheral nerve conduction, both motor and sensory, which is unlikely to be related to OPIDP (e.g. Dési and Nagymajtenyi, 1992). There have been occasional reports of Guillain-Barré syndrome as a sequela to OP poisoning (Fisher, 1977; Adlaka et al., 1987), but in view of the infrequency of such reports, the causal nature of the association is dubious. The question of whether repeated exposure to OPs at low doses causes peripheral nerve changes is controversial. However, the nerve agents soman and sarin, given by multiple sublethal dosing both produced changes in muscle spindle and mechanoreceptor function in cats (Goldstein et al., 1987), but the relevance of this to low-dose exposure is unclear.

1.4.2.14. Non-antiChE Effects of antiChE OPs on the Nervous System

Some effects of OPs do not appear to be mediated by their antiChE action. Thus they can act directly on muscarinic and nicotinic receptors (Bakri et al., 1988; Silveira et al., 1990; Mobley et al., 1990; van den Beukel, et al., 1998), but the concentrations of OP required to do this are generally greatly in excess of that required to inhibit cholinesterases.

There is some evidence of effects of OPs on pathways other than cholinergic ones. A notable example is the effects on GABAergic systems that have been demonstrated with certain OPs. Thus, leptophos affects GABA-regulated chloride channels (Gant *et al.,* 1987) and sarin in the Matsumoto terrorist attack in Japan produced epileptiform EEGs in 2 patients, which may be related to effects on the GABAergic system (Morito *et al.,* 1995).

DFP influences dopaminergic and somatostatinergic pathways in the rat (Naseem, 1990; Smallridge *et al.,* 1991) and moreover, parathion, parathion-methyl and malathion affect calmodulin-dependent phosphodiesterase activity (Pala *et al.,* 1991); however, as is discussed above, cholinergic pathways and pathways using other neurotransmitters interrelate, so that changes in non-cholinergic neurotransmitters after administration of OPs to experimental animals cannot be taken as definite evidence of a direct effect on non-cholinergic systems. The extent to which these non-antiChE effects contribute to acute OP toxicity or to the delayed effects discussed in this book is uncertain

1.4.3. Organ Specific Effects Outside the Nervous System

1.4.3.1 Heart

Effects observed in the heart seem to be due to antiChE effects mainly modulated via the parasympathetic innervation, the parasympathetic effect being to slow the heart. However, this effect is sometimes masked by stimulation of the sympathetic system ganglia. A variety of arrhythmias have been described in severe OP poisoning. Fatal arrhythmias can occur including polymorphous torsade des pointes and ventricular fibrillation (e.g. Wang *et al.,* 1998). It should be noted that pathological changes have been described in experimental animals and humans after exposure to OPs (Pimentel and Carrington da Costa, 1992).

1.4.3.2. Respiratory Tract

The respiratory tract is a target organ for OPs, by peripheral muscarinic actions on the airways, nicotinic actions on the muscles of respiration and effects on the CNS-medullary center.

Indeed, where death occurs in acute OP poisoning, it is commonly due to centrally or peripherally mediated respiratory paralysis, depending on the individual OP. Rhinorrhea and bronchorrhea are prominent in OP poisoning and may interfere with respiratory function as may bronchoconstriction. Effects at the neuromuscular junction may interfere with the action of the muscles of respiration, especially the diaphragm. In severe OP poisoning respiratory failure of central origin may occur, while Intermediate Syndrome generally affects the respiratory musculature (see Chapter 6). Asthmatics are usually advised to avoid contact with OPs, as the possibility that OPs in lower doses might precipitate asthma has given rise to some concern.

The reason for this is that bronchospasm is a feature of both asthma and acute OP poisoning. Nevertheless the mechanisms involved in the two conditions are different and the evidence base for asthmatics avoiding OPs is exiguous. There have been a few case reports of small amounts of OPs precipitating respiratory problems very like allergic asthma e.g. two cases reported by Bryant (1985) of exposure to respectively fenthion used on sheep fleeces and the other to dichlorvos used in a cat flea collar. It was noteworthy that two asthmatic volunteers challenged with fenthion failed to develop symptoms. However, a case of a more persistent asthma-like condition was reported be Deschamps et al. (1994) after exposure of an individual to dichlorvos, probably by inhalation. A major instance of severe respiratory ill-health produced by OPs was that induced by certain trialkyl phosphorothioate impurities of malathion in Pakistani spray men. These impurities produced consolidation in the lungs characterised by injury to type 1 pneumocytes, type 2 cell proliferation and a monocytic infiltrate (Dinsdale, 1992; FAO/WHO, 1998). Unlike the other effects of OPs on the lungs, the effects of these malathion impurities is almost certainly unrelated to antiChE activity.

1.4.3.3. Eyes

Toxicity to the eye is frequently seen in OP poisoning (Grant, 1986; WHO, 1986). Miosis (constriction of the pupil) produces dimming of vision in acute cholinergic OP poisoning. A notable feature of the Tokyo and Matsumoto terrorist attacks using sarin in Japan was painful spasm of the ciliary muscle to a degree not seen with OP insecticide poisoning, producing "glassy eyes" (Masuda et al., 1995). This may be a route specific effect, or possibly a result of other substances in the very impure sarin used in the Japanese attacks.

Largely confined to Japan, changes including myopia, astigmatism, retinal degeneration, constriction of the retinal vessels and papilloedema have been associated with OP exposure and some of these findings have been reproduced in experimental studies in animals (Dementi, 1994). Cortical visual loss has occasionally been reported after OP poisoning (Wang *et al.*, 1999)

1.4.3.4. Gut

The main effects of OPs on the gut are cholinergic effects, such as increased motility, abdominal cramping, involuntary defecation. In very mild poisoning especially by the oral route, abdominal pain may be the main or only symptom. These effects are caused by AChE inhibition and ACh accumulation in the gut wall.

1.4.3.5. Skeletal Muscle

The effects of OPs on skeletal muscle are complex. Initially accumulation of ACh at the neuromuscular junction causes fasciculation, and eventually paralysis. Myopathic changes have been noted in human muscle tissue at autopsy and also in experimental animals, where segmental necrosis of muscle fibres is seen (Ariens *et al.*, 1969) (see also cholinergic syndrome).

1.4.3.6. Other Effects

In regulatory studies of individual OPs, outcomes are often observed which may or may not to be the result of antiChE activity, but which are unrelated to the recognised effects of OPs on esterases and syndromes such as the acute cholinergic or intermediate syndromes or OPIDP. Thus immunotoxicity has been observed while hepatotoxic effects may occur with certain OPs. Effects on the kidney are sometimes seen (Wedin, 1992), while developmental toxicity and or reproductive toxicity is sometimes observed (WHO, 1986; Tyl, 1992; Astroff *et al.*, 1998). As the OPs are neurotoxicants, neurobehavioral teratology is clearly an area of interest (Eskanazi *et al.*, 1999). OPs may give positive results in mutagenicity tests and carcinogenicity studies, for example trichlorfon/metrifonate and dichlorvos. This may be related to the DNA-binding capacity of serine-reactive OPs, which are strongly electrophilic.

It is often unclear to what extent these effects are related to antiesterase or specifically antiChE properties; although not class effects of OPs, these effects may have important consequences in regulatory toxicology,

1.4.4. Clinical Effects of Different antiChE OPs

The relative effectiveness of particular OPs in their effects upon the autonomic nervous system, the neuromuscular junction and CNS depends on dispositional factors as well as factors such as the rate of reaction of the OP with AChE and the rate of reactivation and ageing of the resultant complex. The CNS is, with certain OPs, efficiently protected by the blood brain barrier, however certain OPs may increase the permeability of this barrier and there is considerable variation in the extent to which individual OPs can penetrate the blood brain barrier. Some differences arise because of different routes of exposure: the G type nerve agents are vapour hazards and, as such, the initial symptoms and clinical signs affect the eyes and respiratory tract, with dimming of vision, sneezing and bronchoconstriction. By contrast exposure to insecticides in food initially gives rise to symptoms and signs referable to the gastrointestinal tract.

1.5. OPS USED FOR PROPERTIES OTHER THAN ANTIChE ACTIVITY.

There are a number of OP compounds that have found uses that do not depend upon antiChE activity. They can be divided into three groups. Group 1 comprises fairly typical antiChEs that have been found to have other useful properties, an example being the fungicide pyrazophos. Group 2 includes a number of compounds that have atypical structures and weak antiChE properties. They include the cotton defoliants, tri-S-butyl phosphorotrithioate and tri-S-butyl phosphorotrithioite as well as tri-o-cresyl phosphate, used in jet engines; all three of these are inducers of OPIDP. Ethephon, an agrochemical also belongs to this group but appears not to cause OPIDP (FAO/WHO, 1994). Group 3 comprises a number of compounds, more or less devoid of antiChE activity. Compounds in this group include two important herbicides, glyphosate, a phosphonic acid derivative and glufosinate, a phosphinic acid derivative. The phosphorus-based fire retardants, tetrakis (hydroxymethyl)phosphonium chloride and tris(2,3-dibromopropyl) phosphate must also be included in this group.

The views expressed in this chapter are those of the author and not necessarily those of any UK government agency

References

Adlaka, A., Philip, P.J., Dhar, K.L. Guillain–Barré syndrome as a sequela of organophosphorus poisoning. *Journal of the Association of Physicians of India* 1987;**35**:665–6.

Ahmed, G.M., Davies, D.R. Chronic organophosphate exposure: towards the definition of a neuropsychiatric syndome. *Journal of Nutrition and Environmental Medicine* 1997;**7**:169–76.

Aldridge, W.N. Some properties of specific cholinesterase with particular reference to the mechanism of inhibition of diethyl p-nitrophenyl thiophosphate (11605) and analogues. *Biochemical Journal* 1950;**46**:451–60

Aldridge, W. N., Nemery, B. Toxicology of trialkylphosphorothioates with particular reference to lung toxicity. *Fundamental and Applied Toxicology* 1984;**4**:S215–23.

Ariens, A.T., Wolthuis, O.L., van Benthan, R.M.J. Reversible necrosis at the end plate region in striated muscles of the rat poisoned with cholinesterase inhibitors. *Experientia* 1969;**1**:57–9.

Astroff, A.B., Freshwater, K.S., Eigenberg, D.A. Comparative organophosphate-induced effects observed in adult and neonatal Sprague–Darley rats during the conduct of multigeneration toxicity studies. *Reproductive Toxicology* 1998;**12**:619–45.

Bakry, N.M.S, el-Rashidy, A.H., Eldefrawi, A.T., *et al.* Direct actions of organophosphate antiChEs on nicotinic and muscarinic acetylcholine receptors. *Journal of Biochemical Toxicology* 1988;**3**:235–59.

Boyd, R.T. The molecular biology of neuronal nicotinic acetylcholine receptors. *Critical Reviews in Toxicology* 1997;**27**:99–318.

Carpentier, P., Jacquemond .V., Blanchet, G. EEG, PO2 intracerebrale et périphérique chez le rat intoxiqué par le soman relation avec la pathogenie de l'encephalopathie. *Travail Scientifique* 1988;**9**:109–10

Carpentier, P., Delamanche, I., Le Bert, M., *et al.* Seizure related opening of the blood-brain barrier induced by soman: possible correlation with the acute neuropathology observed in poisoned rats. *Neurotoxicology* 1990;**11**:493–508.

COT. Organophosphates. Report of the Committee on Toxicity. Department of Health. London. 1999.

Davies, D.R. Neurotoxicity of organophosphorus compounds. In: Koelle, G .B. ed. *Handbuch der Experimentellen Pharmakologie*, Berlin: Springer; 1963. p. 860–88

Dementi, B. Ocular effects of organophosphates: a historical perspective of Saku disease, *Journal of Applied Toxicology*. 1984;**14**:119–29.

Dési, I., Nagymajtényi, L. Acute and subchronic neurotoxicity and cardiotoxicity of antiChEs. In:. *Clinical and Experimental Toxicology of Organophosphates and Carbamates*. Ballantyne, B., Marrs, T.C. eds: Butterworth–Heinemann; Oxford 1992. p. 84–9.

Eglen, R.M., Whiting, R.L. Heterogeneity of vascular muscarinic receptors. *Journal of Autonomic Pharmacology* 1990;**10**:233–45.

Eskanazi, B., Bradman, A., Castorina, R. Exposures of children to organophosphate pesticides and their potential adverse health effects. *Environmental Health Perspectives* 1999;**107 Suppl 3**:409–19.

FAO/WHO. Pesticide residues in food-1993. Toxicology evaluation: *World Health Organization,* 1994

Filliat, P., Baubichon, D., Burckhart, M-F. *et al.* Memory impairment after soman intoxication in the rat: correlation with central neuropathology. Improvement with anticholinergic and antiglutaminergic therapeutics. *Neurotoxicology* 1999;**20**:535–50

Fisher, J.R. Guillain–Barré syndrome following organophosphate poisoning. *Journal of the American Medical Association* 1977;**238**:1950–1.

Gallo, M.A., Lawryk, N.J. Organic Phosphorus Pesticides. In: *Handbook of Pesticide Toxicology.* Hayes, W.J., Laws, B.R. eds. :Academic Press; San Diego 1991. p. 917–1123.

Ganong, W.B. Review of Medical Physiology 15th Edition; Appleton, A., Large, A.T. eds. Saddle River, New Jersey: Prentice Hall International Ltd; 1991. p. 35

Gant, D.B., Elderfrawi, M.E., Elderfrawi, T. Action of organophosphates on GABAa receptor and voltage-dependent chloride channels. *Fundamental and Applied Toxicology* 1987;**9**:698–704.

Glickman, A.H., Wing, K.D., Casida, J.E. Profenofos insecticide bioactivation in relation to antidote action and stereospecificity of antiChE inhibition, reactivation and aging. *Toxicology and Applied Pharmacology* 1984;**73**:16–22.

Goldstein, B.D., Fincher, D.R., Searle, J.R. Electrophysiological changes in the primary sensory neuron following subchronic soman and sarin: alterations in sensory receptor function. *Toxicology and Applied Pharmacology* 1987;**91**:55–64

Grant, W.M. *The Toxicology of the Eye*; 3rd Ed. Springfield, Illinois:Charles C Thomas; 1986

Gray, P.J., Dawson, R.M. Kinetic constants for the inhibition of eel and rabbit brain AChE by some organophosphates and carbamates of military significance. *Toxicology and Applied Pharmacology* 1987;**91**:140–4.

Gyrd-Hansen, N., Kraul. I. Obidoxime reactivation of organophosphate inhibited cholinesterase activity in pigs. *Acta Veterinaria Scandinavica* 1984;**5**:86–95.

Heilbron, E. In vitro reactivation and "ageing" of tabun-inhibited blood cholinesterases studies with N-methylpyridinium-2-aldoxime methane sulphonate and N,N'-trimethylene bis (pyridinium-4-aldoxime) dibromide. *Biochemical Pharmacology* 1963;**1**:25–36

Hinz, V.C., Koib, J., Schmidt, B.H. Effects of subchronic administration of metrifonate on cholinergic neurotransmission in rats. *Neurochemical Research* 1998;**3**:931–8

Holmstedt, P. Structure-activity relationships of the organophosphorus antiChE agents In: *Handbuch der Experimentel len Pharmakologie.*. Koelle, G.B. ed. Springer; Berlin:1963. p. 428–85

Inns, R.H., Marrs, T.C. Prophylaxis against antiChE poisonining. In: *Clinical and Experimental Toxicology of Organophosphates and Carbamates*. Ballantyne, B., Marrs, T.C. eds. Butterworth–Heinemann; Oxford:1992. p. 602–10.

ISO. Progress in standardization. Annex 1 ISO common names for pesticides. Annex 3 ISO common names for pesticides. 1965. Geneva: International Organization for Standardization.

ISO. International standard 1750. Geneva: 1981;International Organization for Standardization.

Jamal, G.A. Neurological syndromes of organophosphorus compounds. *Adverse Drug Reactions and Acute Poisonings Review* 1997;**16**:133–70.

Jones, S.V. Muscarinic receptor subtypes: modulation of ion channels. *Life Sciences* 1935;**52**:457–64.

Kadar, T., Shapim, S., Cohen, G. *et al.* Sarin-induced neuropathology in rats. *Human and Experimental Toxicology*. 1995;**14**:252–9.

Keller, H., Müller, T. Erhöhung des Narkoserisikos durch den Einsatz moderner Antihelminthika beim Pferd. *Berlin und München Tierarztliche Wochenschreiben* 1978;**4**:63–5.

Kimura, J. Electrodiagnostic study of pesticide toxicity. In: Xintaras, C., Johnson, B.L., de Groot, I. eds. *Behavioral toxicology: early detection of occupational hazards.* Washington DC, US Department of Health, Education and Welfare; 1974. p. 174–81.

La Du, B.N., Lockridge, O. Molecular biology of human serum cholinesterase. *Federation Proceedings* 1986;**45**:2968–9.

Lim, D.K., Hoskins, B., Ho I. K. Effects of diisopropylfluorophosphate on brain acetylcholinesterase, butyrylcholinesterase, and neurotoxic esterase in rats. *Biomedical Environmental Science* 1989;**2**:295–304

Lebeda, F.J., Wierwille, R.C., VanMeter, W.G. *et al.* Acute ultrastructural alterations induced by soman and hypoxia in rat hippocampal and pyramidal neurones. *Neurotoxicology* 1988;**9**:10–22.

McDonough, J.H., Smith, R.F., Smith, C.D. Behavioral correlates of soman-induced neuropathology: deficits in DRL acquisition. *Neurobehavioural Toxicology and Teratology* 1986;**8**:179–87.

McDonough, J.L., Jaax, N.K., Crowley, A. *et al.* Atropine and/or diazepam therapy protects against soman-induced neural and cardiac pathology. *Fundamental and Applied Toxicology* 1989;**13**:256–76.

McLeod, C.G.. Pathology of nerve agents: perspectives on medical management. *Fundamental and Applied Toxicology* 1988;**5**:S10–S16.

Main, A.R., Iverson, F. Measurement of the affinity and phosphorylation constants governing irreversible inhibition of cholinesterases by diisopropyl phosphorofluoridate. *Biochemical Journal* 1966;**100**:525–31.

Marrs, T.C., Maynard, R.L., Sidell, F. *Chemical Warfare Agents, Toxicology and Treatment.* John Wiley, Chichester. 1996

Marrs, T.C., Dewhurst, L. Toxicology of Pesticides. In: Ballantyne, B., Marrs, T.C., Syversen, T. eds. *General and Applied Toxicology* 2nd edition. London: Macmillan; 1999.

Martin, U., Doebbler, J.A., Shih, T-M. *et al.* Protective effect of diazepam pretreatment on soman-induced brain lesion formation. *Brain Research* 1985;**325**:287–9.

Mason, H.J., Waine, B., Stevenson, A. *et al.* Aging and spontaneous reactivation of human plasma cholinesterase activity after inhibition by organophosphorus pesticides. *Human and Experimental Toxicology* 1993;**12**:497–503

Masson, P., Privat de Garilhe, A., Burnat, P. Multiple molecular forms of human plasma butyrylcholinesterase. II-- study of the C1, C3 and C4 components by means of affinity chromatography. *Biochimica et Biophysica Acta* 1982;**701**:269–84.

Massoulié, J., Bon, S. The molecular forms of cholinesterase and acetylcholinesterase in vertebrates. *Annual Review of Neuroscience* 1982;**5**:57–106

Massoulié, J., Anselmet, A., Bon, S., *et al*. The polymorphism of acetylcholinesterase: post-translational processing, quatenary associations and localization. *Chemico Biological Interactions* 1999;**119/120**:29–42

Masuda, N., Takatsu, M., Morinari, H. *et al*. Sarin poisoning in Tokyo subway. *Lancet* 1995;**345**:1446

Maynard, R.L., Beswick, F.W. Organophosphates as chemical warfare agents. In: Ballantyne, B., Marrs, T.C. eds. *Clinical and Experimental Toxicology of Organophosphates and Carbamates*. Oxford:Butterworth–Heinemann; 1992. p 373–85.

Mobley, P.L. The cholinesterase inhibitor soman increases inositol triphosphate in rat brain. *Neuropharmacology* 1990;**29**:189–91.

Morito, I.I., Yanagisawa, N., Nakajima, T. *et al*. Sarin poisoning in Matsumoto, Japan. *Lancet* 1995;**346**:290–3.

Naseem, S.M. Effect of organophosphates on dopamine and muscarinic receptor binding in rat brain. *Biochemistry International* 1990;**20**:799–806.

Oda, Y. Choline acetyltransferase: the structure, distribution and pathologic changes in the central nervous system. *Pathology International* 1999;**49**:921–37.

Østergaard, D., Jensen, F.S., Viby-Møgensen, J. Pseudocholinesterase deficiency and anticholinesterase toxicity. In: Ballantyne, B., Marrs, T.C. eds. *Clinical and Experimental Toxicology of Organophosphates and Carbamates*. Oxford: Butterworth–Heinemann; 1992. p. 520–7.

Petras, J.M. Soman neurotoxicity. *Fundamental and Applied Toxicology* 1981;**1**:242

Pimentel, J.M., Carrington da Costa, R.B. Effects of organophosphates on the heart In: Ballantyne, B., Marrs, T.C. eds. *Clinical and Experimental Toxicology of Organophosphates and Carbarnates*. Oxford:Butterworth–Heinemann; 1992. p. 145–8

Ray, D.E. Chronic effects of low level exposure to antiChEs – a mechanistic review. *Toxicology Letters* 1998;**102–103**:527–33.

Reiner, E. Spontaneous reactivation of phosphorylated and carbamylated cholinesterases. *Bulletin of the World Health Organisation* 1971;**44**:109–12.

Richter, E. Organophosphorus pesticides, a multinational epidemiological study. WHO Regional Office for Europe, Copenhagen. 1991 Document EUR/RC41/InfDoc.

Savage, E.P., Keefe, T.J., Mounce, L.M. *et al.* Chronic neurological sequelae of acute organophosphate pesticide poisoning. *Archives of Environmental Health* 1988;**43**:38–45.

Senanayake, N., Karalliedde, L. Intermediate syndrome in antiChE neurotoxicity. In:. *Clinical and Experimental Toxicology of Organophosphates and Carbamates.* Ballantyne, B., Marrs, T.C. eds: Butterworth–Heinemann; Oxford 1992. p. 126–134.

Silveira, C.L.P., Eldefrawi, A.T., Eldefrawi, M.E. Putative muscarinic receptors of rat heart have high affinity for organophosphorus antiChEs. *Toxicology and Applied Pharmacology* 1990;**47**;4481.

SIPRI. Stockholm International Peace Research Institute. The problem of chemical and biological warfare. Vol 1 The rise of CB weapons. Stockholm 1963: Almqvist and Wiksell.

Škinjaric-Špoljar, M., Simeon, V., Reiner, E. Spontaneous reactivation and aging of dimethylphosphorylated AChE and cholinesterase. *Biochemica et Biophysica Acta* 1973;**315**:363–9.

Smallridge, R.C., Carr, F.E., Fein, H.G. Diisopropylfluorophosphate (DFP) reduces serum prolactin, thyrotropin, luteinizing hormone, and growth hormone and increases adrenocorticotropin and corticosterone in rats: involvement of dopaminergic and somatostatinergic as well as cholinergic pathways. *Toxicology and Applied Pharmacology* 1991;**108**:284–95.

Stålberg, E., Hilton-Brown, P., Kolmodin-Hedman, B. *et al.* Effect of occupational exposure to organophosphorus insecticides on neuromuscular function. *Scandinavian Journal of Work, Environment and Health* 1978;**4**:255–61.

Talbot, B.O., Anderson, D.R., Harris, L.W. *et al.* A comparison of in vivo and in vitro rates of aging of soman-inhibited erythrocyte AChE in different animal species. *Drug and Chemical Toxicology* 1988;**11**:289–305.

Vale, J.A. Toxicokinetic and toxicodynamic aspects of organophosphorus (OP) insecticide poisoning. *Toxicology Letters* 1998;**102–103**, 649–52.

Van den Beukel, L., van Kleef, R.G.D.M., Oortgiesen, M. Differential effects of physostigmine and organophosphates on nicotinic receptors in neuronal cells of different species. *Neurotoxicology* 1998;**19**:777–88

Wang, F.B., Holst, M.C., Powley, T.L. The ratio of pre- to postganglionic neurons and related issues in the autonomic nervous system. *Brain Research Brain Research Reviews* 1995;**21**:93–115.

Wang, A-G., Lin, R-S., Liu, J-H. *et al.* Positron emission tomography scan in cortical visual loss in patients with organophosphate toxicity. *Ophthalmology* 1999;**106**:1287–91.

Wang, M-H., Tseng, C-D., Bair, S.Y. Q-T interval prolongation and pleomorphic ventricular tachyarrhythmia (torsade de pointes) in organophosphate poisoning: report of a case, *Human and Experimental Toxicology* 1998;**17**:587–90.

Wedin, G.P. Nephrotoxicity of antiChEs, In: Ballantyne, B., Marrs, T.C. eds. *Clinical and Experimental Toxicology of Organophosphates and Carbamates.* Oxford:Butterworth–Heinemann; 1992. p. 195–202

Wehner, J.M., Smolen, A., Smolen, T.N. Recovery of acetylcholinesterase activity after acute organophosphate treatment of CNS re-aggregate cultures. *Fundamental and Applied Toxicology* 1985;**5**:1104–9

WHO Environtmental Health Criteria No 63. *Organophosphorus Insecticides: a General Introduction.* Geneva World Health Organization. 1986

Wilson, B.W., Hooper, M.J., Hansen, E. *et al.* Reactivation of organophosphorus inhibited AChE with oximes. In Chambers, J.E., Levi, P.E. eds. *Organophosphates, chemistry, fate and effects.* New York:Academic Press; 1992

Wilson, L.B., Ginsberg, S. Reactivation of AChE inhibited by acetylphosphates. *Arch Biochem Biophys* 1955;**54**:569–71.

Worek, P., Diepold, C., Eyer, P. Dimethylphosphoryl-inhibited human cholinesterases: inhibition, reactivation, and aging kinetics. *Archives of Toxicology* 1999;**7**:7–14.

CHAPTER 2

Socio-Economics, Health Issues and Pesticides

Lakshman Karalliedde and Tim Meredith

2.1. Introduction

In the mind of the general public, the introduction of new chemicals into the environment is associated with potential risks and, especially, concern regarding possible impacts on human health and ecosystems. The current state of the science means that only rarely can categorical answers be given concerning the presence or absence of such effects. That being so, it is inappropriate to dismiss such public concern as being ignorant, irrational or even hysterical, as sometimes happens, and it behoves scientists and policy makers to identify research needs and to fill data gaps. Pesticides in general and organophosphorus insecticides in particular represent good cases in point where, despite widespread and longstanding usage for the public good, there are important data gaps in relation to impacts on human health, particularly within vulnerable population subgroups such as children.

Organophosphorus (OP) compounds, of which there are more than 50,000, are usually esters of phosphoric, phosphonic, phosphorothioic or phosphoramidic acids (see Chapter 1). OP compounds have important biological effects and are used principally in agriculture as pesticides, usually as insecticides. They are important for the well being of food-producing animals but in addition they are used to treat ectoparasitic infections in non-food-producing animals such as horses, and in pets such as cats and dogs. Some OP compounds are used in human medicine, for example malathion, in the treatment of louse infestations and trichlorfon in the treatment of *Schistosoma haematobium* infestation. Others are used in industry as lubricants, plasticisers and flame-retardants. Still others are used in horticulture, for example, to prevent insect damage to timber. OP compounds have also gained notoriety as agents of chemical warfare.

Formulations of OP compounds are tailored to their intended use, but their toxicity is essentially non-selective. As a consequence, their worldwide usage is associated with significant, but as yet poorly defined, morbidity and mortality as a result of occupational exposure, accidental poisoning and intentional ingestion with suicidal intent.

This chapter examines socio-economic aspects of OP compound usage, including those related to known adverse health effects. Socio-economic aspects are of special relevance in developing countries where OP compounds are used extensively in agriculture and in public health programmes (Jeyaratnam, 1985). In some developing countries, 60% of the workforce is employed in agriculture where, without pesticides, one third of crops would be destroyed by pests.

2.2. Role in Control of Vector Borne Diseases

Pathogens (viruses, rickettsiae, bacteria, protozoa and nematode worms) responsible for many human diseases themselves make use of insect, tick or mite vectors for the purpose of transmission to their human hosts. Their impact on human health worldwide is not inconsiderable (see Table 2.1.).

There are also many arthropod-borne viruses (arboviruses), most of which are of importance only sporadically and in local areas. In addition, there are arthropods that are not vectors but which cause harm by means of stings (e.g. scorpions, wasps), allergenic faeces that cause asthma (e.g. house dust mites) or which act as irritating nuisances (e.g. head lice, biting mosquitoes and *Culicoides* midges).

In a few instances, vector-borne diseases may be controlled by vaccines (e.g. yellow fever, Japanese and tick borne encephalitis, Lyme disease). For all of these diseases except those of viral aetiology, there are drug treatments available for human patients. However, there are considerations of expense in developing countries and the problem of the development of drug resistance. Vector control therefore plays, or ought to play, an important part in the control of most vector-borne diseases.

Mosquitoes (*Anopheles*) are important as vectors of malaria, various forms of filariasis and numerous arboviruses, the best known being dengue and yellow fever. In many temperate climates, mosquitoes are of little or no importance as disease vectors. Nevertheless, they can still cause considerable annoyance because of their bites (subfamily *Culicine*). The greatest numbers of mosquitoes are found in the northern areas of the temperate regions especially near or within the Arctic Circle, where, at certain times of the year, the number of insects biting can be so huge as to make any outdoor activity virtually impossible.

For all these reasons, greater efforts have been made to control mosquitoes than any other biting insect.

Table 2.1. Summary of the available information on the human impact of the vector borne diseases (By permission Prof C. Curtis 2000).

Disease (pathogen genus and class)	Vectors (generic and common name)	Route of infection of vector	Affected areas of the World	Human impact
Malaria (4 spp. of *Plasmodium*, protozoa)	*Anopheles* mosquito	By biting humans	Tropical Africa, South Asia, tropical America, Melanesia, formerly in temperate zone	c. 300x10^6 clinical cases and 10^6 deaths/year
Chagas disease (*Trypanosoma cruzi*, protozoan)	*Triatoma, Rhodnius.* Triatomine bugs	By biting humans, or animals	Tropical Americas	4th most important parasitic disease
Lymphatic filariasis (*Wuchereria, Brugia,* nematodes)	*Culex quinque-fasciatus, Anopheles, Mansonia, Aedes,* mosquitoes	By biting humans (rarely monkeys)	Trop. Africa, south Asia, Polynesia, NE Brazil	Elephantiasis is 2nd largest cause of disablement
Diarrhoeal diseases, (*Shigella* etc., bacteria)	*Musca domestica,* houseflies, (as well as non vector routes)	By contact with faeces	All warm countries	3x10^6 deaths/year
Trachoma (*Clamydia,* bacterium)	*Musca sorbens,* (as well as contagion)	By contact with eye secretions	Tropics (formerly temperate zone also)	Largest single cause single cause of preventable blindness
Dengue (virus)	*Aedes,* mosquitoes	By biting humans	SE Asia, tropical America, Polynesia	50x10^6 infections/year; 250,000 severe cases/year

Table 2.1. Summary of the available information on the human impact of the vector borne diseases (By permission Prof C. Curtis 2000). - continued

Disease (pathogen genus and class)	Vectors (generic and common name)	Route of infection of vector	Affected areas of the World	Human impact
Leishmaniasis (several spp. of *Leishmania*, protozoa)	*Phlebotomus*, (Old world), *Lutzomyia* (New World), sandflies	By biting rodents, dogs or humans	Warm countries	1.5×10^6 cutaneous and 0.5×10^6 visceral cases/year
Onchocerciasis (*Onchocera*, nematode)	*Silmulium*, black flies	By biting humans	Tropical Africa, tropical America	Millions blinded or with severe itching
Sleeping sickness (*Trypanosoma brucei* group, protozoa)	*Glossina*, tsetse flies	By biting humans or animals	Tropical Africa	Disastrous epidemics in early 20th century and recent resurgence
Typhus (*Rickettsia prowazeki*, rickettsia)	*Pediculus*, body louse	By biting humans	Tropics formerly temperate zone also	2×10^6 killed during Russian Civil War
Bubonic plague (*Yersinia*, bacteria)	*Xenopsylla*, rat flea (also contagion)	By biting rodents	Foci in tropics and temperate zone	One third of population of Europe killed in 14th century
Japanese encephalitis (virus)	*Culex tritaeniorhynus* mosquitoes	By biting pigs and birds	East Asia	40,000 cases/year, 11,000 deaths/year

Table 2.1. Summary of the available information on the human impact of the vector borne diseases (By permission Prof C. Curtis 2000). - continued

Disease (pathogen genus and class)	Vectors (generic and common name)	Route of infection of vector	Affected areas of the World	Human impact
Yellow fever (virus)	*Aedes, Haemogogus*, mosquitoes	By biting monkeys	Tropical Africa, tropical America (not Asia)	Disastrous epidemics in 18th century in Caribbean
Lyme disease (*Borrelia burgdorferi*, spirochaete)	*Ixodes*, hard ticks	By biting field mice	Temperate zone	Now the only important vector human disease in USA
Relapsing fever (*Borrelia duttoni* and *B. recurrentis*, spirochaete)	*Orinthodoros*, soft ticks and *Pediculus*, body lice	Transovarial or by biting humans	Foci in Africa and Middle East	
Loiasis (*Loa*, nematode)	*Chrysops*, deer flies	By biting humans	West and Central Africa	c. 10^6 people affected
Scrub typhus *Rickettsia tsutsugamushi*	*Leptotrombidium*, chigger mites	Transovarial or by biting	Western Pacific	

Attempts at biological control were popular during the early part of the 20th century, but these were replaced by insecticidal control in the latter half.

Recently, however, there has been renewed interest in biological control because of the development of resistance to insecticides and a greater concern regarding environmental impacts. Unfortunately, biological control is difficult to implement and maintain and its effects are not rapid. For example, if predators, such as larvivorous fish, are used, it is unlikely that they will prey solely on larvae and pupae, thus affecting harmless and beneficial insects.

Alternatives to insecticides that have been employed are genetic control (e.g. release of sterile male mosquitoes into the field), physical control (eradication of breeding places), and application of oils (diesel and kerosene) or fine dusts (copper acetoarsenite) on to water surfaces.

So far as insecticides are concerned, OPs (malathion, primiphos-methyl, fenitrothion, temephos) are considered most suitable because they are less persistent and more biodegradable than organochlorines. Pyrethroids (e.g. permethrin) tend to kill other aquatic insects, crustaceans and even fish. Fenthion and chlorpyrifos are recommended for use in organically polluted waters where insecticides such as malathion are relatively ineffective. Chlorpyrifos is more toxic to mosquito larvae than most other insecticides but it causes higher mortality among fish and other aquatic organisms and therefore needs to be used cautiously. These insecticides are typically delivered by spray at 10–14 day intervals. Temephos has very low mammalian toxicity and this has been used successfully to control *Aedes aegypti* mosquitoes.

Eradication programmes are estimated to have prevented the occurrence of more than 2000 million cases of malaria during 1961–1971. They are also estimated to have prevented 15 million persons from dying. In Sri Lanka, between 1968 and 1970 there were 1.5 million cases of malaria, out of a total population of 12 million. As a result of mosquito eradication programmes, there were only 18 cases in 1973.

Ground-based or aerial ultra-low volume (ULV) applications of malathion, fenitrothion and primiphos-methyl are used in disease epidemic situations (for example, involving dengue fever or yellow fever), where one of the main objectives is to kill infected adult vectors as quickly as possible so as to halt the epidemic.

Because of the prevalence and severity of river blindness in the Volta River Basin area of West Africa and its devastating effect on rural life, the World's most ambitious and largest vector control programme was initiated in 1974 by WHO (the Onchocerciasis Control Programme or OCP). This programme originally involved Benin, Burkina Faso, Côte d'Ivoire, Ghana, Mali, Niger and Togo.

Since 1986, it has also involved parts of Guinea, Guinea Bissau, Senegal and Sierre Leone. Approximately 50,000 km of rivers over an area of 1.3 million km^2 that were breeding the *S. damnosum* complex were dosed at weekly intervals with temephos. Because of the appearance of temephos resistance in 1980, some rivers were treated with other insecticides or with *Bacillus thuringiensis*, subspecies *israeliensis*. To hinder the emergence of further resistance, rotation of different insecticides was introduced in 1982. Since 1988, the OCP has been undertaking large-scale distribution of the microfilaricide, ivermectin, which is administered orally to patients once or twice a year. Results achieved by the OCP have been spectacular, and transmission of river blindness has ceased over most of the OCP area (Service, 2000).

Houseflies can transmit the viruses of polio, trachoma, Coxsackie and infectious hepatitis, as well as rickettsia, such as Q fever, and the bacteria of numerous diseases, mainly those of an enteric nature, such as bacillary dysentery, cholera, typhoid and paratyphoid. They are known to transmit enterotoxic *Escherichia coli* (ETEC) and campylobacter, as well as a variety of staphylococci and streptococci. They may also be vectors of protozoan parasites such as those causing amoebic dysentery. Houseflies carry eggs and cysts of a variety of helminths (e.g. *Taenia, Hymenolepsis, Dipylidium, Diphyllobothrium, Necator, Ancylostoma, Ascaris*) and can be carriers in the tropical Americas of the eggs of *Dermatobia hominis*, a myiasis-producing fly. To control houseflies, diazinon, bromophos, fenchlorphos, fenitrothion and fenthion have been used as larvicides to spray the inside of dustbins and over garbage and refuse heaps, and manure piles. Dichlorvos (0.5%), malathion (2–4%), pirimiphos-methyl (2%) and fenchlorphos (0.1–0.5%) are used to kill adult flies (through aerosol applications, insecticidal cords and space-spraying). It is important to note that in many parts of the world, houseflies have become resistant to many organochlorine insecticides and to some organophosphorus insecticides.

OPs have been used to spray inside the surfaces of walls and ceilings (particularly against *Anopheles* mosquitoes and sand flies), against adult insects in the form of ULV space sprays (against dengue vector *Aedes*), and in aerial spraying (against Tsetse flies).   However, the use of these insecticides is not without disadvantage in the control of vectors because recent work has shown the development of resistance in some insects, especially mosquitoes.

Vector-borne diseases have serious economic implications as a result of lost working hours, and the high costs of treating the sick and controlling the vectors of disease. For example, the total economic impact of schistosomiasis was estimated to be around $US 642 million per annum in the 1970s.

Schistosomiasis is caused by a flat worm—a fluke (*Schistosoma mansoni* in Africa and South America, *Schistosoma haematobium* in Africa and Middle East and *Schistosoma japonicum* in Asia). The vectors are fresh water snails.

2.3. Role in Food Production and Storage

Pesticides, including OPs, are used both on arable crops (rice, wheat, etc.) and on food-producing livestock.

2.3.1. Arable Crops

Historically, the rate of world population growth has tended to exceed the World's ability to produce sufficient food and when, for example, large-scale droughts or outbreaks of disease or crop destruction by pests occur, famine results. Current population figures are salutary. The world population grows by approximately 1.6% per annum with an accompanying increase in food requirements of 2–3% per annum. The area of land available for growing crops decreases by at least one per cent each year as a result of soil erosion and salinisation. As a percentage of the total world population, that in developing countries will increase from 77% in 1990 to 88% in 2100 (World Bank). At present, there are nearly 650 million people who are considered to be undernourished—of these, 35% are in sub-Saharan Africa, 22% in Asia and 14% in Latin America. Rice, wheat, maize and potatoes represent the principal staple foods of the world.

Table 2.2. Production data and losses due to pests 1988–1990

	Asia	Africa	America
Attainable production (Mt)	962.7	24.1	51.1
Production at present (Mt)	466.6	11.1	25.5
Production without crop protection (Mt)	169.1	4.3	7.8
Estimated losses due to: diseases	20%	18%	22%
animal pests	30%	18%	18%
weeds	33%	46%	45%

adapted from Oerke EC *et al., Crop Production and Crop Protection,* Elsevier 1994

2.3.1.1. Rice

Rice is the staple food for more than 50% of the World's population. In 1990, almost 520 million tonnes (Mt) of rice were grown on 146 million hectares of land, with more than 90% being produced in Asia. Most was for home consumption— only 3–5% entered the world market. World reserves of rice are estimated to be sufficient for two months consumption only. Yet rice as a staple crop is vulnerable to disease and attack by pests. In the 1990s, 12 bacterial, 58 fungal and 17 viral or mycoplasma-like pathogens were known to cause disease in rice.

Animal pests include more than 30 species of nematode and, in South-East Asia alone, 100 species of insect are known to attack rice plants. Worldwide, rice crops are damaged by nearly 1800 species of weeds as well as by rodents and birds.

Farmers spend approximately $US 2.4 billion on pesticides in rice fields, of which about 80% are employed in Asia (http://www.american.edu/projects/mandala/TED/vietpest.htm). Over 90% of the pesticides sprayed were insecticides, and approximately half of them were OP compounds including parathion-methyl, monocrotophos and methamidophos (PANUPS, 1995).

2.3.1.2. Wheat

Wheat is the staple food for about 35% of the World's population. Wheat and rice each account for about 20% of calories in the food consumed by the peoples of the world. States of the Former Soviet Union (FSU) grow by far the largest areas of wheat in the world, with the other major producers being USA, China, India, France, Canada, Australia, Argentina and Turkey.

2.3.1.3. Cotton

In 1990, the estimated loss due to animal pests in the production of cotton, an important cash crop for many developing countries, was 15%. Arthropod pests, above all bollworms, the boll weevil and leaf worms, are the major crop protection problems for cotton. The potential loss rates in a "no protection scenario" due to arthropod pests, and nematodes and weeds, are estimated to be 37% and 36%, respectively.

The effectiveness of crop protection in cotton is much higher than in food crops, and insect control is a high priority.

Table 2.3. Production data and losses due to pests 1988-1990 in relation to wheat

	Europe	Former USSR	Africa	Asia	North America
Attainable production (Mt)	171.7	162.4	21.8	290.2	125.4
Production at present (Mt)	127.7	94.9	13.3	191.8	83.9
Production without crop protection (Mt)	81.2	72.5	10.3	145.2	3.1
Estimated losses due to:					
diseases	9%	17%	8%	12%	12%
animal pests	7%	10%	12%	9%	11%
weeds	9%	14%	19%	13%	11%

adapted from Oerke EC *et al.*: Crop Production and Crop Protection Elsevier 1994

2.3.1.4. Maize

Animal pests cause nearly a 20% loss in production of maize in South America where it is a staple food, and nearly a 28% loss in production in South East Asia. Losses in Europe and the FSU range from 5 to 15%. The average loss sustained in 1990 worldwide despite the use of crop protection was estimated to be 38%. The European corn borer (*Ostrinia mibilalis*) causes damage amounting to $US 350 million annually to maize crops in the US (New Scientist, 22.4.2000).

2.3.1.5. Potato

The losses worldwide in potato produce are 16% due to disease, 16% due to animal pests and 9% due to weeds. The losses due to animal pests are greatest in the tropics. In developed countries such as the USA, the Colorado beetle ravages millions of dollars worth of potato crops every year. In the Russian Federation, the problem is of such severity that the growth of potatoes has become extremely difficult (New Scientist, 19.2.2000).

2.3.1.6. Coffee

In the 1990s, approximately 40% of the attainable harvest of coffee was lost—14% due to diseases, 15% due to animal pests and 10% due to weeds. Animal pests cause the greatest damage in Asia and Latin America. Crop protection can almost double the yield of coffee.

The various figures cited above do not take account of the impact on food production caused by disability of workforces due to vector borne diseases and external and internal parasites. The same considerations apply to livestock production (see below).

2.3.1.7. Complications of Pesticide Usage in Arable Crop Production

The use of pesticides in agriculture is certainly not problem free. In Indonesia in 1986, an outbreak of brown plant hopper devastated rice output, destroying enough rice to feed three million people (Science News, 1992). Neither pesticides nor modified strains of rice were able to stop the infestation of the plant hopper and the plant virus it carried. Subsequent research showed that pesticides had exaggerated the problem by encouraging the development of resistant plant hopper strains and by killing the natural predators of the insect (Science News, 1992) which made one researcher comment "trying to control population outbreaks with insecticides is like pouring kerosene on a house fire" (Science News, 1992). Subsequent introduction of an Integrated Pest Management (IPM) system enabled a 75% reduction in pesticide use in Indonesia in the mid-1990s with a significant increase in rice production.

However, implementation of IPM programmes involves substantial cost and it is therefore necessary to demonstrate their cost-effectiveness to farmers, to overcome the scepticism of conservative rural societies. Farmers in Asia view pesticides as products with medicinal-like qualities that cure the ailments of their crops. As a result, application of pesticides has been indiscriminate and liberal (Ecology, 1996).

More than 900 species of insects, weed and plant pathogens worldwide have now developed some resistance to at least one pesticide—up from 182 in 1965. At least 17 insect species have shown some resistance to all major insecticide classes. In 1980–1990, there were only a dozen herbicide-resistant weeds. Today there are 84.

The 'Green Revolution' introduced high-yielding plant varieties, particularly of rice and wheat.

Although this resulted in considerable increases in crop production, these varieties were found to be more susceptible than conventional varieties to pathogens and to attack by plant hoppers and leafhoppers and to the virus diseases that they transmit. It has taken time to breed plants that are totally or partially resistant to these pests. Indiscriminate use of broad-spectrum insecticides has also led to the development of resistance and to the killing of insect predators, both of which have increased the problems caused by pests.

In Asia, high temperatures and humidity predispose crops to damage. Losses due to animal pests in Asia are almost double those in developed countries. Thus, in a region where population growth is relatively uncontrolled, where vector-borne disease contributes significantly to population mortality, where economies are struggling to provide health care, where malnutrition affects millions, pests destroy most crops and the high temperatures predispose to post-harvest losses. Asia is perhaps most affected by insecticide-related human ill health, yet arguably it is the region, which can least afford not to use insecticides.

Africa, Latin America, Asia, East Europe and the FSU account for nearly 77% of the actual production of food, and losses reach 45%. In Western Europe, farmer's harvest nearly 77% of the produce yet contribute only 8% to the actual global production of the eight crops :rice, wheat, maize, barley, coffee, cotton, soya bean, potato.

Globally, the overall loss of attainable arable crop production was 41% in 1990. Without the use of physical, chemical or biological measures to protect crops, it is estimated that this loss would be nearer 70%. The measures taken to protect crops therefore prevented production losses to the value of $US 160,000 million. Some believe that every dollar expended on pesticides generated four dollars of additional sales. In the absence of crop protective measures, prices would likely be 50–100% higher for foodstuffs made from crops such as fruit, vegetables and non-staple commodities.

2.3.2. Livestock

From early times, man has used domestic animals to provide food and manure, clothing and leather, transport and power, employment and protection, company and recreation. Farm animals can suffer infestations of external parasites with subsequent risk of spread of infection to humans. Parasitic populations reduce the economic performance of livestock.

For these several reasons, it has become obligatory to protect farm animals in the UK from infestations (Farm Animal Welfare Codes). OPs used to treat animals there include diazinon, fenthion, phosmet, cythioate, dichlorvos, fenitrothion, propetamphos and tetrachlorvinphos. These OPs were chosen based on their effectiveness and relative lack of toxicity, that is, an ability to target specific pests without causing harm to host animals. Although alternatives to OPs have always been present, OPs continue to be used widely because they are both efficacious and cost-effective in the control of a wide range of pests. In many countries, for example the UK, animal medicine authorisations are routinely and continuously reviewed by law and permission for their use may be revoked, should a need for revocation be demonstrated. Under such laws, manufacturers and veterinary surgeons are typically obliged to report to licensing authorities any adverse reactions to animal medicines, both in animals and man. Sales outlets for such medications are staffed by trained and qualified personnel in the UK and EU. Precautions such as the 'withdrawal period'—when an animal or its produce cannot enter the food chain until a specified period has passed—are in use in many developed countries. As regards availability to the public, licensing authorities in most countries determine whether an insecticide should be available by general sale or restricted to sale by qualified personnel or even by prescription by a veterinarian only.

Parasites reduce the economic performance of livestock. Losses of millions of dollars have followed babesiosis (a protozoal disease disseminated by tick infested cattle), trypanosomiasis, sheep scab and fluke infections. Tick infestations cause itching and scratching which often leads to secondary infection, thus reducing the quality of hide with consequent losses in leather production, as well as leading to animal distress.

Thus, at present, the role of insecticides in the livestock industry appears unarguable until cost-effective alternatives become available. Pesticides have become an integral part of the production process. Wholesale banning of their use would have an impact on the consumer, farmer and society as a whole.

2.3.2.1. Other uses

OP pesticides are used on non-food producing animals, including horses and pets such as cats and dogs, to treat ecto-parasitic infestations. Pets are often an important source of companionship and comfort and provide protection and sometimes transport in many differing communities in the world.

Pets in good health, free from parasitic infestations, contribute to the well being of humans. However, the use of OPs on pet animals presents particular opportunities for exposure of children.

Stable flies (*Stomoxys calcitrans*) inflict painful bites in cattle, horses and pets, especially dogs. Adult flies of this species do not transmit diseases to humans, but they appear to transmit *Trypanosoma evansi*, the causative agent of Surra, a disease that infects camels, horses and many other animals in tropical countries. OPs have been used to spray breeding places and insecticidal spraying is carried out inside horse stables, animal shelters, barns and other farm buildings.

Certain species of fleas are important vectors of disease but the most widespread complaint concerns the annoyance caused by their bites. Fleas are difficult to catch and insecticides remain the main tool for flea control. Malathion (2–5%), diazinon and dichlorvos can be either applied to the fur of animals or used as flea collars. There is increasing reliance on the use of insect growth regulators (IGRs), such as cyromazine or lufenuron, for effective control of fleas.

One of the commonest causes of poisoning in dogs and cats is insecticide poisoning. This often follows overenthusiastic use or disregard of safety precautions.

2.4. Pesticide-Associated Human Ill-Health

Human exposure to OPs can result from inhalation, ingestion, eye or skin contact. Oral intake may be either accidental or suicidal. Reportedly, in the first half of the 1990s, as many as 2–5 million cases of pesticide poisoning occurred, of which 400,000 were said to be fatal.

Some 2–3% of agricultural workers in developing countries are believed to have suffered some form of intoxication of which 10–12% suffered fatal consequences. However, the impact on human health of OP insecticides in terms of death, illness or dysfunction is not known with certainty at present (see Chapter 17). The earlier reported figures need to be checked and studies to that end are being undertaken by WHO.

The effect of acute OP exposure has been relatively well studied even though there remain many uncertainties regarding pathogenesis and optimal management. The effects of low-dose, long-term OP exposure have aroused much debate in both scientific and public circles. While there is a large number of prospective, controlled epidemiological studies on the sequelae of acute OP poisoning, most of those on long-term low-dose poisoning are cross-sectional in design. Moreover, the design of the studies has not been sufficiently similar for metanalysis to be practicable. The fact that many of the studies on the sequelae of acute poisoning have taken place in developing countries, whereas those on long-term low dose exposure have taken place in developed ones, reflects the differing priorities of these different groups of countries.

Occupational exposure, particularly in developing countries, is primarily the result of protective clothing not being available, or being unsuitable because of climatic conditions, and the use of faulty sprayers and cheap and toxic OPs (see Chapter 17). Occupational exposures and deliberate oral intake with suicidal intent in developing countries affects individuals during a productive phase of their lives. Ill health and/or loss of work-years associated with such incidents represents an additional strain on the health services and economies of poor countries. The increasing incidence of accidental exposures both in developing, and also developed, countries needs to be addressed.

Despite the advances in medical care, particularly critical and intensive care, the morbidity and mortality associated with acute OP poisoning has not decreased over the years. The lack of clinical trials studying newer antidotal agents, particularly those that have been found to be effective in animals, is disappointing.

This is particularly so because there are controversies as to the effectiveness of the antidotes that have been used for the past three decades.

2.5. Effects on the Environment and Wild Life

Robert Costanza, Director of the University of Maryland Institute for Ecological Economics and his colleagues have estimated that the market value of "services" provided for us by nature is approximately $US 33 trillion per year. Many natural services are impossible to price. Soil, for example, is a living biosystem. One cubic metre of soil contains thousands of tiny creatures and billions of micro-organisms, each of which may be affected by use of non-selective insecticides and fungicides. The consequences of disturbing nature cannot be disregarded economically.

Numerous reports and publications have highlighted the adverse effects insecticides have had on the environment.

These include:

- The decline of farmland birds such as the skylark, corn bunting and grey partridge by 59% and 82%, respectively over the past 30 years.
- The destruction of lug worms, an important source of food for wild fish
- The decline of nearly 1200 wild vertebrate pollinators, which are held responsible for decreasing yields of blueberries in New Brunswick, cherries in Ontario, pumpkins in New York, cashew nuts in Borneo and Brazil nuts in Bolivia and Brazil (New Scientist, 14.2.1998).

Bees play an essential role as pollinators in addition to being kept for honey production. In some parts of Tanzania and Kenya, bee keeping has become non-existent as a result of insecticide use (Bull). It has been estimated that pollination losses due to pesticides come to at least $US 80 million. Adding the cost of reduced pollination to the direct environmental costs of the effect of pesticides on honey bees and wild bees, result in a total annual loss calculated to be about $US 135 million.

2.6. Insecticide-Related Disease and Global Health Priorities

The relative global burden of disease attributable to non-communicable diseases (NCDs) compared to that attributable to communicable diseases (CDs) is uncertain. Christopher Murray and Alan Lopez, using the "disability-adjusted life year" (DALY) concept, predicted that by the year 2020, NCDs would be causing nearly 73% of all deaths worldwide.

On the other hand, AIDS, malaria and dengue continue to affect millions and none of these diseases has a vaccine developed for prevention. People in developing countries now have healthier childhoods, and live longer as a result of global health developments, thus increasing the likelihood of NCDs affecting more and more individuals in developing countries.

Pesticide-related ill health represents a NCD with high mortality and morbidity, especially in poorer developing countries. Unfortunately, the requirements for pesticides in these countries is high. Pesticide-induced ill health in such countries mainly affects the younger age groups (18–30 years) as a result of oral intake with suicidal intent. The emphasis Global Health Authorities place on this unique NCD is awaited with interest.

2.7. Role of Industry

The pesticide industry employs high technology and is research-intensive. However, the implementation of safety controls in countries vary from those that are very stringent to those that are completely absent. Nevertheless, over the years, industry has developed strategies to prevent ill health associated with insecticides. These include labelling of products with details of constituents, guidelines for use including the wearing of protective gear, and therapeutic procedures to follow in the event of exposures occurring. Work has also been undertaken to provide information on the effects of differing climatic conditions and safe time limits for work involving insecticides. Industry has trained medical personnel in some developing countries, provided literature on toxicity and management, and provided hospitals with therapeutic agents. In addition, industry has supported research on OP poisoning and, through in-house research programmes, it has attempted to develop safer products.

Despite all of these measures, though, there remain important problems associated with the use of OP insecticides and pesticides. A significant proportion of the labour force that uses pesticides, particularly in developing countries, is illiterate, thus limiting the effectiveness and usefulness of labelling. Many dialects are in use and the most effective language for communication cannot always be easily identified. In one country, for example, industry has found the need to print labels in 12 languages.

Protective clothing is more suited to workers in temperate climates and it is often uncomfortable and impractical in hot tropical climates. Guidelines for treatment cannot always be followed because health services show wide variation in capacity and distribution in different districts and countries. Lack of clean water to wash off contaminated skin or clothes is a major cause of ill health associated with insecticides. Economies where insecticides need to be used intensively often cannot afford the safer but more expensive insecticides or equipment for spraying (see Chapter 17).

2.8. Environmental Changes: Effect on Food and Disease

2.8.1. Global Warming

The expected increase in temperature of 1.6°C from 1990 values over a 60-year period has serious implications for food production and disease. The greatest effect could be in the tropics where there will be less rainfall and higher evaporation rates, which will in turn seriously impede farming.

In consequence, it has been estimated that there would be an increase of 20–22 million in the numbers of people at risk of starvation.

The El Niño effect caused a resurgence of malaria in Venezuela, Guyana and Colombia. With global warming, the increase in temperature will increase the incidence of malaria and dengue fever. Malaria is generally confined to areas with a minimum winter temperature of 16°C and a humidity of at least 55%. Higher temperatures would result in the spread of malaria from low-lying lands to higher altitudes and there would be more regions favouring persistence of the vector mosquitoes.

With higher temperatures and/or higher relative humidity, certain illnesses (e.g. related to *Fusarium* spp., *Ustilago maydis*) and insects (e.g. *Ostrinia* spp., mites etc.) will become more prevalent north to south and west to east.

Staple crops would also be affected by changes in temperature. For example, highest yields of potatoes are achieved when they are grown at temperatures of between 15°C and 18°C. Night-time temperatures above 20°C reduce tuber development and temperatures above 30°C suppress it altogether and losses in potato production due to *Ohytophthora infestans* are greatest in regions with higher temperatures.

2.9. Alternatives

2.9.1. Biological Control and Environmental Management

Altering breeding sites of vectors, filling of ponds and marshes, and the use of living organisms or their products to control vectors or pest insects have all been used over the decades. These measures are most effective when used in combination.

Bacterial larvicides (e.g. *Bacillus thuringiensis* [Bt] strain H-14) produce toxins very effective in killing mosquito and black fly larvae. At normal doses, the toxins are harmless to man and they are effective against insects that have developed resistance to chemical larvicides.

The dried spores of the bacteria have been used as a pesticide for more than 30 years and they represent one of the very few insecticides sanctioned for use on organic crops in Europe. In certain circumstances, Bt H-14 can be harmful to organisms other than larvae.

Thus, Bt strain H-34 destroyed tissue in the wounds of a French soldier in Bosnia, it infected wounds in immuno-suppressed mice, and it can kill mice with intact immune systems if they inhale spores. Françoise Ramisse *et al.* (Le Bouchet army research laboratories, France) have reported that healthy mice inhaling 10^8 spores of Bt H-34 died within 8 hours as a result of internal bleeding and tissue damage (New Scientist, 29.5.1999).

Biological products have technical limitations. These include extreme specificity, sensitivity to environmental factors and problems with robustness of the formulations. However, this may prevent the consequence of resistance in insects (because there is no continuous exposure). Even so, after over two decades of Bt use without problems, a number of reports of resistance in insects are now appearing.

Genetic modification of crops can be used to cause them to produce insecticidal toxins. However, these can in turn poison beneficial insects—such as lacewings and ladybirds. Pollen from maize engineered to make Bt insecticide appears to be toxic to the Monarch butterfly.

Many of these methods of biological control are held under patents and licensing agreements. Scientific bodies (National Scientific bodies of India, Mexico, Brazil and China along with the Royal Society in the UK and the US National Academy of Sciences) have requested those bodies that dominate agricultural biotechnology to make available genetically modified crops to the 800 million people of the poor countries of the world (Andy Coghlan, New Scientist, 15.7.2000). In the meantime, there are reports of failures of biological control (e.g. failure of weevils to eradicate water hyacinths in Lake Victoria) and of risk of transfer of resistant genes to related weeds.

2.9.2. Mechanised Farming

Recent years have seen the development of precision farming systems using global positioning system satellites to draw detailed maps of each field complete with information about persistent weeds, soil chemistry and yields to ensure that pesticides and fertilisers are automatically applied to a field in precisely the right places and quantities. This ensures greater profit and reduced use of chemicals.

A tractor-mounted video and computer system that recognises weeds between rows of crops and uses mechanical hoes to dig them up has been developed (Silsoe Research Institute).

Nevertheless, satellite and video technologies are too expensive for most farmers, at least for the time being.

2.9.3. Integrated Crop Management

There is a host of combination techniques for integrated crop management. One of the most vigorous of these is Linking Environment and Farming (LEAF) which incorporates the best of traditional and modern techniques, for example constant monitoring of soils and crops, applying fertiliser when it will be taken up by the growing crop and only spraying chemicals when pests reach a threshold level above which they will cause real problems. A 30–40 % reduction in pesticide use is achievable by this means, which may involve a small yield penalty, but profitability is at least as high as from conventional farming and it actually reduces farmers' risks.

There are other techniques of "new agriculture" which involve abandonment of autumn ploughing, direct drilling of seeds, spraying herbicide only once to decrease soil erosion, and the leaching of plant nutrients and pesticides. These technologies and techniques to help farmers improve the environment without cutting profits.

Notably, Sharma (New Scientist, 8.7.2000) reported that the land in Punjab and Haryana states (which produces 80% of the food surplus in India) has not been able to support the burden of intensive agriculture. "Intensive farming practices have virtually mined nutrients from the soil and 50 million people in West and Central India are short of water. Debts amongst farmers are increasing and more than 250 farmers have committed suicide in the past two years."

2.10. Conclusions

The need for pesticides cannot be questioned at present. Their removal at this point of time without practical and economically viable alternatives would be likely to result in famine and vector-borne disease epidemics. The increasing populations of the world require food and millions need protection from vector-borne disease.

On the other hand, there is increasing evidence that human health may be put at risk as the result of the introduction of chemicals into the environment. A particular concern is that we have failed to identify with precision the health risks associated with long-term, low-dose exposure to these chemicals.

In this and other areas, it is necessary for clinicians, toxicologists, environmental scientists and occupational physicians to co-operate with industry to develop a realistic and accurate view of benefits, health hazards and environmental sequelae.

Acknowledgements

The data for this script has been obtained primarily from

- several issues of the New Scientist, Ecology and Science news
- *The Pesticide Hazard* by Barbara Dinham
- *Cultivating Crisis* by Douglas L Murray
- *Pesticides and Human Welfare* by D.L. Gunn and J.G.R. Stevens
- *Saving the Planet with Pesticides and Plastic* by Dennis Avery
- *Medical Entomolgy for Students* by Mike W. Service
- *Crop Production and Crop Protection* by E-C Oerke, H-W. Dehne, F. Schonbeck and A. Weber
- *Pesticides and the Third World Poor* by David Bull.
- *Public Health Impact of Pesticides used in Agriculture.* World Health Organization and United Nations Environment Programme 1990
- *Vector control.* Prepared by Jan A Rozendaal. World Health Organization, Geneva 1997

Other sources of information

Committee on Toxicity of Chemicals in Food, Consumer Products and the Environment. Organophosphates. Department of Health, UK 1999

Headley, J.C. Economics of agricultural pest control. *Annual Reviews of Entomology* 1972;**17**:273–86.

Hemingway, J., Karunaratne, S.H. Mosquito carboxylesterases: a review of the molecular biology and biochemistry of a major insecticide resistance mechanism—A Review. *Medical and Veterinary Entomology* 1998;**12**:1–12

Jeyaratnam, J. ed. *Occupational Health in Developing Countries.* Oxford Medical Publications; 1992.

Jeyaratnam, J. Health problems of pesticide usage in the third world. Editorial. *British Journal of Industrial Medicine* 1985;**42**:505–6.

Jeyaratnam, J., Chia, K.S. eds. *Occupational Health in National Development.* World Scientific Singapore; 1994.

Thanks

- Pesticide Trust UK (Peter Beaumont and Alison Craig) for providing access to their data
- Professor Chris Curtis of the London School of Hygiene and Tropical Medicine for advice and literature on vector borne diseases
- Dr Ivor Tittawella of University of Umeå, Sweden for literature and advice on vector borne diseases.
- Dr Tim Marrs for reading the script.

CHAPTER 3

Factors Influencing Organophosphate Toxicity in Humans

Philippa Edwards

3.1. Introduction

Organophosphates (OPs) represent a group of chemicals with a diverse range of chemical structures and activities. However, the OPs which have been most associated with toxicity in humans are those compounds which have a rapid effect on the function of the nervous system by inhibiting the enzyme acetylcholinesterase (AChE) (see Chapter 1). Interest in these compounds arises from this property, whether the target was AChE in insects in the development of pesticides, or humans in the case of chemical warfare agents. The intended use of the OP will determine the characteristics selected by the development chemists. Volatile OPs, such as soman, have been selected for anti-human nerve gases and non-volatile OPs are usually selected for pesticide use. Most pesticidal OPs have vapour pressures between 10^{-8} and 10^{-4} mm Hg; dichlorvos is the exception, having a vapour pressure of 10^{-2} mm Hg (Racke, 1992). In addition, pesticidal OPs are selected on the basis of preferential toxicity to insects as opposed to mammals. In general, this preferential toxicity is related to a more rapid metabolic detoxification in mammals compared to insects. Pesticidal OPs have been developed that require metabolic activation for maximal activity and this can add a further differential toxicity between insects and mammals. Such pesticides contain a P=S group in place of a P=O group. The parent compound is often referred to as the "thion" and the oxygenated derivative formed by metabolism as the "oxon", as shown for parathion and paraoxon below (Fig. 3.1.).

The intended use of individual OPs thus results in the development of cholinesterase inhibiting OPs with different characteristics and resulting differences in the human toxicity. Some OPs, including the defoliants, fire retardants and lubricants, were developed for commercial uses unrelated to cholinesterase inhibition. These compounds generally have low anticholinesterase activity but some, such as the tricresyl phosphate lubricants, are potent inhibitors of neuropathy target esterase (NTE) and are used experimentally as typical inducers of delayed neuropathy (see Chapter 7).

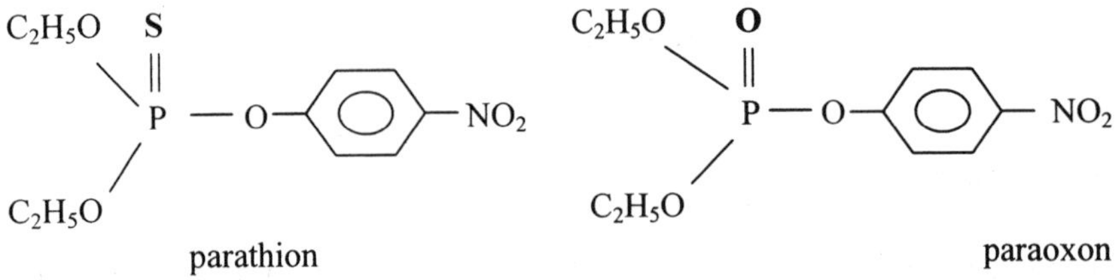

Figure 3.1. Parathion and paraoxon

Whilst the majority of the health effects resulting from exposure to OPs developed as pesticides or chemical warfare agents can be attributed directly or indirectly to inhibition of AChE, the possibility that other potential sites might be responsible for some of the actions of certain OPs cannot be excluded.

Whatever the eventual biological target for the OP, the agent must first enter the body and reach that target at a concentration sufficient to exert a toxic effect. This will depend on the route of exposure, the dose, the distribution of the toxin in the body, the metabolism to more toxic and to less toxic derivatives, removal from the body, the affinity and the rate of reaction of the OP with its target and the reversibility of that reaction. The affinity and rate of reaction of OPs with their targets and the reversibility of the reaction are dealt with in more detail in Chapter 1. The other factors affecting toxicity are discussed in this chapter in relation to the inhibition of AChE, although the same considerations would also apply to actions at other known or potential targets.

3.2. Route of Exposure and Absorption

Although dermal, oral or inhalation routes of exposure can result in systemic toxicity, the dose required may differ. In addition, the balance of signs may be affected by the route, as cholinergic systems exposed directly to the OP, prior to dilution in the circulation and metabolism in the liver, receive a higher initial dose. Thus gastrointestinal signs are more common following oral ingestion whereas respiratory signs and miosis, probably by direct action on the eye, are more frequent following exposure to airborne contamination.

3.2.1. Oral

Most serious poisoning cases are the result of deliberate intake with suicidal intent. The route is normally oral, although an unusual case of intravenous injection has also been reported (Güven et al., 1997). Pesticide OPs are usually used for this purpose because of their widespread availability. Ingestion of significant amounts can also occur accidentally as a result of mistaken identity of improperly stored pesticides (Fang et al., 1995) and of small amounts arising from transfer of pesticide from hands to mouths as a result of poor hygiene procedures during the use of pesticides (Niven et al., 1993). The major route of exposure of the general population is also oral, as a result of ingestion of pesticide residues in foods and in drinking water. Regulatory controls on pesticide use are designed to ensure that this exposure is insufficient to result in adverse health effects but rare instances where the pesticides have been used inappropriately have resulted in poisoning (Chaudhry et al., 1998). Pesticide OPs, including metrifonate (trichlorfon) given orally in humans in the treatment of schistosomiasis, are rapidly and extensively absorbed in the gastrointestinal tract. Metabolism occurs in the gut lumen and gut wall and more extensively in the liver before the compound reaches the systemic circulation, allowing activation of thio-compounds and detoxification.

3.2.2. Dermal

Occupational exposure to pesticides predominantly occurs as a result of dermal contamination (IPCS, 1986; Leonard and Yeary, 1990). Absorption is very variable and highly dependent of the solvent carrying the pesticide. Solvents that permeate the skin readily, such as acetone, result in a higher uptake than suspensions of OPs in water (El-Sebae, 1980). Dermal penetration also varies with the site on the body and other factors, such as temperature and degree of hydration of the skin (Riviere and Chang, 1992). Furthermore, exposure to a pesticide that has reached the inside of protective clothing, such as gloves, will be absorbed much more extensively than from open skin, particularly if the skin is sweaty. The enzyme systems responsible for the activation and detoxification of OPs are present in the skin but these have been less extensively studied than liver enzymes.

An in vitro study on pig skin indicated that absorbed parathion was present largely as the paraoxon derivative, with less than 20% of the absorbed material being as the parent parathion (Carver et al., 1990).

Studies of urinary excretion following dermal application of malathion and diazinon in studies in human volunteers indicated rates of absorption of less than 5% (Wester *et al.*, 1993; Krieger and Dinoff, 2000). However, the urinary excretion was prolonged and not all the applied material was accounted for. A depot of absorbed material may have formed in the skin or fat and this would result in underestimation of the absorption. An *in vitro* study indicated about 14% absorption of diazinon across human skin over 24 hours. Some rodent studies have indicated prolonged systemic absorption from skin depots, with total distribution from a dermal site of uptake of parathion-methyl being 50% complete within 1 h but requiring a further 95 h for complete absorption (Abu-Qare *et al.*, 2000).

The relatively low absorption of most OPs following dermal contamination generally reduces the toxicity by this route. For example, the dermal LD_{50} in rats for omethoate is 860–1020 mg/kg body weight (bw) whereas the oral LD_{50} is 25–28 mg/kg bw (FAO/WHO, 1978). However, this may be offset by the fact that absorbed OPs pass directly to the systemic circulation without being subject to metabolism in the liver. For example, the OPs DEF and EPN are at least as toxic by the dermal as by the oral route (IPCS, 1986).

3.2.3. Inhalation

Inhalation of OPs may result from exposure to volatile OPs developed as nerve gases, as occurred in the terrorist attack in the Tokyo subway. However, it can also occur as a result of the use of sprays, powders, and mists of less volatile pesticide products, although, as noted above, overall this route of exposure appears to be less than the dermal route in practice. Absorption following inhalation is rapid and almost complete. Limited metabolism occurs in the lungs and the absorbed OPs will reach the systemic circulation without first passing through the liver. Exposure to air-borne OPs also results in relatively high exposures of the eyes and the respiratory mucous membranes.

3.3. Dose

There is often confusion between the extent of contamination (i.e. the amount of OP that reaches the site of potential uptake into the body), the internal exposure (i.e. the total amount of OP that is taken up) and the toxic exposure (i.e. the concentration reaching the target).

The dose reaching the target enzyme is affected by the factors discussed in this chapter and is often very poorly characterised. In addition, because the reaction with cholinesterase results in the formation of a covalent bond, rather than a rapidly reversible binding to a receptor molecule, the duration of exposure of the target is important as well as the concentration of the OP. Bearing these factors in mind, suicide attempts generally involve high doses, whereas occupational exposures result in relatively low doses. The intention of chemical warfare agents is to deliver high doses but there is the potential for a wide range, as seen in the Tokyo terrorist attack (Okumura *et al.*, 1996). Most animal experiments are carried out with relatively high doses. *In vitro* studies often feature high concentrations and the relevance of any effects found is therefore questionable in relation to human toxicity. Particular care is needed in evaluating the role of various metabolic pathways to toxicity, as the significance of each pathway depends on the dose. Some enzymes only come into play at high concentrations of the OP, whilst others may be operating well below maximum capacity at low concentrations. Thus, whilst the potential role of various metabolic pathways may have been established experimentally, their contribution to the toxicity observed in real human exposure scenarios remains uncertain.

3.4. Distribution

Following uptake, OPs are distributed widely in the body and readily cross the placenta. Most anticholinesterase OPs are lipophilic and therefore pass the blood-brain barrier and can also form depots in fat and skin. The extent to which this occurs varies with the degree of lipophilicity and can alter the time-course and the severity of the poisoning. In rhesus monkeys given an intravenous dose of radiolabelled diazinon, 40% of the dose was eliminated in the urine within 24 h (Wester *et al.*, 1993). This was followed by a slow and almost constant excretion at 5% of the dose per day between 3 and 7 days. A similar profile of prolonged excretion was reported in humans following dermal exposure. This would suggest a potential for accumulation of OP in depots, presumably in fat tissue and/or skin on repeated exposure. However, a study of excretion of metabolites following repeated low dermal exposure of 2 sheep handlers to diazinon over 10 weeks showed no evidence of this (CVL, 1993), possibly because of a long interval (2 weeks) between each exposure.

Studies in experimental animals have not indicated significant storage of OPs in tissues. However, this varies with different compounds and has in some cases been shown to influence the time-course of the toxic response in poisoned humans. In a case of human poisoning by dichlorofenthion, steadily decreasing concentrations of the pesticide were found in serial fat biopsy samples up to 48 h after a single intoxication. The decline matched a return in blood cholinesterase towards normal and recovery from the symptoms of cholinergic poisoning (IPCS, 1986). A similar phenomenon may explain the protracted inhibition of cholinesterase in a patient following fenitrothion ingestion (Ecobichon et al., 1977).

3.5. Metabolism

Although many tissues, including the gut, skin, lung, kidney and the nervous system, contain enzymes that can activate and/or detoxify OPs, the liver and blood are the main sites for modifying the total body burden of toxic forms. Mammalian metabolism of OPs involves a number of distinct enzyme systems and the pathway that predominates varies with the compound, the dose and the route of exposure. The potential reactions are discussed below:

3.5.1 A-esterases

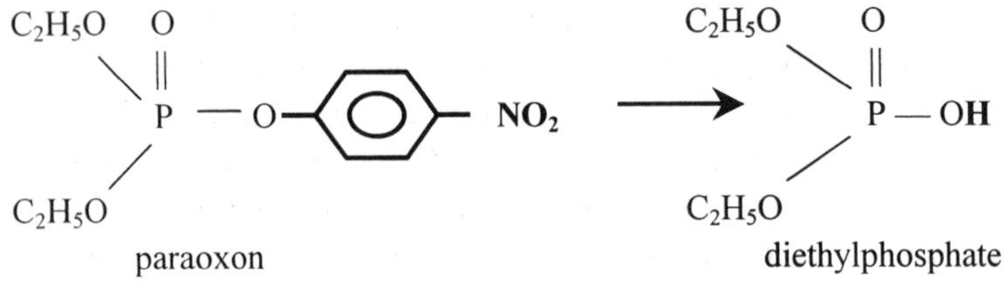

C_2H_5O O C_2H_5O O

P — O — ⬡ — NO_2 → P — OH

C_2H_5O C_2H_5O

           paraoxon   diethylphosphate

Figure 3.2. Hydrolysis of paraoxon

The A-esterases are a group of enzymes capable of hydrolysing a broad range of substrates, including OPs as shown above for paraoxon. Parathion and similar thion compounds are not substrates for these enzymes. They are present in a range of tissues, including liver and intestine and in the serum. In serum, the activity is associated with high density lipoproteins. The paraoxon-hydrolysing activity of A-esterase (known as paraoxonase activity) has been extensively studied.

The human serum paraoxonase activity shows a wide variation between individuals (Mutch *et al.*, 1992; Playfer *et al.*, 1976). In British and Indian subjects, there was a clear bimodal distribution of activity, with 40–50% of the population having low serum paraoxonase activity. The difference is due in part to polymorphism in the structural gene *(PON1)* coding for the enzyme, one isoform being more active against paraoxon than the other. However, this difference is substrate-specific. The A-esterase activity in human serum does not display polymorphism when malaoxon or chlorpyrifos oxon are used as the substrate (Sams and Mason, 1999) and the relative activities of the 2 forms with diazoxon, soman or sarin as the substrate is the reverse of that for paraoxon (Davies *et al.*, 1996). Differences in the level of expression of the paraoxon gene also contribute to the observed inter-individual differences (Richter and Furlong, 1999). In experimental animals, injection of purified paraoxonase enzyme has been shown to reduce the toxicity of high (lethal) doses of paraoxon. However, the affinity of the enzyme for paraoxon is relatively low and it is only a good substrate for paraoxonase *in vitro* at concentrations above 200 µM, whereas paraoxon inhibits AChE at sub-micromolar concentrations (Mutch *et al.*, 1999). This may explain why 'knock-out' mice devoid of paraoxonase activity in liver and plasma showed increased sensitivity to chlorpyrifos oxon and diazoxon but no change in sensitivity to paraoxon (Furlong *et al.*, 2000).

The products of hydrolysis of OPs by A-esterases are excreted in the urine. Insecticidal OPs differ most in the leaving group removed in the hydrolytic process therefore common products (dimethylphosphate, diethylphosphate, dimethylphosphorothioate and diethylphosphorothioate) are found in the urine of individuals exposed to a number of different OPs. These metabolites have therefore been used to monitor occupational exposure. Given the individual variation and the influence of the compound on the extent of hydrolysis, care should be exercised in any quantitative interpretation of such results. However, in a study of formulation workers exposed to a variety of OPs, excretion of diethylphosphate and diethylphosphorothioate paralleled changes in plasma cholinesterase activity (Nutley and Cocker, 1993) indicating that under these circumstances, urinary metabolites gave a good measure of systemic exposure to cholinesterase inhibitory agents.

3.5.2. Carboxylesterases (including B-esterases)

Carboxylesterase (CaE) enzymes that have a normal physiological role in lipid metabolism can contribute to detoxification of OPs by 2 mechanisms: hydrolysis of carboxyl ester side chains and irreversible binding of the OP without hydrolysis. In general, thions are hydrolysed but the corresponding oxons bind and inhibit enzyme activity. The products of hydrolysis are carboxylic acid derivatives, which are less toxic and more water-soluble and therefore more rapidly excreted in the urine. Both mechanisms reduce the concentration of free active compound available for binding to AChE.

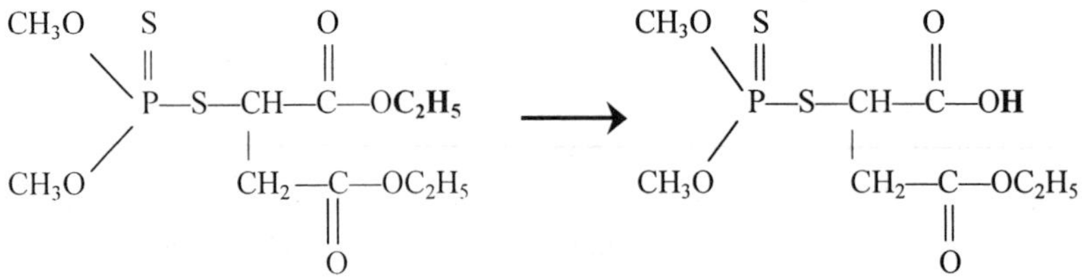

Figure 3.3. Hydrolysis of the carboxyl ester side chain of malathion

Carboxylesterases (CaEs) have also been classified as B-esterases if they are inhibited by OPs but this classification is not absolute since the enzymes are inhibited by some OPs but hydrolysed others. The enzymes are active in mammalian plasma and many tissues including lung, liver, kidney, brain, intestines, muscle and gonads, although molecular cloning of the enzymes has indicated that the enzymes found in different tissues are different gene products and hence may have different characteristics (Wallace *et al.,* 1999). This is a significant route for detoxifying some OPs as shown, for instance, by an increased toxicity of malathion when CaE activity is abolished. The rat oral LD_{50} for malathion is decreased from 10000 to 100 mg/kg bw by inhibition of CaE (IPCS, 1986).

The plasma enzyme can also play a significant role as a binding site rendering the OP unavailable for inhibition of tissue AChE even if the OP is not hydrolysed by the enzyme. This route is particularly significant for the more toxic OPs, soman, sarin and tabun, used as chemical warfare agents. For instance, inhibition of CaE *in vivo* with cresyl benzodioxaphosphorin prevents soman binding and decreases the rat LD_{50} of soman by 50 to 90% although soman is not hydrolysed by CaE (Maxwell *et al.,* 1987).

The sensitivity of rats to the lethal effects of repeated doses of soman is largely predicted by the return of CaE activity and thus soman binding sites in the plasma, which occurs with a half-life of 17.1 hours (Maxwell, 1992). Differences in levels of plasma CaE also contribute to species differences in the toxicity of soman among mammals. Carboxylesterases have a low capacity to remove OPs by binding alone and do not play a significant role in detoxifying less potent OPs unless the enzymes are also capable of hydrolysing the OP, as is the case with malathion.

OPs that bind to, but are not hydrolysed by the CaE enzyme known as egasyn, cause a release of hepatic microsomal β-glucuronidase, with which egasyn is normally complexed. The resulting increase in plasma glucuronidase activity has been shown to be a more sensitive marker of OP exposure than plasma cholinesterase activity for these OPs (Satoh et al., 1999).

3.5.3. Fluorohydrolases

A number of enzymes that hydrolyse the P-F bond in DFP, and the nerve agents soman and tabun, have been described in a range of tissues, including human plasma.

These enzymes are not involved in the metabolism of pesticidal OPs but can hydrolyse the phosphoric anhydride bond in tetraethyl pyrophosphate, a highly toxic potential impurity in some pesticidal OPs, notably inadequately stabilised preparations of diazinon. The products of the reactions are inactive against AChEs.

3.5.4. Amidases

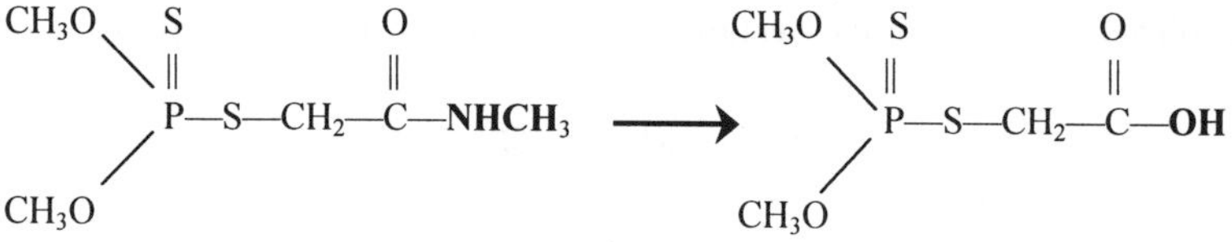

Dimethoate

Figure 3.4. Amidases catalyse the hydrolytic cleavage of carboxylamide bonds

Amidases present in the liver catalyse the hydrolytic cleavage of carboxylamide bonds if these are present in phosphorothioates (Chen and Dauterman, 1971).

Oxon derivatives of dimethoate (omethoate) and other amide-containing OP compounds, such as dicrotophos, are not substrates for the enzymes but inhibit the activity.

3.5.5. Microsomal Oxygenases

Microsomal oxygenases catalyse a range of oxidative reactions with OPs. The most important microsomal enzymes involved in the initial metabolism of OPs are the family of enzymes that contain cytochrome P450. However, the family of enzymes containing flavin (FMOs) also make a significant contribution. Many of the reactions catalysed are the same, although the P450 systems are capable of a more extensive range of reactions. The relative contribution of these two enzyme systems varies with the OP, the tissue, the species and the sex (Levi and Hodgson, 1992).

These enzymes are found in most tissues but the predominant activity in relation to the body burden of OPs is found in the liver. In the lung and kidney, the FMOs are generally predominant. The P450 enzymes show extensive genetic polymorphism in the human population with important genetic differences in reaction rates. This is much less extensive among the FMOs. The P450 enzymes are inhibited and/or induced by a large number of xenobiotics whereas this phenomenon has not been reported for the FMO enzymes. For simplicity, the microsomal oxidative reactions occurring as a result of either system have been described here together.

The activity of these enzymes results in oxidative desulphuration (conversion of thions to the more active oxon forms), N-dealkylation of substituted amide side chains, O-dealkylation and side-chain oxidation of alkyl, aryl and thioether substituents. Examples of these reactions are shown in Fig. 3.5. to 3.10. The significance of each reaction for the overall toxicity of OPs is discussed below.

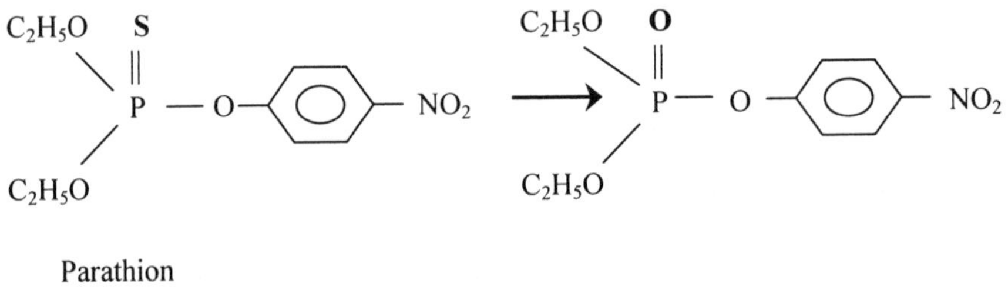

Parathion

Figure 3.5. Oxidative desulphuration

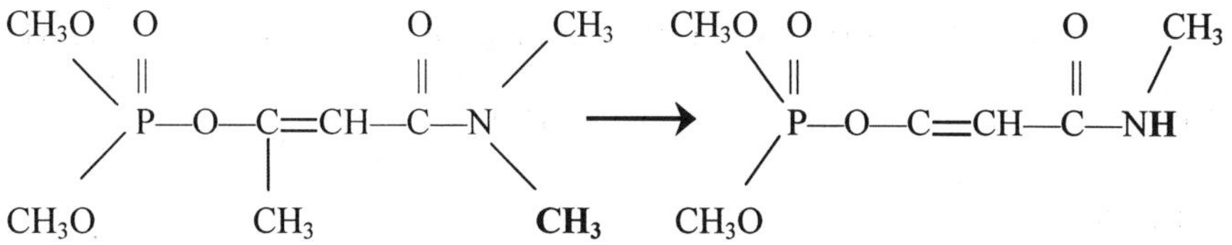

Dicrotophos

Figure 3.6. Oxidative N-dealkylation

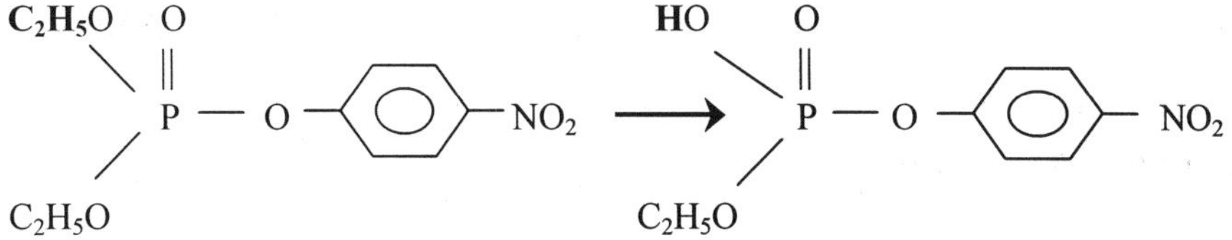

Paraoxon

Figure 3.7. Oxidative O-dealkylation

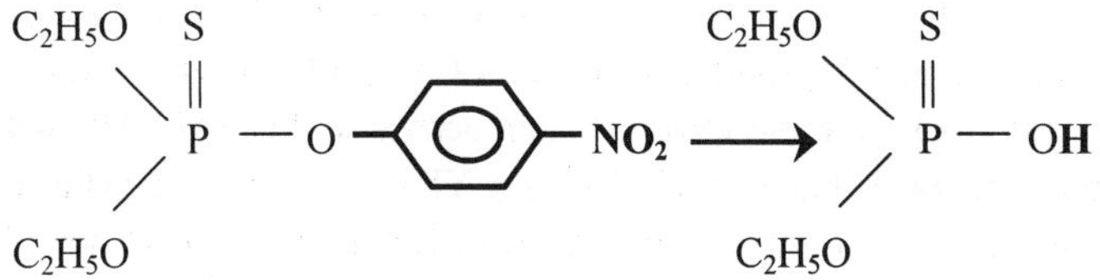

Parathion

Figure 3.8. Oxidative O-dearylation

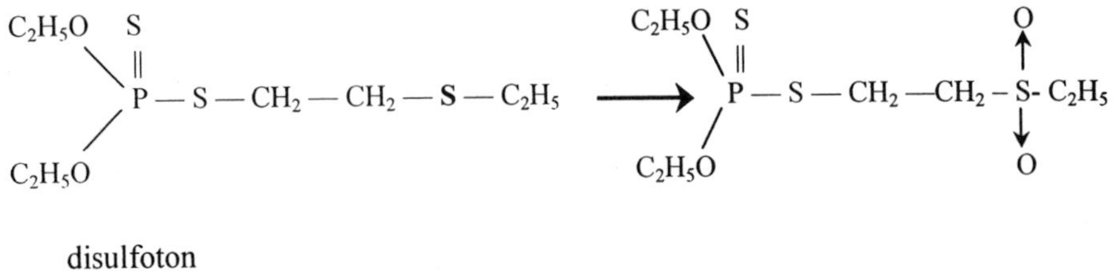

disulfoton

Figure 3.9. Thioether oxidation

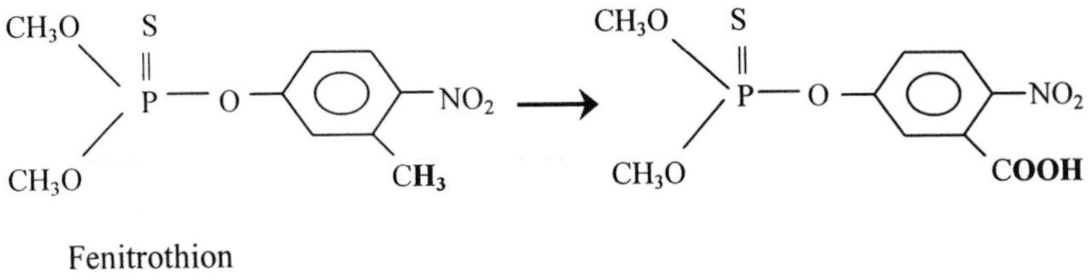

Fenitrothion

Figure 3.10. Side chain oxidation

Oxidative desulphuration (Fig. 3.5.)

Oxidative desulphuration of OPs can be catalysed by both the P450 and the FMO systems. The anticholinesterase activity of the oxon products is higher than that of the parent thions but the scale of the difference varies. The inhibitory activity of paraoxon against AChE is almost a thousand times greater than that of parathion. This reaction therefore results in an increase in toxicity. The specific cytochrome P450 responsible for activation of parathion in mice is CYP3A4. In human liver, microsomal CYP3A4 and 3A5 were the most efficient activators but lAl, 2B6 and 2C8 also catalysed the reaction (Mutch *et al.*, 1999). CYP3A4 shows wide (up to 15-fold) inter-individual variation in activity and ethnic differences have been found (Ahsan *et al.*, 1993). In addition to its high activity in the liver, CYP3A4 is also found in the intestine but not in the lung or skin. In the skin another enzyme must be responsible for the observed conversion of parathion to paraoxon (Carver *et al.*, 1990).

CYP3A4 is responsible for the metabolism of many therapeutic drugs in common medicinal use and its activity in the liver can be inhibited or increased by exposure to a number of therapeutic agents. CYP3A4, together with CYP2C8, is capable of activation of chlorpyrifos to its oxon form. These enzymes also catalyse the oxidative detoxification of chlorpyrifos and chlorpyrifos oxon. The effect of a change in the activity of these enzymes therefore depends on the balance between the activation and detoxification reactions. Studies *in vitro* indicate that in the liver, hydrolysis by A-esterase is the most important route of metabolism of chlorpyrifos.

Oxidative O- and N-dealkylation, and dearylation (Fig. 3.6. to 3.8.)

These reactions all result in an increased water-solubility and a consequent decrease in toxicity

Thioether oxidation (Fig. 3.9.)

This reaction can result in an increase in toxicity. The oxidation of the thio-ether bond in disulfoton results in an increased potency for *in vitro* inhibition of AChE by about 30-fold.

Side chain oxidation (Fig. 3.10.)

The carboxylic acid product of the side-chain oxidation of fenitrothion is more water-soluble than the parent molecule and therefore can be eliminated more readily in the urine. This contributes to the 50-fold reduction in oral toxicity of fenitrothion in rats as compared to parathion-methyl. The structure of parathion-methyl is identical to fenitrothion except for the absence of a methyl group on the ring structure and therefore parathion-methyl is not a substrate for this enzyme. Side-chain oxidation usually results in decreased toxicity but this is not always the case. Oxidation of profenofos changes the leaving group and the resulting inhibited enzyme undergoes ageing whereas the product of the non-oxidised form undergoes hydrolysis. This is shown below (Fig. 3.11.).

In this instance, the side chain oxidation of profenofos therefore leads to an increase in toxicity.

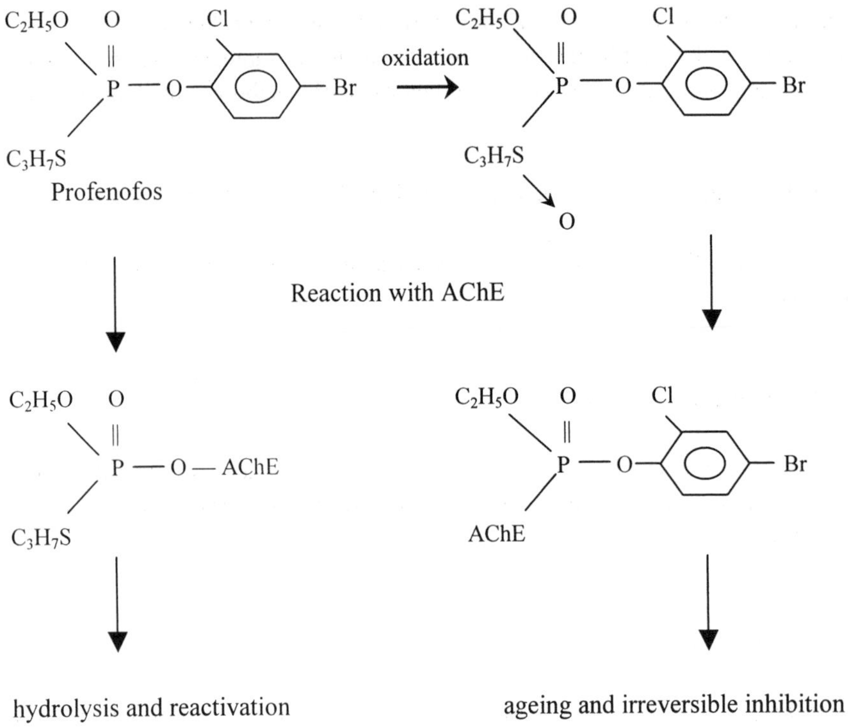

C₂H₅O O   Cl   C₂H₅O O   Cl

$$C_2H_5O \quad O \quad Cl$$

C_2H_5O O Cl

P — O —⟨benzene⟩— Br   oxidation ⟶   P — O —⟨benzene⟩— Br

C_3H_7S
Profenofos

C_3H_7S
O

Reaction with AChE

C_2H_5O O
P — O — AChE
C_3H_7S

C_2H_5O O Cl
P — O —⟨benzene⟩— Br
AChE

hydrolysis and reactivation   ageing and irreversible inhibition

Figure 3.11. Oxidation of profenofos changes the leaving group and the resulting inhibited enzyme undergoes ageing whereas the product of the non-oxidised form undergoes hydrolysis.

3.5.6. *Conjugation*

Conjugation with sugars, sulfate and glutathione are all implicated in the metabolism of OPs, but the latter is probably the most significant (Dauterman, 1971).

Glutathione S-transferases are a family of enzymes that have the potential to catalyse conjugation of a wide range of chemicals, including intact OPs, with glutathione. Liver enzymes with overlapping specificities for individual compounds *in vitro* have been described. However there is no evidence that this is a significant pathway *in vivo*. Many of the metabolites (carboxylic acids, phenols, amino, imino and sulfhydryl compounds) formed by hydrolysis or oxidation of the parent compounds are conjugated by this route and this aids the elimination via the urine. At high doses, this can lead to depletion of tissue glutathione, which may render the animals more susceptible to other toxins.

3.6. Tissue binding

OPs react covalently with broad spectrum of proteins in tissues, including the CaE. Binding is principally in liver and muscle. The number of binding sites is relatively low but this can nonetheless remove a significant proportion of the dose for highly toxic OPs, such as chemical warfare agents (Lauwerys and Murphy, 1969). Some of these proteins may be enzymes and the OP binding may inhibit normal activity and cause effects independent of cholinesterase inhibition. Such an inhibition has recently been shown for the action of metrifonate on N-acyl peptidase in rat brain (Ray, 1998) and egasyn (see above). The inhibition of N-acyl peptidase is highly compound-dependent and the biological significance of the inhibition is unknown. The inhibition of AChE and pseudocholinesterase (BuChE) in the blood can also be included because, although they have been used as markers for exposure, it is not thought that inhibition of these enzymes in blood has any adverse effects. BuChE shows significant genetic polymorphism in humans, with 24% of the population having at least one genetic variant allele. Most variants have a decreased enzyme activity, which is clinically important because individuals with low activity are highly sensitive to succinylcholine. However, the significance of the polymorphism for OP toxicity is not known (Lockridge and Masson, 2000).

3.7. Elimination

As indicated in the foregoing sections, most OPs are rapidly degraded in the body and the products are excreted largely in the urine. Urinary excretion of metabolites usually peaks within 2 days of exposure then falls rapidly.

However, excretion rates do not fall to zero probably because of depots of parent molecule in fat. Release from these depots can give rise to continuing toxicity. Some residues remain in the body as covalently bound forms and these will not give rise to further toxicity.

3.8. Alterations in Metabolism

Many therapeutic compounds are also metabolised by microsomal P450 systems and these can both inhibit and induce enzyme activity. CYP3A enzymes are known to be inhibited by cimetidine and activity can also be altered by dietary components, such as naringenin found in grapefruit juice. Because OPs can undergo a variety of different reactions, which can either increase or decrease toxicity, no general rules can be used to predict the overall effect of changes in microsomal enzyme activity on toxicity. The net effect will vary depending on the profile of changes brought about in enzyme activity, the particular OP and the dose and route of exposure. For instance, pre-treatment of mice with piperonyl butoxide, which inhibits microsomal enzymes, increased the intraperitoneal toxicity of parathion by 2-fold but decreased that of parathion-methyl by 40-fold (Gallo and Lawryk, 1991).

As discussed above, inhibition of tissue CaE by some OPs occurs at doses lower than those required to inhibit AChE. Of itself, this inhibition is not known to have any adverse effect but it could increase the sensitivity to other OPs, such as malathion, and other xenobiotics, such as the synthetic pyrethroids which are significantly metabolised via this route. Toxic impurities in poorly produced malathion increase the toxicity of malathion by this mechanism (Aldridge et al., 1979.).

Similarly, carboxylamide pesticides (e.g. EPN) and other amidase inhibitors increase the toxicity of some OPs such as dimethoate, (El-Sebae, 1980). Several of the enzymes involved in OP metabolism are developmentally regulated (Atterbury et al., 1997). Newborn rodents have low PON1 and CaE activity and this probably explains the higher sensitivity of newborn rats to lethal doses of certain OPs, such as chlorpyrifos. The differential sensitivity of newborn rodents is not, however, absolute. Young rats are not more sensitive to methamidophos at high doses (Padilla et al., 2000) nor to chlorpyrifos at low doses (Sheets, 2000).

The activities of the cytochrome P450 enzymes also show developmental changes but the contribution of these developmental changes to overall sensitivity to chlorpyrifos is less clear because these enzymes contribute to the generation of the more toxic oxon derivative of chlorpyrifos as well as to detoxification.

3.9. Racemic Mixtures

Many OPs contain one or more centres of asymmetry at the phosphate group or at carbon groups in the side chains. For each centre of asymmetry, there are a pair of chemically identical enantiomers differing only in the steric conformation of the groups around the asymmetric centre. The enantiomers are designated + or - depending on their optical properties or R and S. Most of these OPs are synthesised as a mixture containing equal quantities of the 2 enantiomers. Although they are chemically identical the enantiomers may show significant differences in biological activity because of the stereospecificity of biological systems. This includes both the target sites and the enzymes involved in metabolism For example, the isomers of soman that contain the (-) conformation at the P group are toxic whereas the P(+) isomers are not toxic. Carboxylesterases are about 70 times more reactive with the toxic P(-) isomers of soman than with the P(+). In contrast, the hydrolases act preferentially on the P(+) isomers and therefore contribute little to the detoxification of the mixture of isomers (Maxwell, 1992).

3.10. Concluding Remarks

The toxicity of any OP is dependent on the physical and chemical characteristics of the poisonous substance, the form to which a person is exposed, the route of exposure and the susceptibility of the individual, which may vary depending on genetic factors, age, sex and exposure to other agents. For oral doses, the toxicity of an OP depends on the amount of the toxic form, be it the parent compound or an intermediate, that escapes detoxification in the liver. For parathion, this dose in rats is about 10 mg/kg bw. At this dose, paraoxon elutes from the liver and toxic signs are observed (Becker and Nakatsugawa, 1990). At doses of 15 mg/kg, parathion also appears in the circulation and this may be activated in target tissues to the toxic oxon.

The concentration of parathion to which hepatic enzymes are exposed at these doses are in the order of 10^{-7}M. Enzymes active at these low concentrations will therefore make the major contribution to the biotransformation. Metabolic activities demonstrated using optimal substrate concentrations *in vitro* may therefore not be significant in modulating toxicity in human poisoning incidents. Likewise, the high affinity, low capacity carboxylesterase system is of importance in modulating the toxicity of highly potent chemical warfare OPs but is not a major component in the detoxification of low potency pesticides.

With increasing knowledge of the genetic makeup of humans, it may be possible to deduce more about the relative importance of individual metabolic pathways and the contribution of genetic factors, as compared with other variables

The views expressed in this chapter are those of the author and not necessarily those of any UK government department.

References

Abu-Qare A.W., Abdel-Rahman, A.A., Kishk, A.M., *et al.* Placental transfer and pharmacokinetics of a single dermal dose of [^{14}C]methyl parathion in rats. *Toxicological Sciences* 2000;**53**:5–12

Ahsan, C.H., Renwick A.G., Waller, D.G., *et al.* The influences of dose and ethnic origins on the pharmacokinetics of nifedipine. *Clinical Pharmacology and Therapeutics* 1993;**54**:329–38.

Aldridge, W.N., Miles, J.W., Mount, D.L., *et al.* The toxicological properties of impurities in malathion. *Archives of Toxicology* 1979;**42**:95–106.

Atterberry, T.T., Burnett, W.T., Chambers, J.E. Age-related differences in parathion and chlorpyrifos toxicity in male rats: Target and nontarget esterase sensitivity and cytochrome P450 mediated metabolism. *Toxicology and Applied Pharmacology* 1997;**147**:411–8.

Becker, J.M., Nakatsugawa, T. Hepatic breakthrough thresholds for parathion and paraoxon and their implications to toxicity in normal and DDE-pretreated rats. *Pesticide Biochemistry and Physiology* 1990;**36**:83–98.

Carver, M.P., Levi, P., Riviere, J.E. Parathion metabolism during percutaneous absorption in perfused porcine skin. *Pesticide Biochemistry and Physiology* 1990;**38**:245–54.

Chaudhry, R., Lall, S. B., Mishra, B., *et al.* A foodborne outbreak of organophosphate poisoning. *British Medical Journal* 1998;**317**:268–9.

Chen, P.R.S., Dauterman, W.C. Studies on the toxicity of dimethoate analogs and their hydrolysis by sheep liver amidase. *Pesticide Biochemistry and Physiology* 1971;**1**:340–8

CVL. Central Veterinary Laboratory. Diazinon: post dipping exposure in humans. Report CVLS 50/93 Addlestone: CVL 1993

Dauterman, W.C. Biological and non-biological modifications of organophosphorus compounds. *Bulletin of the World Health Organization.* 1971;**44**:133–50

Davies, H.G., Richter, R.J., Keifer, M., *et al.* The effect of the human serum paraoxonase polymorphism is reversed with diazoxon, soman and sarin. *Nature Genetics* 1996;**14**:334–6

Ecobichon, D.J., Ozere, R.L., Reid, E., *et al.* Acute fenitrothion poisoning. *Canadian Medical Association Journal.* 1977;**116**:377–9

El-Sebae, A.H. Biochemical challenges in future toxicological research. *Journal of Environmental Science and Health, part B* 1980;**15**:689–721.

Fang, T-C., Chen, K-W., Wu, M-H., *et al.* Coumaphos intoxications mimic food poisoning. *Clinical Toxicology* 1995;**33**:699–703.

FAO WHO. Joint Meeting on Pesticide Residues. Pesticide Residues in food 1978. Report of the Joint Meeting of the FAO Panel of Experts on Pesticide Residues in Food and the Environment and the WHO Expert Group on Pesticide Residues. Rome: 1978 WHO/FAO.

Furlong, C.E. PON1 status and neurologic symptom complexes in Gulf War veterans. *Genome Research* 2000;**10**:153–5.

Furlong, C.E., Li, W-F., Richter, R.J. *et al.* Genetic and temporal determinants of pesticide sensitivity: role of paraoxonase (PON1). *Neurotoxicology* 2000;**21**:91–100.

Gallo, M.A., Lawryk, N.J. Organic phosphorus pesticides. In: *Handbook of Pesticide Toxicology.* Volume 2. Classes of Pesticides. Hayes, W.J., Jr., Laws, E.R., Jr. eds. Academic Press; San Diego. 1991. p. 917–1123.

Güven, M., Ünlühızarcı, K., Göktaş, Z., *et al.* Intravenous organophosphate injection: an unusual way of intoxication. *Human and Experimental Toxicology* 1997;**16**:279–80.

International Programme on Chemical Safety. *Environmental Health Criteria, Document No 63*, 1986, Geneva: World Health Organization.

Krieger, R.I., Dinoff, T.M. Malathion deposition, metabolite clearance, and cholinesterase status of date dusters and harvesters in California. *Archives of Environmental Contamination and Toxicology* 2000;**38**:546–53.

Lauwerys, R.R., Murphy, S.D. Interaction between paraoxon and tri-o-tolyl phosphate in rats. *Toxicology and Applied Pharmacology* 1969;**14**:348–57.

Leonard, J.A., Yeary, R.A. Exposure of workers using hand-held equipment during urban application of pesticides to trees and ornamental shrubs. *American Industrial Hygiene Association Journal* 1990;**51**:605–9.

Levi, P.E., Hodgson, B. Metabolism of organophosphorus compounds by the flavin-containing monoxygenase. In: *Organophosphates: Chemistry, Fate and Effects*. Chambers, J.E., Levi, P.E. eds. Academic Press; San Diego. 1992. p. 141–54.

Lockridge, O., Masson, P. Pesticides and susceptible populations: people with butyrylcholinesterase genetic variants may be at risk. *Neurotoxicology* 2000;**21**:113–26.

Maxwell, D.M. Detoxication of organophosphorus compounds by carboxylesterase. In: *Organophosphates: Chemistry, Fate and Effects*. Chambers, J.E., Levi, P.E. eds. Academic Press; San Diego.1992. p. 183–99.

Maxwell, D.M., Brecht, K.M., O'Neill, B.L. The effect of carboxylesterase inhibition on interspecies differences in soman toxicity. *Toxicology Letters.* 1987;**39**:35–42.

Mutch, E., Blain, P.G., Williams, F.M. Interindividual variations in enzymes controlling organophosphate toxicity in man. *Human and Experimental Toxicology* 1992;11:109–16.

Mutch, E., Blain, P.G., Williams, F.M. The role of metabolism in determining susceptibility to parathion toxicity in man. *Toxicology Letters.* 1999;**107**:177–87.

Niven, K.J.M., Scott, A.J., Hagen, S., *et al.* Report TM/93/03 from the Institute of Occupational Medicine. Edinburgh: Institute of Occupational Medicine. *Occupational hygiene assessment of sheep dipping practices and processes.* 1993

Nutley, B.P., Cocker, J. Biological monitoring of workers occupationally exposed to organophosphorus pesticides. *Pesticide Science* 1993;**38**:315–22

Okumura, T., Takasu, N., Ishimatsu, S., *et al.* Report on 640 victims of the Tokyo subway sarin attack. *Annals of Emergency Medicine.* 1996;**28**:129–35.

Padilla, S., Buzzard, J., Moser, V.C. Comparison of the role of esterases in the differential age-related sensitivity to chlorpyrifos and methamidophos. *Neurotoxicology* 2000;**21**:49–56.

Playfer, J.R., Eze, L.C., Bullen, M.F. et al. Genetic polymorphism and inter-ethnic variability of plasma paroxonase activity. *Journal of Medical Genetics.* 1976;**13**:337–42.

Racke, K.D. Degradation of organophosphorus insecticides in environmental matrices. In: *Organophosphates: Chemistry, Fate and Effects.* Chambers, J.E., Levi, P.E. eds. Academic Press; San Diego. 1992. p. 47–78.

Ray, D.E. Chronic effects of low level exposure to anticholinesterases—a mechanistic review. *Toxicology Letters.* 1998;**102-103**:527–33

Richter, R.J., Furlong, C.E. Determination of paraoxonase (PON1) status requires more than genotyping. *Pharmacogenetics* 1999;**9**:745–53.

Riviere, J.E., Chang, S-K. Transdermal penetration and metabolism of organophosphate insecticides. In: *Organophosphates: Chemistry, Fate and Effects.* Chambers, J.E., Levi, P.E. eds. Academic Press; San Diego. 1992. p. 241–53.

Sams, C., Mason, H.J. Detoxification of organophosphates by A-esterases in human serum. *Human and Experimental Toxicology* 1999;**18**:653–8.

Satoh T, Suzuki S, Kawai N, *et al.* Toxicological significance in the cleavage of esterase-β-glucuronidase complex in liver microsomes by organophosphorus compounds. *Chemico Biological Interactions* 1999;**119–120**:471–8.

Sheets, L.P. A consideration of age-dependent differences in susceptibility to organophosphorus and pyrethroid insecticides. *Neurotoxicology* 2000;**21**:57–64.

Wallace, T.J., Ghosh, S., Grogan, W.M. Molecular cloning and expression of rat lung carboxylesterase and its potential role in the detoxification of organophosphorus compounds. *American Journal of Respiratory and Cell Molecular Biology* 1999;**20**:1201–8.

Wester, R.C., Sedik, L., Melendres, J., *et al.* Percutaneous absorption of diazinon in humans. *Food and Chemical Toxicology* 1993;**31**:569–72.

CHAPTER 4

Organophosphorus Chemical Warfare Agents

Timothy C Marrs and Robert L Maynard

4.1. Introduction

The OP nerve agents, commonly and almost always erroneously called nerve gases, are chemically and toxicologically related to the OP pesticides and their history together with that of the OP insecticides has already been discussed in Chapter 1. Despite the similarity of OP insecticides and nerve agents, the latter differ in several crucial respects from the OP pesticides, notably by having much greater acute toxicity to mammals, particularly via the percutaneous route. Furthermore, most have notable vapour pressures and consequently present inhalation hazards. Nevertheless, qualitatively the toxicology of the OP nerve agents and pesticides is similar, both groups of compounds being anticholinesterases and, in general, treatment modalities are alike. Tabun, sarin, and soman were developed in Germany before and during World War II (UK Ministry of Defence 1972, see also Chapter 1), but they were not used by the Germans. Allied countries learnt of German work on nerve agents at the end of the war and rapidly introduced their own research and development programmes. Very large stocks of nerve agents were built up particularly by the United States and the, then, Soviet Union. These stockpiles are now decades old and present difficult problems of disposal. Degradation of weapons stored in bombs and shells may be a significant problem. The extreme toxicity of agents such as VX (1 mg might well kill a man) should be borne in mind when considering the size of the stockpiles. In 1999, Munro *et al.* published a comprehensive review of degradation products of chemical warfare agents. The authors pointed out that VX is stored in 1ton containers. If we take 1ton as approximately 1000 kg then each container encloses about 1×10^9 lethal doses of VX. It is, in some ways, encouraging that the authors record that these 1ton containers are stored on Johnston Island in the Pacific Ocean at an Army Depot. Other nerve agents were developed subsequently (see Chapter 1) and stocks are believed to be held by the USA, Russia and possibly other successor states of the former USSR, France and Iraq. However, nerve agents have rarely been used in warfare, the only notable instance being by Iraq in Iraqi Kurdistan (le Chêne, 1989). Chemical warfare agents are sometimes referred to as the poor man's atomic bomb.

The OP nerve agents are relatively easy and cheap to synthesize, especially tabun and the V agents (see below). Many of the precursors required are widely used industrial chemicals, raising difficulties about the control of dissemination. Control, of export of precursors, which is by end-user certification, is not always effective. The use of sarin, albeit impure, in terrorist attacks in Japan, demonstrates that a large chemical infrastructure is not necessary for the manufacture of these compounds, hence it is unlikely that disarmament agreements will render knowledge of nerve agent toxicity redundant.

4.2. Physical properties

The nerve agents are commonly divided into two groups, the G-agents and the V-agents, the former being, with the exception of tabun, phosphonofluoridates, generally methylphosphonofluoridates with a branched chain alkoxy group. In the case of soman, the alkoxy group is a bulky pinacoloxy group, which gives this G-agent special properties (see ageing below). GF has a cyclic group replacing the alkoxy group and is sometimes known as cyclosarin. The V-agents are mostly S-alkyl phosphonothioates (see Table 4.1.).

The G and V agents differ in physical properties (Tables 4.2. and 4.3.). Consequently the G agents are both percutaneous and respiratory hazards, the V agents, unless aerosolised, are contact poisons. Furthermore, the physical properties, may affect the way these substances are deployed. Nerve agents can be delivered by rockets bombs and shells. Spraying from low flying aircraft is also possible - and likely to be effective against poorly protected troops with inadequate air defences. GB and GA are comparatively volatile agents (the vapour pressure of GB being 2.10 mmHg and its volatility i.e. maximum vapour concentration being 22,000 mg/m^3) and disappear fairly rapidly after use. VX, on the other hand, can be used to contaminate ground. Field studies with VX have shown a decline in ground concentrations of 3 orders of magnitude in 17–52 days (Small, 1984). GD can be thickened with methyl methacrylate to increase its persistence. In its thickened form GD is a sticky substance that can be difficult to remove from surfaces - including protective clothing.

Table 4.1. G and V agents

Code	Name	Formula
GA	Tabun (ethyl-N,N-dimethyl phosphoramidocyanidate)	$(CH_3)_2N-\overset{\displaystyle O}{\underset{\displaystyle CN}{P}}-OCH_2CH_3$
GB	Sarin (isopropylmethyl phosphonofluoridate)	$F-\overset{\displaystyle CH_3}{\underset{\displaystyle O}{P}}-OCH(CH_3)_2$
GD	Soman (pinacolylmethyl phosphonofluoridate)	$H_3C-C(CH_3)_2-CH(CH_3)-O-\overset{\displaystyle O}{\underset{\displaystyle CH_3}{P}}-F$
GE	Isopropylethyl phosphonofluoridate	$(CH_3)_2CHO-\overset{\displaystyle O}{\underset{\displaystyle F}{P}}-CH_2CH_3$
GF	Cyclosarin (cyclohexylmethyl phosphonofluoridate)	cyclohexyl$-O-\overset{\displaystyle O}{\underset{\displaystyle CH_3}{P}}-F$
VE *	O-Ethyl-S-[2-(diethylamino)ethyl]ethyl phosphonothioate	$CH_3CH_2O-\overset{\displaystyle CH_2CH_3}{\underset{\displaystyle O}{P}}-S(CH_2)_2N(CH_2CH_3)_2$
VG *	O,O-Diethyl-S-[2-(diethylamino)ethyl] phosphorothioate	$CH_3CH_2O-\overset{\displaystyle OCH_2CH_3}{\underset{\displaystyle O}{P}}-S(CH_2)_2N(CH_2CH_3)_2$
VM *	O-Ethyl-S-[2-(diethylamino)ethyl]methyl phosphonothioate	$CH_3CH_2O-\overset{\displaystyle CH_3}{\underset{\displaystyle O}{P}}-S(CH_2)_2N(CH_2CH_3)_2$
VX *	O-Ethyl-S-[2-(diisopropylamino)ethyl]methyl phosphonothioate	$CH_3CH_2O-\overset{\displaystyle CH_3}{\underset{\displaystyle O}{P}}-S(CH_2)_2N(CH(CH_3)_2)_2$

Adapted from Maynard and Beswick (1992) with the permission of the authors and Butterworth–Heinemann.

Note * Sometimes referred to as A or F agents

The G agents and V agents differ in physical properties, the latter being less volatile (Tables 4.2., 4.3.).

Table 4.2. Physicochemical properties of nerve agents. Volatility and vapour pressure

	Tabun		Sarin		Soman		VX		GF	
°C	VP MmHg	Vol^a Mg/m^3	VP MmHG	Vol Mg/m^3	VP MmHg	Vol Mg/m^3	VP MmHg	Vol Mg/m^3	VP MmHg	Vol Mg/m^3
0	0.004	38	0.52	4279	0.044	470.9			0.006	63
10	0.013	119.5	1.07	8494	0.11	1135.5			0.017	173
20	0.036	319.8	2.10	16101	0.27	2692.1	0.00044	5.85^b	0.044	434
25	0.07	611.3	2.9	21862	0.40	3921.4	0.0007	10.07	0.068	659
30	0.094	807.4	3.93	29138	0.61	5881.4			0.104	991
40	0.23	1912.4	7.1	60959	-	-			0.234	2159
50	0.56	4512.0	12.3	83548	2.60	23516.0			0.501	4480

Adapted from Maynard and Beswick (1992) with the permission of the authors and Butterworth–Heinemann.

a. Volatility = concentration of saturated vapour at specifies room temperature

Volatility calculated from PV = nRT

$$Vol = \frac{VP \times 101\,325 \times MW}{760 \times 8.3143 \times °A} = \frac{VP \times MW \times 16.035}{°A}$$

(4.1.)

°A = Absolute temperature

b. Some authorities quote values as low as 0.1–1.0 mg/m^3

4.3. Toxicology

The toxic actions of all the nerve agents are very similar, but some differences have been observed with certain OPs, particularly with respect to their relative central and peripheral effects (Ligtenstein, 1984; Misulis *et al.*, 1987).

The reaction of OPs with cholinesterases has been dealt with in Chapter 1 and the same considerations (reactivity of OP with enzyme, reactivation rate of the phosphorylated enzyme, synthesis *de novo* of the inhibited enzyme and ageing) are important in determining the severity and duration of effects. The main difference between nerve agents and OP pesticides is that the nerve agents inhibit AChEs at much lower concentrations and are thus several orders of magnitude more acutely toxic than most OP pesticides. With soman a further difference has already been alluded to: ageing of AChE occurs so fast after inhibition with that nerve agent that spontaneous reactivation does not occur, nor can oximes bring about reactivation. Failure of post-exposure therapy has led to the development of various means of prophylaxis and pretreatment to oppose the effects of nerve agents.

Since the most obvious pharmacological effect of nerve agents is the same as that of the OP insecticides, namely to cause accumulation of acetylcholine, their effects on the cholinergic muscarinic and nicotinic receptors (see chapter 1) are very similar and will not be discussed in detail here. Unlike the insecticide OP compounds, G-type nerve agents are likely to be encountered in the form of vapour. The eyes are affected and miosis and a dimness of vision are early symptoms: this is not the case following ingestion of OP pesticides. Spasm of the ciliary muscles is followed by severe headache. The recent use of GB by terrorists in the incident in the Tokyo subway has provided first hand accounts of the effects of this compound. More details are provided below but attention is drawn to a detailed article in the The Observer newspaper, of 14 May 2000, entitled "Doomsday on the Tokyo tube" by Haruki Murukami.

A first hand account by a patient records early weakness of the legs and a feeling that his "head was spinning". Collapse followed rapidly.

4.3.1. Non-Anticholinesterase Effects

The important toxicological effects of OP nerve agents are almost entirely a result of their anticholinesterase activity. However there is evidence that some OPs, including nerve agents, can interact directly with cholinergic receptors (Bakri *et al.*, 1988; Silveira *et al.*, 1990).

However unlike some other OP anticholinesterases, there is little evidence that nerve agents can cause delayed polyneuropathy (see below). Although there are reports that OPs, including nerve agents, can affect non-cholinergic neurotransmitter systems in the CNS, it is likely that most such perturbations are secondary to effects on cholinergic pathways. Non-cholinergic pathways that may be affected include GABAergic, dopaminergic, glutaminergic and somatostatinergic pathways (Sivam *et al.*, 1984; Valdes *et al.*, 1985; Smallridge *et al.*, 1999; Rocha *et al.*, 1999; Chechabo *et al.*, 1999; Lallement *et al.*, 1999). It has been suggested that components of these pathways might be involved in the psychiatric consequences of nerve agent exposure (Valdes *et al.*, 1985) and that disturbances of glutaminergic neurotranmission may be involved in nerve agent induced seizures (Lallement *et al.*, 1999). See also below.

4.4. General Toxicity

4.4.1. Acute Toxicity

4.4.1.1. Acute Toxicity in Experimental Animals: Figures for the acute toxicity of the main nerve agents, sarin, soman, tabun and VX are given in Table 4.4. Figures for the acute toxicity of other nerve agents are not readily available, but the intramuscular LD50 for GF was 80 µg/kg in rats (Kassa and Cabal, 1999), and 47 µg/kg in rhesus monkeys (Young and Koplovitz, 1995). Qualitatively, as discussed above, the acute toxicity of nerve agents in animals is very similar to that of OP insecticides (see chapter 1).

Table 4.3. Physicochemical properties of nerve agents. Molecular weight etc.

	Tabun	Sarin	Soman	VX	GF
Molecular weight (Daltons)	162.3	140.1	182.18	267.36	180.14
Specific gravity at 25°C	1.073	1.0887	1.022	1.0083	1.133 (20°C)
Boiling point °C	246	147	167	300	-
Melting point °C	-49	-56	-80	-20	-12

Adapted from Maynard and Beswick (1992) with the permission of the authors and Butterworth–Heinemann

4.4.1.2. Acute Toxicity in Man

The clinical signs and symptoms to be expected in man have largely been inferred from OP pesticide poisoning of accidental or suicidal origin in man or from experimental studies with nerve agents or pesticides in animals.

Table 4.4. Comparative acute toxicity of nerve agents I

Species	Route	Term	Unit	Tabun	Sarin	Soman	VX
Man	pc	LD50	mg/kg		28[1]		
	pc	LCLO	µg/kg				86[2]
	pc	LDLO	mg/kg	23[1]		18[1]	
	inhal	LDLO	mg/m³	150[1]		70[1]	
	inhal	LD50	mg/m³		70[1]		
	inhal	LDLO	µg/m³		90[3]		
	iv	TDLO	µg/kg	14[1]			
	iv	TDLO	µg/kg				1.5[4]
	oral	TDLO	µg/kg		2[5]		4[4]
	sc	LDLO	µg/kg				30[6]
	im	TDLO	µg/kg				3.2[6]
Rat	pc	LD50	mg/kg	18[1]			
	inhal	LC50	mg/m³/ 10 min	30[4,7]	150[3]		
	iv	LD50	µg/kg	66[7]	39[8]	44.5[1]	12[12]
	oral	LD50	µg/kg	3700[7]	550[7]		
	sc	LD50	µg/kg	193[9]	103[10]	75[11]	
	im	LD50	µg/kg	800[5]	108[13]	62[13]	
	ip	LD50	µg/kg		218[8]	98[14]	
Mouse	pc	LD50	mg/kg	1[7]	1.08[7]		
	inhal	LC50	mg/m³/ 30 min	15[7]	5[15]	1[15]	
	iv	LD50	µg/kg	150[7]	113[7]	35[17]	
	sc	LD50	µg/kg	250[18]	60[15]	40[15]	22[18]
	sc	LD50	µg/kg		172[30]		
	im	LD50	µg/kg	440[7]	222[7]		
	ip	LD50	µg/kg		420[20]	393[20]	50[2]

Table 4.4. Comparative acute toxicity of nerve agents - contd

Species	Route	Term	Unit	Tabun	Sarin	Soman	VX
Dog	pc	LD50	mg/kg	30[7]			
	inhal	LC50	mg/m³/ 10 min	400[7]	100[7]		
	iv	LD50	µg/kg	84[21]	19[21]		
	oral	LD50	µg/kg	200[15]			
	sc	LD50	µg/kg	284[11]		12[22]	
Monkey	pc	LD50	µg/kg	9300[7]			
	inhal	LC50	mg/m³/ 10 min	250[7]	100[7]		
	sc	LD50	µg/kg			13[23]	
	im	LD50	µg/kg		22.3[24]	9.5[25]	
Cat	Inhal	LC50	mg/m³/ 10 min	250[7]	100[21]		
	iv	LD50	µg/kg		22[7]		
Rabbit	pc	LD50	µg/kg	2500[7]	925[7]		
	inhal	LC50	mg/m³ 10 min	840[7]	120[7]		
	iv	LD50	µg/kg	63[7]	15[26]		
	oral	LD50	µg/kg	16300[7]			
	sc	LD50	µg/kg	375[27]	30[27]	20[22]	14[29]
	ip	LD50	µg/kg				66[29]
Guinea Pig	pc	LD50	mg/kg	35[7]			
	inhal	LC50	mg/m³ 2min	393[7]			
	sc	LD50	mg/kg				
	sc	LD50	µg/kg	120[28]	30[27]	24[28]	8.4[28]
Hamster	sc	LD50	µg/kg	245[31]	95[27]		
Farm animal	pc	LD50	µg/kg	1100[7]			
	inhal	LC50	mg/m³/ 14min	400[7]			
Chickens	sc	LD50	µg/kg			50[14]	
	ip	LD50	µg/kg			71[22]	
Frog	ip	LD50	µg/kg			251[14]	

Adapted and reproduced from Table 5 in Chapter 34 Organophosphorus Compounds as Chemical Warfare agents by Maynard and Beswick In: Ballantyne, B. and Marrs, T.C. eds *Clinical and Experimental Toxicology of Organophosphates and Carbamates* with the permission of the publishers, Butterworth–Heinemann and the authors.

Key to Table 4.4.

1. Robinson (1967)
2. WHO (1970)
3. Rengstorff (1985)
4. Sidell (1974)
5. Grob and Harvey (1958)
6. National Academy of Sciences (1982)
7. Gates and Renshaw (1946)
8. Fleisher (1963)
9. Pazdernik et al (1983)
10. Brimblecombe et al. (1970)
11. Bosković et al. (1984)
12. Jovanović (1982)
13. Schoene et al. (1985)
14. Chattopadhyay et al (1986)
15. Lotts (1960)
16. Schoene and Oldiges (1973)
17. Brezenoff et al (1984)
18. Maksimović et al. (1980)
19. Fredriksson (1957)
20. Clement (1984)
21. O'Leary et al. (1961)
22. Berry and Davies (1970)
23. Clement et al (1981)
24. D'Mello and Duffy (1985)
25. Lipp (1972)
26. Wills (1961)
27. Coleman et al. (1968)
28. Gordon and Leadbeater (1977)
29. Leblic et al. (1981)
30. Bright et al. (1991)
31. Coleman et al. (1966)

Poisoning with nerve agents (as opposed to OP pesticides) had only rarely been observed (Sidell, 1974, Maynard and Beswick, 1992; Marrs et al., 1996), although recent events in Iraqi Kurdistan and Japan have largely confirmed the view that qualitatively, OP pesticide poisoning and nerve agent poisoning does not greatly differ. A further source of information has been low dose volunteer studies with nerve agents, and, again, these do not suggest any major differences between man and other animals (see Marrs et al., 1996). (See Table 4.5.)

Despite this toxicological similarity, the physical properties by which the nerve agents differ from most pesticides, especially the volatility of the G agents may influence clinical presentation. Thus, as noted above, after the use of sarin at Matsumoto, the eye signs (constricted pupils) and symptoms (dim vision, eye pain) were comparatively severe (Nohara and Segawa, 1996), presumably because of contact of the vapour with the eyes, whereas symptoms and signs of such severity are rarely observed with OP pesticides.

Nozaki et al. (1995) have recorded clinical details of patients likely to have been exposed to VX. Confirmation of use of VX is lacking: though, apparently, those under arrest with regard to terrorist acts have confessed to using this nerve agent. Those casualties treated by Nozaki and colleagues were exposed to nerve agent some 10 weeks before the terrorist attack on the Tokyo subway (January 4 1995 as compared with March 20 1995). The authors, who were involved in treating the sarin casualties, reported that in the case of sarin poisoning, nicotinic responses dominated the cardiovascular findings whereas in the VX cases bradycardia, a classical muscarinic response, was found.

Table 4.5. Main effects of nerve agents at various sites in the body

Receptor	Target Organ	Symptoms and Signs
Central	Central Nervous System	Giddiness, anxiety, restlessness, headache, tremor, confusion, failure to concentrate, convulsions, respiratory depression
Muscarinic	Glands	
	a) nasal mucosa	rhinorrhea
	b) bronchial mucosa	bronchorrhea
	c) sweat	sweating
	d) lachrymal	lachrymation
	e) salivary	salivation
	Smooth Muscle	
	a) iris	miosis
	b) ciliary muscle	failure of accommodation
	c) gut	abdominal cramp, diarrhoea
	d) bladder	frequency, involuntary micturition
	e) heart	bradycardia
Nicotinic	Autonomic ganglia	sympathetic effects: pallor, tachycardia, hypertension
	Skeletal muscle	weakness, fasciculation

The patient exposed, probably by the percutaneous route, to VX did not show miosis on admission though this sign developed 3 hours later. The authors recorded a rapid response to intravenous atropine in the case of VX poisoning: the pulse rate increased from 43 per minute to 125 per minute within 2 minutes of giving the atropine. Blood pressure also improved rapidly. Diazepam, but not phenytoin, was effective in controlling convulsions. It is interesting to note that the patient's serum cholinesterase concentration returned to normal over a period of 20 days (normal: 258 IU/l, concentration on day following attack: 14 IU/l). Neuropathy (not defined) recovered over 6 months but antegrade and retrograde amnesia persisted. The predominantly nicotinic effects on the cardiovascular system referred to above are noted by Nozaki and Aikawa (1995): in only 1 of 15 patients was bradycardia recorded.

4.4.2. Delayed Effects on the Central Nervous System

Some studies involving the effects of nerve agents on the CNS are summarised in Table 4.6. Behavioral effects together with subtle EEG changes were described in man by Duffy *et al.* (1979) after sarin exposure severe enough to cause symptoms and clinical signs. The EEG changes were mild and only apparent after computer analysis. Furthermore, exclusion criteria were unclear. In a study in rhesus monkeys, Burchfiel *et al.* (1976) described changes, persisting for a year, after a single large dose or repeated small doses of sarin. The observation of abnormalities after the large dose was not unexpected as the animals had convulsions, but the lower dose used was 1µg, given by 10 weekly injections (total dose 10 µg = 7% LD_{50}). The significance of these changes is unclear in view of the small group size (three per test group; two controls). Furthermore some similar electroencephalographic changes were seen after the organochlorine pesticide, dieldrin, viz. a relative increase in beta activity. Pearce *et al.* (1999) carried out a study in marmosets in which the animals were exposed to a single low dose of sarin (3µg/kg), which produced cholinesterase inhibitions of 36–67%. No effect was observed on the EEG nor were deleterious effects on performance of neuropsychological test end points. The two terrorist incidents in Japan, where sarin was used, have given conflicting evidence on the long term effects of exposure to that compound, and their interpretation is complicated by the impure nature of the material used: there being clear evidence that fluoride- and isopropyl alcohol-containing by-products were present in the Tokyo subway incident (Hui and Minami, 2000). A follow-up of affected rescuers from the incident at Matsumoto, provided little evidence of sequelae (Nakajima *et al.*, 1997), although epileptiform EEGs were found in one case series (Sekijima *et al.*, 1997). On the other hand after the Tokyo incident, there was evidence of postural disturbances (Yokoyama *et al.*, 1996) and EEG abnormalities (Murata *et al.*, 1997). Sekijima *et al.* (1997) reported a 1 and 2 year follow-up of patients exposed to sarin in the Tokyo subway incident. Of 6 severely poisoned patients 4 were found to show EEG changes. Sensory polyneuropathy was found in one patient 7 months post-exposure and, surprisingly, one patient showed visual field disturbances at 1 year post-exposure. Hypoxia may play a part in inducing CNS changes and convulsions after exposure to nerve agents may be, in part, due to poor cerebral oxygenation. Delayed effects include amnesia (Hatta *et al.*, 1996). Murata *et al.* (1997) have stressed the occurrence of asymptomatic sequelae following exposure to sarin. Changes included: increased latencies in event-related and visual-evoked potentials and increase heart rate variability (R-R interval variability: CV_{RR}). The latter was related to the serum cholinesterase activity.

Table 4.6. Published work on long term effects of nerve agents

Exposed Group	Result	OP	Reference
Workers	+ve(EEG) multivariate	Sarin	Duffy et al., 1979
Rhesus monkeys	+ve(EEG)	Sarin	Burchfiel et al., 1976
Workers	+ve(EEG)	Sarin DFP	Holmes and Gaon, 1956
Rats	Behavioral decrement; also pathological changes in the CNS	Soman	McDonough et al., 1986
Marmoset	-ve(no change in EEG, no decrement on CANTAB test Battery)	Sarin	Pearce et al., 1999

4.4.3. Peripheral Effects

The acute peripheral effects of nerve agents are similar to those of insecticides, namely effects at sympathetic and parasympathetic ganglia, at autonomic effector sites and at sweat glands (see chapter 1). These are often the most prominent effects observed in nerve agent poisoning. The nicotinic effects at the neuromuscular junction are also important, causing as they do, fasciculation and, in severely affected subjects, paralysis including of respiratory musculature.

4.4.4. Delayed Effects

4.4.4.1. Myopathy and Intermediate Syndrome

In 1987, Senanayake and Karalliedde described a new form of delayed neurotoxicity following intoxication by organophosphorus insecticides. The recovery period in the "Intermediate Syndrome" was relatively brief, viz. 4–18 days. This syndrome has not been described in cases of accidental nerve agent poisoning, however this may simply be a reflection of the infrequency of properly observed nerve agent poisoning. As discussed above, a connection between the "Intermediate Syndrome" and OP-induced myopathy has been considered (see Karalliedde and Henry, 1993).

A number of studies have demonstrated myopathy in experimental animals with nerve agents such as sarin, VX and GF (Bright *et al.*, 1991; Gupta *et al.*, 1991; Young and Koplovitz, 1995). It has further been shown that pretreatment regimes with mementine, D-tubocurarine and atropine, that prevent fasciculation, but do not prevent AChE inhibition, prevented myonecrosis in rats, induced by soman, sarin, tabun or VX (Gupta and Dettbarn, 1992). On the other hand, considerable increases in creatine phosphokinase were observed in rhesus monkeys pretreated with pyridostigmine, poisoned with GF and treated with atropine and either 2-PAM chloride or HI-6.

4.4.4.2. OPIDP

The possibility that OP nerve agents might cause OPIDP has occasionally been considered (Hodgetts, 1991; Maynard and Beswick, 1992), but experimental studies, have generally not shown any propensity of nerve agents to cause this syndrome (e.g. Anderson and Dunham, 1985; Parker *et al.*, 1988; Henderson *et al.*, 1992). Concentrations of nerve agent required to produce AChE inhibition are low compared to those required for inhibition of NTE, the opposite of the case with the neuropathic OPs, such as mipafox or DFP. Thus, Gordon *et al.* (1983) measured the concentrations (IC_{50}) of various OPs required to produce 50% inhibition *in vitro* of, respectively, AChE and NTE. The ratio IC_{50} for acetyl cholinesterase/IC_{50} for NTE was 1.8 for mipafox, 1.1 for DFP, but 0.0056 for sarin, 0.0012 for soman, 0.0005 for tabun, and 10^{-6} for VX. Moreover, Johnson *et al.* (1985) reported that soman-dosed birds do not develop OPIDN and that soman protected hens against the neuropathic effects of DFP. It has also been shown that only that a negligible proportion of soman-inhibited NTE from hen brain and spinal cord undergoes the ageing reaction believed to be an essential preliminary to the development of OPIDP. Additionally, structure-activity considerations would not lead one to expect nerve agents to be neuropathic (Aldridge *et al.*, 1969). Thus, soman demonstrably lacks neuropathic potential. Advances in therapy have produced concerns that patients might survive supralethal doses of nerve agents only to develop OPIDN, this scenario seeming least unlikely with sarin (Willems *et al.*, 1983). Thus it is entirely improbable that OPIDP represents any real problem in nerve agent poisoning in nerve agent toxicity except, perhaps, in extraordinary circumstances.

4.5. Effects of Subchronic or Longterm Exposure to Nerve Agents

In the early days of study of nerve agents comparatively little attention was paid to any long term effect that OPs might have, although the possibility of delayed effects from high doses has long been recognised. Oak Ridge National Laboratory prepared health risk assessments for many nerve and these have been published (Oak Ridge National Laboratory, 2000). In general the effects of prolonged administration to experimental animals of tabun, sarin, soman and VX are what would be anticipated with compounds whose effects are those of almost purely anticholinesterase materials. Critical endpoints in the studies were generally reduced plasma, red cell or brain cholinesterase activity or reduced growth rates. Specific neurological effects typical of OPIDP were not seen. In some studies histopathological changes have been observed in the central nervous system. Although no evidence has been seen that tabun, sarin, soman or VX are carcinogenic, studies have generally been of insufficient duration to exclude the possibility of tumorigenicity.

5. Diagnosis

The diagnosis of nerve agent poisoning on the battle field would depend upon a combination of clinical acumen, nerve agent detection systems and circumstantial evidence. Off the battlefield plasma butyrylcholinesterase and red cell AChE would have the same limitations as in pesticide poisoning. The well established clinical rule of treating on the basis of the patient's clinical condition rather than on the basis of enzyme levels should be recalled. For more definitive detection of exposure to specific nerve agents, plasma or urine alkylphosphates can be used. Thus an anion exchange liquid chromatography tandem electrospray mass spectrometry method for O-isopropyl methylphosphonic acid (IMPA), a metabolite of sarin has been developed (Noort et al., 1998) and gas-liquid chromatography methods have also been described (Nakajima et al., 1998).

6. Treatment

The mainstay of treatment of OP nerve agent poisoning is the concomitant use of an anticholinergic drug, in practice virtually always atropine, and an oxime enzyme reactivator such as pralidoxime or obidoxime (Marrs, 1991; Heath and Meredith, 1992; Bismuth et al., 1992).

A central nervous system depressant, usually diazepam, is used to treat convulsions and/or muscle fasciculations (Sellström, 1992). Atropine eye drops have been used to reverse the miosis produced by nerve agent exposure and to reduce the pain produced by ciliary muscle paralysis. Nozaki and Aikawa (1995) used atropine eye drops in treating patients exposed to sarin in the Tokyo subway incident though not immediately post-exposure. The authors argued that miosis was a valuable sign in assessing the systemic effects of sarin and used it as a basis for judging their systemic treatment with atropine. This approach has not generally been considered to be reliable, miosis being difficult to reverse with intramuscular atropine in cases of sarin exposure. Nozaki and colleagues reported that atropine eyedrops used 3–5 days post-exposure to sarin produced pupillary dilation but that their continued use was rejected by patients on the grounds that inability to accommodate led to poorer rather than better vision. There are some international differences in the oxime favored, the USA using pralidoxime chloride, France the methylsulfate and the UK the methanesulfonate ("mesylate"). Germany favours the use of obidoxime which unlike pralidoxime salts is effective against tabun, but to be weighed against that advantage there is the possible hepatotoxicity of obidoxime. Although the pralidoxime salts will be of equal efficacy on a molar basis, the product literature reveals disconcerting differences in doses advised (See Ayerst, 1986; SERB, 1988). From a purely military point of view, the Hagedorn oximes, especially HI-6 and HLö-7 are attractive as they are effective against nearly all nerve agents, including tabun and GF (Worek et al., 1998a; 1998b; Kassa and Cabal, 1999). Indeed HLö-7 comes near to being a universal antidote. But the most serious gap in the therapeutic efficacy of combinations of atropine and an oxime in the acute cholinergic phase is poisoning with soman, where ageing (see Chapter 1) of the inhibited cholinesterase renders oximes ineffective. There have been two main approaches to this problem: 1) the use of prophylaxes such as the carbamate drugs pyridostigmine or physostigmine (see below and Inns and Marrs, 1992). 2) the study of newer oximes such as HI-6 and HLö-7 (see Bismuth et al., 1992; Kassa, 1995; Worek et al., 1997; Kassa and Bajgar, 1998; Worek et al., 1998b): here there is some indication of efficacy most notably in the periphery, although whether any substantial antidotal effectiveness occurs, particularly in the central nervous system, is not known. Moreover and of greatest practical importance, the usefulness of these oximes in the field is not well established. In the past other approaches that have been considered for the problem of soman poisoning include the injection of cholinesterase and the use of soman antibodies (see Inns and Marrs, 1992; Ci et al., 1995; Liao and Rong, 1995). Pralidoxime salts, but not obidoxime, seem ineffective in tabun poisoning.

The reason for this is not connected to ageing, but probably that the P-N bond causes the phosphorus in the phosphonylated enzyme to be less prone to nucleophilic attack as a result of back donation of electrons (Bismuth *et al.*, 1992). (see Weinbaum *et al.*, 2000, for a review of critical care aspects of management of nerve agent poisoning).

7. Prophylaxis of nerve agent poisoning

One possible answer to the problem of ageing of the soman-inhibited AChE is the use of prophylactic therapy (Table 4.7.). Of these approaches pretreatment with oximes and with anticholinesterases are the only ones that have been seriously considered. Before the advent of carbamate prophylaxis, pralidoxime methanesulfonate tablets were issued to the British military.

Table 4.7. Prophylaxis for OP poisoning

Type of compound	Examples		Reference
Anticholinergics	Atropine		DeCandole and
	Scopolamine		McPhaill, 1957
	Pentamethonium		Anderson *et al*, 1991
			Gupta and Dettbarn, 1992
Oximes	Pralidoxime salts		Brimblecombe *et al*, 1970
Anticonvulsants	Diazepam		Lundy *et al*, 1978
Cholinesterases	Fetal bovine AChE		Wolfe *et al*, 1987
Anticholinesterases	Organo-Phosphates	TEPP Paraoxon	Berry *et al.*, 1971
	Carbamates	Physostigmine, Pyridostigmine, Mobam, Decarbofuran	Gordon *et al*, 1978

7.1. Carbamate Prophylaxis

Most recent work on the prophylaxis of soman poisoning has been undertaken using the carbamate drugs, physostigmine or pyridostigmine.

These compounds inactivate AChE by carbamylating the active site in much the same way as OPs phosphorylate the active site. However the carbamylated enzyme reactivates much more quickly than does the phosphorylated one. Furthermore, that fraction of the enzyme that is carbamylated is unavailable for phosphorylation. In fact successful carbamate prophylaxis requires a fairly stable proportion of the AChE to be carbamylated, sufficient that its unavailability for phosphorylation will protect against soman poisoning, but not so much as to interfere with military performance. The action of pyridostigmine, unlike that of physostigmine is almost entirely peripheral, but the action of the latter is shorter in duration and it is pyridostigmine that has generally been adopted for the protection of soldiers.

A number of studies have showed the efficacy of pyridostigmine in animal species, generally in combination with post-exposure treatment with an anticholinergic and an oxime and often diazepam in poisoning by soman (Gordon et al., 1978; Inns and Leadbeater, 1983; Leadbeater et al., 1985; Anderson et al., 1991). A problem recognised early with carbamate prophylaxis is the possibility that dosing with a carbamate anticholinesterase might inactivate sufficient enzyme to interfere with military activity. This was addressed in some of the studies cited above to some extent, but in the main the possibility has been addressed using primates or human volunteers. A recent study in marmosets has suggested that physostigmine pretreatment at a dose causing approximately 30% blood ACh depression, was both free of effects on behavioural parameters, EEG and cortical evoked visual response and effective, with post-poisoning atropine treatment, in protection against the lethal effects of twice the lethal dose of soman (Phillipens et al., 2000).

In field conditions the dose of pyridostigmine is 30 mg/8 h as pyridostigmine bromide tablets. After about 24 h the red cell AChE stabilizes at about 20% inhibited. The first large scale use of pyridostigmine bromide tablets as a pre-treatment for nerve agent poisoning took place during the Gulf War. As expected, the use of pyridostigmine produced side effects. Sharabi et al. (1991) recorded nausea, abdominal pain, frequent urination and rhinorrhoea. The authors reported that the side effects were generally mild and occurred about 1.6 hours after each dose. Interestingly, no association between cholinesterase depression and symptoms was discovered. Cholinesterase depression (AChE) of about 20% (18.8 ± 3.5 in the symptomatic group, N = 9, and 19.3 ± 6.6 in the asymptomatic group, N = 12) was observed.

The level of cholinesterase depression recorded here is appropriate as regards the use of pyridostigmine as a pre-treatment for nerve agent poisoning. The use of pyridostigmine bromide has been suggested as a possible cause of the so-called Gulf War Syndrome.

Detailed discussion of the syndrome is not possible here and the reader is referred
to a series of papers that appeared in 1997 (Haley *et al.*, 1997a; Haley *et al.*, 1997b;
Haley and Kurt, 1997; Iowa Persian Gulf Study Group, 1997). Hyams *et al.* (1996)
have published an interesting account of war syndromes and place evidence for the Gulf
War Syndrome in an historical context.

This chapter reflects the views of the authors and not necessarily those of any UK
Government Department or Agency.

References

Aldridge, W.N., Barnes, J.M., Johnson, M.K. Studies on delayed neuropathy produced
    by some organophosphorus compounds. *Annals of the New York Academy of
    Sciences* 1969;**160**:314–22.
Anderson, R.J., Dunham, C.B.   Electrophysiologic changes in peripheral nerve
    following repeated exposure to organophosphorus agents. *Archives of Toxicology*
    1985;**58**:97–101.
Anderson, D.R., Harris, L.W., Lennox, W.J., *et al.* Effects of subacute pretreatment
    with carbamate together with acute adjunct pretreatment against nerve agent
    exposure. *Drug and Chemical Toxicology* 1991;**14**:1–19.
Ayerst. Protopam chloride brand of pralidoxime chloride. Ayerst Laboratories, New
    York. 1986.
Bakri, N.M.S., El-Rashidy, A.H., Eldefrawi, A.T., *et al.* Direct actions of
    organophosphate anticholinesterases on nicotinic and muscarinic acetylcholine
    receptors. *Journal of Biochemical Toxicology* 1988;**3**:235–9.
Benschop, H.P., Bijleveld, E.C., de Jong, L.P.A., *et al.* Toxicokinetics of the four
    stereoisomers of the nerve agent soman in atropinized rats—influence of a soman
    simulator. *Toxicology and Applied Pharmacology* 1987;**90**:490–500.
Berry, W.K., Davies, D.R. Use of carbamates and atropine in the protection of animals
    against poisoning by 1,2,2-trimethylpropyl phosphonofluoridate. *Biochemical
    Pharmacology* 1970;**19**:927–34.
Berry, W.K., Davies, D.R., Gordon, J.J. Protection of animals against soman (1,2,2-
    trimethylpropyl methylphosphonofluoridate) by pretreatment with some other
    organophosphorus compounds, followed by oxime and atropine. *Biochemical
    Pharmacology* 1971;**20**:125–34.

Bismuth, C., Baud, F., Conso, F., et al. Toxicologie Clinique, Paris: Flammarion; 1987. p. 667.

Bismuth, C., Inns, R.H., Marrs, T.C. Efficacy, toxicity and clinical use of oximes in anticholinesterase poisoning. In:. *Clinical and Experimental Toxicology of Organophosphates and Carbamates*. Ballantyne, B., Marrs, T.C. eds Butterworth–Heinemann; Oxford.1992. p. 555–77.

Bosković, B., Kovacević, V., Jovanović, D. 2-PAM chloride, HJ-6 and HGG-12 in soman and tabun poisoning. *British Journal of Pharmacology* 1984;**39**:822–30.

Brezenoff, H.E., McGee, J., Knight, V. The hypertensive response to soman and its relation to brain AChE inhibition. *Acta Pharmacologica Toxicologica* 1984;**55**:270–7

Bright, J.E., Inns, R.H., Tuckwell, N.J. et al. A histochemical study of changes observed in the mouse diaphragm after organophosphate poisoning. *Human and Experimental Toxicology* 1991;**10**:9–14.

Brimblecombe, R.W., Green, D.M., Stratton, J.A. et al. The protective actions of some anticholinesterase drugs in sarin poisoning. *British Journal of Pharmacology*, 1970;**L9**:822–30.

Burchfiel, I.L., Duffy, F.H., van Sim, M. Persistent effects of sarin and dieldrin upon the primate electroencephalogram. *Toxicology and Applied Pharmacology* 1976;**35**:365–79.

Chattopadhay, D.P., Dighe, K., Nashikkar, A.B. et al. Species differences in the *in vitro* inhibition of brain AChE and carbaoxyl esterase by mipafox, paraoxon and soman. *Pesticide Biochemistry and Physiology* 1986;**L6**: 202–8.

Chechabo, S.R., Santos, M.D., Albuquerque, E.X. The organophosphate sarin, at low concentrations, inhibits the evoked release of GABA in rat hippocampal slices. *Neurotoxicology* 1999;**20**:871–82.

Ci, Y., Zhou, Y., Guo, Z., et al. Production, characterization and application of monoclonal antibodies against the organophosphorus nerve agent, VX. *Archives of Toxicology* 1995;**69**:565–7.

Clement, J.G. Role of antiesterase in organophosphate poisoning. *Fundamental* and *Applied Toxicology* 1984;**4**:S96–S1O5.

Clement, J.G., Hand, B.T., Shilloff, J.D. Differences in the toxicity of soman in various strains of mice. *Fundamental and Applied Toxicology* 1981;**1**:419–20.

Coleman, I.W., Little, F.E., Patton, G.E. et al. Cholinolytics in the treatment of anticholinesterase poisoning. IV The effectiveness of five binary combinations of cholinolytics with oximes in the treatment of organophosphorus poisoning. *Canadian Journal of Physiology and Pharmacology* 1966;**44**:743–64.

Coleman, I.W., Patton, G.E., Bannard, R.A. Cholinolytics in the treatment of anticholinesterase poisoning V. The effectiveness of parpanit with oximes in the treatment of organophosphorus poisoning. *Canadian Journal of Physiology and Pharmacology* 1968;**46**:109–17.

DeCandole, C.A., McPhaill, M.K. Sarin and paraoxon antagonism in different species. *Canadian Journal of Biochemistry and Physiology* 1957;**35**:1071–83.

D'Mello, G.D., Duffy, E.A.M. The acute toxicity of sarin in marmosets (*Callithrix jacchus*): a behavioral analysis. *Fundamental and Applied Toxicology* 1985;**5**:S169–74.

Duffy, F.H., Burchfiel, J.L., Bartels, P.H., *et al.* Long-term effects of an organophosphate upon the human electroencephalogram. *Toxicology and Applied Pharmacology* 1979;**47**:161–76.

Fleisher, B. Effects of p-nitrophenyl phosphonate (EPN) on the toxicity of isopropyl methyl phosphonofluoridate (GB). *Journal of Pharmacology and Experimental Therapeutics* 1963;**139**:390.

Fredriksson, T. Pharmacological properties of methyl fluorophosphonylcholines, two synthetic cholinergic drugs. *Archives Internationales de Pharmacodynamie et de Therapie* 1957;**113**:101–4.

Gates, M., Renshaw, B.C. Fluorophosphates and other phosphorus-containing compounds. Summary technical report of Division 9, vol 1, parts I and II, 1946. p. 131–55. Washington DC, Office of Scientific Research and Development

Gordon, J.J., Inns, R.H., Johnson, M.K. *et al.* The delayed neuropathic effects of nerve agents and some other organophosphate compounds. *Archives of Toxicology* 1983;**51**:71–82

Gordon, J.J., Leadbeater, L., Maidment, M.P. The protection of animals against organophosphate poisoning by pre-treatment with a carbamate. *Toxicology and Applied Pharmacology* 1978;**43**:207–16.

Gordon, J.J., Leadbeater, L.L. The prophylactic use of 1-methyl 2-hydroxyiminomethylpyridinium methanesulfonate (P25) in the treatment of organophosphate poisoning. *Toxicology and Applied Pharmacology* 1977;**40**:109–14.

Grob, D., Harvey, A.M. Effects in man of the anticholinesterase compound sarin (isopropyl methyl phosphonofluoridate). *Journal of Clinical Investigation* 1958;**37**:350–68.

Gupta, R.C., Dettbarn, W.D. Potential of memantine, D-tubocurarine, and atropine in preventing acute toxic myopathy induced by organophosphate nerve agents: soman, sarin, tabun and VX. *Neurotoxicology* 1992;**13**:649–61.

Gupta, R.C., Patterson, G.T., Dettbarn, W.D. Comparison of cholinergic and neuromuscular toxicity following acute exposure to sarin and VX in rat. *Fundamental and Applied Toxicology* 1991;**16**:449–58.

Haley, R.W., Kurt, T.L., Horn, J. Is there a Gulf War Syndrome? Searching for syndromes by factor analysis of symptoms. *Journal of the American Medical Association* 1997a;**277**:215–22.

Haley, R.W., Horn, J., Roland, P.S., et al. Evaluation of neurologic function in Gulf War veterans. A blinded case-control study. *Journal of the American Medical Association* .1997b;**277**:223–30.

Haley, R.W., Kurt, T.L. Self-reported exposure to neurotoxic chemical combinations in the Gulf War. A cross-sectional epidemiologic study. *Journal of the American Medical Association* 1997;**277**:231–7.

Hatta, K., Miura, Y., Asukai, N., et al. Amnesia from sarin poisoning. *Lancet* 1996;**347**:1343.

Heath, A.J.W., Meredith, T. Atropine in the management of anticholinesterase poisoning. In: *Clinical and Experimental Toxicology of Organophosphates and Carbamates.* Ballantyne, B., Marrs, T.C. eds. Butterworth–Heinemann; Oxford.1992. p. 543–54.

Hodgetts, T.J. Update box. *British Medical Journal* 1991;**302**:398.

Hui, D., Minami, M. Monitoring of fluorine in urine samples of patients in the Tokyo sarindisaster. *Clinica Chimica Acta* 2000;**302**:171–88

Hyams, K.C., Wignall, F.S., Roswell, R.R. War syndromes and their evaluation: from the U.S. Civil War to the Persian Gulf War. *Annals of Internal Medicine* 1996;**125**:398–405.

Inns, R.H., Leadbeater, L. The efficacy of bipyridinium derivatives in the treatment of organophosphate poisoning in the guinea pig. *Journal of Pharmacy and Pharmacology* 1983;**35**:427–33.

Inns, R.H., Marrs, T.C. Prophylaxis against anticholinesterase poisoning. In: *Clinical and Experimental Toxicology of Organophosphate and Carbamates.* Ballantyne, B., Marrs, T.C. eds. Butterworth–Heinemann; Oxford.1992. p. 602–10.

Iowa Persian Gulf Study Group. Self-reported illness and health status among Gulf War veterans. A population-based study. *Journal of the American Medical Association* 1997;**277**:238–45.

Johnson, M.K., Willems, J.L., de Bisschop, H.C., et al. Can soman cause delayed neuropathy? *Fundamental and Applied Toxicology* 1985;**5**:S180–1.

Jovanovic, D. The effect of bis-pyridinium oximes on neuromuscular blockade induced by highly toxic organophosphates in the rat. *Archives Internationales de Pharmacodynamie et de Therapie* 1982;**262**:231–41.

Karalliedde, L., Henry, J.A. Effects of organophosphates on skeletal muscle. *Human and Experimental Toxicology* 1993;**12**:289–96.

Kassa, J. Comparison of the efficacy of two oximes (HI-6 and obidoxime) in soman poisoning of rats. *Toxicology* 1995;**101**:167–74.

Kassa, J., Bajgar, J. Changes of AChE activity in various parts of brain following nontreated and treated soman poisoning in rats. *Molecular and Chemical Neuropathology* 1998;**33**:175–84.

Kassa, J., Cabal, J. A comparison of the efficacy of actylcholinesterase reactivators against cyclohexyl methylphosphonofluoridate (GF agent) by *in vitro* and *in vivo* methods. *Pharmacology and Toxicology* 1999;**84**:41–5.

Lallement, G., Clarençon, D., Galonnier, M., *et al.* Acute soman poisoning in primates neither pretreated nor receiving immediate therapy: value of gacyclidine (GK-11) in delayed medical support. *Archives of Toxicology* 1999;**73**:115–22.

Leadbeater, L., Inns, R.H., Rylands, J.M. Treatment of poisoning by soman. *Fundamental and Applied Toxicology* 1985;**5**:S225–31.

Leblic, C., Cox, H.M., le Moan, L. Etude de la toxicité, de l'eserine, VX et le paraoxon, pour établir un modèle mathematique de l'extrapolation à être humain. *Archives Belges de Médecine Sociale, Hygiene, Médecine du Travail et Médecine Légale* 1977;**Suppl**:226–42.

le Chêne, E. *Chemical and biological warfare—Threat of the future.* Mackenzie Paper. Toronto, Canada: The Mackenzie Institute; 1989

Liao, W.-G., Rong, K.-T. An explanation on the limited efficacy of detoxication against VX toxicity by purified specific antibodies. *Fundamental and Applied Toxicology* 1995;**27**:90–4.

Ligtenstein, D.A. On the synergism of the cholinesterase reactivating bispyridinium-aldoxime HI-6 and atropine in the treatment of organophosphate intoxications in the rat. MD Thesis. University of Leyden, the Netherlands. 1984

Lipp, S.A. Effect of diazepam upon soman induced seizure activities and convulsions. *Electroencephalography and Clinical Neurophysiology* 1972;**32**:557–60.

Lotts, von K. Zur Toxicologie und Pharmakologie organische Phosphosäurester. *Deutsche Gesundheitsweren* 1960;**15**:2133–79.

Lundy, P.M., Magor, G., Shaw, R.K. Gamma aminobutyric acid metabolism in different areas of rat brain at the onset of soman-induced convulsions. *Archives Internationales de Pharmacodynamie et de Therapie* 1978;**234**:64–73.

Maksimović, M., Bosković, B., Rodović, L. Antidotal effects of bis pyridinium 2 mono oxime carbonyl derivatives in intoxication with highly toxic organophosphorus compounds. *Acta Pharmaceutica Jugoslavica* 1980;**30**:151–60.

Marrs, T.C. Toxicology of oximes used in the treatment of organophosphate poisoning. *Adverse Drug Reactions and Acute Poisonings Reviews.* 1991;**10**:61–73.

Marrs, T.C., Maynard, R.L., Sidell, F.R. *Chemical Warfare Agents Toxicology and Treatment.* Chichester: John Wiley and Sons; 1996.

Maynard, R.L., Beswick, B.W. Organophosphorus compounds as chemical warfare agents. In: *Clinical and Experimental Toxicology of Organophosphates and Carbamates.* Ballantyne, B., Marrs, T.C. eds. Butterworth–Heinemann; Oxford. 1992. p. 373–85.

Maynard, R.L., Marrs, T.C., Johnson, M.K. Organophosphorus poisoning [Letter]. *British Medical Journal* 1991;**302**:963.

Maxwell, D.M., Lenz, D.E. Structure-activity relationships and anticholinesterase activity. In: *Clinical and Experimental Toxicology of Organophosphates and Carbamates.* Ballantyne, B., Marrs, T.C. eds. Butterworth–Heinemann; Oxford. 1992. p. 47–58.

McDonough, J.H., Smith, R.F., Smith, C.D. Behavioral correlates of soman-induced neuropathology: deficits in DRL acquisition. *Neurobehavioral Toxicology and Teratology* 1986;**8**:179–87.

Metcalfe, D.R., Holmes, J.H. EEG, psychological and neurological alterations in humans with organophosphorus exposure. *Annals of the New York Academy of Sciences* 1969;**160**:357–65.

Millis, R.M., Archer, P.W., Whittaker, J.A., et al. The role of hypoxia in organophosphorus intoxication. *Neurotoxicology* 1988;**9**:273–86.

Misulis, K.E., Clinton, M.E., Dettbarn, W-D., et al. Differences in central and peripheral neural actions between soman and diisopropyl fluorophosphate, organophosphorus inhibitors of AChEs. *Toxicology and Applied Pharmacology* 1987;**89**:391–8.

Mobley, P.L. The cholinesterase inhibitor soman increases inositol triphosphate in rat brain. *Neuropharmacology* 1990;**29**:189–91.

Munro, N.B., Talmaage, S.S., Griffin, G.D., et al. The sources, fate, and toxicity of chemical warfare agent degradation products. *Environmental Health Perspectives* 1999;**107**:933–74.

Murata, K., Araki, S., Yokoyama, K., et al. Asymptomatic sequelae to acute sarin poisoning in the central and autonomic nervous system 6 months after the Tokyo subway attack. *Journal of Neurology* 1997;**244**:601–6.

Nakajima, T., Sasaki, K., Ozawa, H., *et al.* Urinary metabolites of sarin in a patient of the Matsumoto sarin incident. *Archives of Toxicology* 1998;**72**:601–3.

Nakajima, T., Sato, S., Morita, H., *et al.* Sarin poisoning of a rescue team in the Matsumoto sarin incident in Japan. *Occupational and Environmental Medicine* 1997;**54**:697–701.

Naseem, S.M. Effect of organophosphates on dopamine and muscarinic receptor binding in rat brain. *Biochemistry International* 1990;**20**:799–806.

National Academy of Sciences. Possible long-term health effects of short term exposure to chemical agents, Vol 1, anticholinesterases and anticholinergics, Washington DC, National Academy of Sciences. 1982. p. 1–6.

Nohara, M. Segawa, K. Ocular symptoms due to organophosphorus gas (sarin) poisoning in Matsumoto. *British Journal of Ophthalmology* 1996;**80**:1023.

Noort, D., Hulst, A.G., Platenburg, D.H.J.M., *et al.* Quantitative analysis of O-isopropyl methylphosphonic acid in serum samples of Japanese citizens allegedly exposed to sarin: estimation of internal dosage. *Archives of Toxicology* 1998;**72**:671–5.

Nozaki, H., Aikawa, N. Sarin poisoning in Tokyo subway. *Lancet* 1995;**345**:1446–7.

Nozaki, H., Aikawa, N., Fujishima, S., *et al.* A case of VX poisoning and the difference from sarin. *Lancet* 1995;**346**:698–9.

Oak Ridge National Laboratory. Appendices A-D. *Journal of Toxicology and Environmental Health Part A* 2000;**59**:361–469.

O'Leary, T.F., Kunkel, A.M., Jones, A.H. Efficacy and limitations of oxime-atropine treatment of organophosphorus anticholinesterase poisoning. *Journal of Pharmacology and Experimental Therapeutics* 1961;**132**:50–2.

Pazdernik, T.L., Cross, R., Nelson, S. Soman-induced depression of brain activity in TAB-pretreated rats: 2-deoxyglucose study. *Neurotoxicity* 1983;**4**:27–34.

Pearce, P.C., Crofts, H.S., Muggleton, N.G., *et al.* The effects of acutely administered low dose sarin on cognitive behaviour and the electroencephalogram in the common marmoset. *Journal of Psychopharmacology* 1999;**13**:128–35.

Phillippens, I.H., Vanwersh, R.A., Groen, B., *et al.* Subchronic physostigmine pretreatment in marmosets: absence of side effects and effectiveness against soman poisoning with negligible post intoxication incapacitation. *Toxicological Sciences* 2000;**53**:84–91.

Rengstorff, H.H. Accidental exposure to sarin: vision effects. *Archives of Toxicology* 1985;**56**:201–3.

Robinson, J.P. Chemical warfare. *Science Journal* 1967;**3**:33–40.

Rocha, E.S., Santos, M.D., Chechabo, S.R., *et al.* Low concentrations of the organophosphate VX affect spontaneous and evoked transmitter release from hippocampal neurones: toxicological relevance of cholinesterase-independent actions. *Toxicology and Applied Pharmacology* 1999;**159**:31–40.

Schoene, K., Hochrainer, D., Oldiges, H. The protective effect of oxime pretreatment upon the inhalative toxicity of sarin and soman in rats. *Fundamental and Applied Toxicology* 1985;**5**:584–8.

Schoene, K., Oldiges, H. Efficacy of pyridinium salts against tabun and sarin poisoning *in vivo* and *in vitro*. *Archives Internationales de Pharmacodynamie et de Therapie* 1973;**204**:110–23.

Sekijima, Y., Morita, H., Yanagisawa, N. Follow-up of sarin poisoning in Matsumoto. *Annals of Internal Medicine* 1997;**127**:1042.

Sellström, Å. Anticonvulsants in anticholinesterase poisoning. In:. *Clinical and Experimental Toxicology of Organophosphates and Carbamates*. Ballantyne, B., Marrs, T.C. eds Butterworth–Heinemann; Oxford.1992. p 578–86

Senanayake, N., Karalliedde, L. Neurotoxic effects of organophosphorus insecticides. An intermediate Syndrome. *New England Journal of Medicine* 1987;**316**:761–3.

Senanayake, N., Karalliedde, L. The intermediate syndrome in anticholinesterase neurotoxicity. In: *Clinical and Experimental Toxicology of Organophosphates and Carbamates*. Ballantyne, B., Marrs, T.C. eds. Butterworth–Heinemann; 1992. Oxford: p. 126–34.

SERB. Data sheet Contrathion, pralidoxime pralidoxima. Laboratoires SERB, 53 Rue de l'Isle Adam, Paris. 1987

Sharabi, Y., Danon, Y.L., Berkenstadt, H., *et al.* Survey of Symptoms following intake of pyridostigmine during the Persian Gulf War. *Israel Journal of Medical Sciences* 1991;**27**:656–8.

Sidell, F.R. Soman and Sarin: Clinical manifestations and treatment of accidental poisoning by organophosphates. *Clinical Toxicology* 1974;**7**:1–17.

Silveira, C.L.P., Eldefrawi, A.T., Eldefrawi, M.E. Putative M2 muscarinic receptors of rat heart have high affinity for organophosphorus anticholinesterases. *Toxicology and Applied Pharmacology* 1990;**103**:474–81.

Sivam, S.P., Hoskins, B., Ho, I.K. An assessment of comparative acute toxicity of diisopropyl-fluorophosphate, tabun, sarin, and soman in relation to cholinergic and GABAergic enzyme activities in rats. *Fundamental and Applied Toxicology* 1984;**4**:531–8.

Small, M.J. Compounds formed from the chemical decontamination of HD, GB and VX and their environmental fate. Tech Rpt 8304; AD A149515. Fort Detrick, MD; US Army Medical Bioengineering Research and Development Laboratory. 1984

Smallridge, R.C., Carr, F.E., Fein, H.G. Diisopropylfluorophosphate (DFP) reduces serum prolactin, thyrotropin, luteinizing hormone and increases adrenocorticotropin and corticosterone in rats: involvement of dopaminergic and somatostatinergic as well as cholinergic pathways. *Toxicology and Applied Pharmacology* 1991;**108**:284–5.

Valdes ,J.J., Chester, N.A., Menking, D. *et al.* Regional sensitivities of neuroleptic receptors to subacute soman poisoning. *Brain Research Bulletin* 1985:**14**:117–21.

Weinbrown, A.A., Rudick, V., Paret, G. *et al.* Anaesthesia and critical care considerations in nerve agent warfare trauma casualties. *Resuscitation* 2000;**47**:113–23.

WHO. Report of a group of experts. Geneva. World Health Organization 1970.

Wills, J.H. Anticholinergic compounds as adjuncts to atropine in preventing lethality by sarin in the rabbit. *J Med Pharmacol Chem* 1961;**3**:353–9.

Worek, F., Widmann, R., Knopff, O., *et al.* Reactivating potency of obidoxime, pralidoxime, HI 6 and HLö 7 in human erythrocyte AChE inhibited by highly toxic organophosphorus compounds. *Archives of Toxicology* 1998a;**72**:237–43.

Worek, F., Eyer, P., Szinicz, L. Inhibition, reactivation and ageing kinetics of cyclohexylmethylphosphonofluoridate-inhibited human cholinesterases. *Archives of Toxicology* 1998b;**72**:580–7.

Worek, F., Backer, M., Thiermann, H., *et al.* Reappraisal of indications and limitations of oxime therapy in organophosphate poisoning. *Human and Experimental Toxicology* 1997;**16**:466–72.

Young, G.D., Koplovitz, I. Acute toxicity of cyclohexylmethylphosphonofluoridate (CMPF) in rhesus monkeys: serum biochemical and hematologic changes. *Archives of Toxicology* 1995;**69**:379–83.

CHAPTER 5

The Acute Cholinergic Syndrome

Lakshman Karalliedde and John Henry

5.1. Introduction

The acute cholinergic syndrome is responsible for the initial symptoms and signs following acute exposure to OP agents. The clinical picture is attributed mainly to accumulation of acetylcholine (ACh) resulting from inhibition of cholinesterases (ChE) (see Chapter 1). Ingestion is the main route of exposure for the general population and arises from contamination of food and water, usually with trace amounts of insecticide. Ingestion of large volumes of insecticide with suicidal intent is a major cause of acute poisoning particularly in developing countries (Senanayake, 1998; Karalliedde and Senanayake, 1986). Occupational exposure may be by dermal absorption, by inhalation, or by the oral route. Iatrogenic toxicity may also occur. When malathion is used in the treatment of head lice, sufficient dermal absorption may take place to cause toxicity (Opawoye and Haque, 2000). Acute poisoning with OP agents has also been described following subcutaneous (Serrano and Fedriani, 1997), intramuscular (Zoppellari et al., 1997) and intravenous injection (Güven et al., 1997). In recent years acute cholinergic symptoms have followed accidental foodborne poisonings in families (Greenaway and Orr, 1996; Chaudhry et al., 1998).

Inhaled OPs (as vapour, dusts or droplets) are usually absorbed more rapidly than after skin contamination. However, in workers involved in the manufacture of OPs or spraying orchards, transdermal absorption is often the major route of exposure. The blood levels arising from skin contamination in workers at an OP formulation plant and in workers involved in spraying OPs may be 100–400 fold higher than those following inhalation (IPCS, 1986; Health and Safety Executive, 1998). Dermal absorption is greater if solutions contaminate cotton clothing.

During the course of intoxication, the OP compounds enter the circulation and are subsequently transferred to body tissues where they phosphorylate and inhibit the ChEs—neural, red cell, and plasma. Free serum OP compounds are rapidly metabolised by serum and hepatic microsomal enzymes (e.g. P450 enzymes and A-esterases) to less toxic metabolites and excreted in the urine (see Chapter 3).

A-esterases (e.g. paraoxonase) are a group of enzymes which hydrolyse OP esters but are not inhibited by them. In contrast B-esterases (e.g. acetylcholinesterase (AChE)) are inhibited by OP compounds (Mutch *et al.,* 1992).

The severity of the poisoning and time of onset of symptoms depend mainly on the dose of OP agent and the mode of intoxication. Following massive ingestion, symptoms arise within minutes. Death has occurred within 5 minutes of ingestion of concentrated tetra-ethyl pyrophosphate (TEPP). However, in most instances, symptoms appear within 30 minutes of ingestion and almost always in less than 12 h (Karalliedde and Senanayake, 1989). Delayed cholinergic manifestations occur with the fat-soluble OPs, such as fenthion and chlorfenthion and similar compounds requiring metabolic conversion to active agents (e.g. parathion which undergoes hepatic conversion to paraoxon) (Mahieu *et al.,* 1982). In the experimental animal, compounds such as fenitrothion, merphos and mevinphos were found to be more toxic by the dermal route when compared to the oral route (Gaines, 1969). This may reflect the metabolism of the compounds by the gastrointestinal tract.

Accumulation of ACh at different functional sites enables grouping of the symptoms of the acute cholinergic syndrome on a physiological basis.

5.1.1. Muscarinic Effects

The **muscarinic** actions are due to accumulation of the neurotransmitter at nerve terminals of the parasympathetic nervous system. The effects on glands are predominant. Rhinorrhoea, bronchorrhoea, sweating, lachrymation, and salivation produce a clinical scenario of increased secretions. Constriction of the bronchial smooth muscle produces tightness of the chest, wheezing and difficulty in breathing. The combination of bronchoconstriction and increased secretion often leads to severe impairment in oxygenation (hypoxaemia) and patients may present with cyanosis.

In the eye, parasympathomimetic contraction of smooth muscle causes miosis, failure of pupillary accommodation and blurring of vision. A feature of acute intoxication following the Tokyo subway incident was the occurrence of severe pain in the eyes. Excessive activity in the gastro-intestinal and genito-urinary systems give rise to nausea, vomiting, abdominal cramps, diarrhoea, frequency of micturition and urinary incontinence. The muscarinic effect on the heart produces bradycardia and cardiac arrhythmias which can lead to ventricular fibrillation or asystole; these will be aggravated by hypoxaemia.

5.1.2. Nicotinic Effects

The **nicotinic** effects are due to stimulation of the nicotinic receptors at autonomic ganglia, at the neuromuscular junction and the adrenal medulla. The nicotinic features pallor, tachycardia and hypertension are due to stimulation of the autonomic ganglia of the sympathetic nervous system. The overall effect on the heart depends on whether muscarinic or nicotinic effects predominate and thus both bradycardia and tachycardia may be observed, often at different times in the same patient. The nicotinic effects at the neuromuscular junction produce fasciculations and muscle weakness. The fasciculations are frequently observed in the eyelid and oro-facial musculature after systemic absorption.

The accumulation of ACh at the neuromuscular junction may be of sufficient intensity to produce muscle paralysis. Muscle weakness and paralysis of muscles of respiration may occur very early as a result of severe depression of the central nervous system along with cardiovascular depression. The muscle weakness which sets in after fasciculations has been attributed to depolarisation neuromuscular block. The danger with muscle weakness is respiratory failure and death (Karalliedde and Henry, 1993; Karalliedde and Senanayake, 1989).

5.1.3. Central Effects

Central effects are attributed mainly to cholinergic stimulation in the brain. The accumulation of ACh in the central nervous system produces giddiness, anxiety, restlessness, tremor, headache, failure to concentrate, confusion and convulsions. Other symptoms reported are sleep disturbances, slurred speech, emotional lability and excessive dreaming (Wadia et al., 1974). Mild exposure may lead to very subtle central nervous system disturbances such as impaired vigilance and memory, reduced information processing and psychomotor speed, irritability and insomnia (Whorton and Obrinsky, 1983). These subtle disturbances are of importance in warfare and amongst pilots undertaking aerial spraying. Following severe intoxication, depression of the centres of respiration (Stewart and Anderson, 1968) and circulation (e.g. vasomotor centre) may occur causing hypotension, dyspnoea, Cheyne—Stokes respiration and cyanosis.

As OPs are known to vary in their potency to induce seizures, some workers believe that this clinical manifestation may not be entirely related to AChE inhibition.

Unusual CNS clinical features of acute OP poisoning have also been reported. They include extrapyramidal symptoms (Senanayake and Sanmuganathan, 1995) and atypical ocular bobbing (Hata *et al.*, 1986).

An important effect of OPs is to increase the permeability of the blood brain barrier (BBB) which facilitates the access of other chemicals to the brain including oximes. This is considered to have important therapeutic implications (Firemark *et al.*, 1964). In 10-day-old rats, Gupta *et al.*, (1999) observed that repeated exposure (over 8 days) to the OP quinalphos increased the permeability of the blood brain barrier by approximately 130% which lasted up to 13 days after the exposure. They also observed that a single dose exposure to $1/100^{th}$ of the LD 50 caused changes. This raises the possibility that the developing BBB could be highly vulnerable to single or repeated low doses of OP pesticides.

Electroencephalographic (EEG) abnormalities can be detected at the onset of symptoms and are characterised by irregularities in rhythm, variation and increase in potential and intermittent bursts of abnormally slow waves of elevated voltage similar to those seen in epilepsy.

Exposure levels that are toxic but too low to threaten life are usually accompanied by marked desynchronisation of the EEG, and a triad of changes, consisting of increased high frequency activity, decreased low frequency activity and lowered back-ground voltage (Burchfiel and Duffy, 1982). At higher dose levels, OPs cause slowing of the EEG followed by the development of spike wave discharges which accompany clinical convulsions (Burchfiel and Duffy, 1982). There is some evidence that long-term EEG sequelae may follow a single exposure to OP (Duffy *et al.*, 1979; Vale, 1999), but the significance of these changes remains unclear. However, a follow-up of 100 patients with previously documented acute OP poisoning in Colorado and Texas revealed no significant abnormalities on EEG when compared to an unexposed group (Savage *et al.*, 1988).

The CNS pathology after severe acute OP poisoning in humans or animals is non-specific, although the vascular damage commonly seen is attributed to increased permeability of the vessel walls. Other histopathological features have been related either to seizure activity and/or to hypoxia. Yilmazlar and Ozyurt (1997) observed perfusion defects especially in the parietal lobe in patients during the first week after OP poisoning.

Approximately 90% of 37 patients showed abnormal CT scans when performed between 3rd and 10th day following poisoning with OPs (Pach *et al.*, 1997). Some of the common changes were generalised atrophy of the cortex and sub-cortex and areas of low density in the sub-cortical nuclei.

The severity of the abnormality was related to severity of poisoning and changes were more frequent among older patients.

They suggested that AChE also has a neuromodulatory role in the nervous system, involved in inducing long-term changes in synaptic efficacy. The delayed effects of poisoning were attributed to the loss of this non-enzymatic neuromodulatory role.

5.2. Acute Cholinergic Syndrome and Cardiovascular Effects

The ECG may display a variety of abnormalities in acute OP poisoning (See Chapter 10). Classically a phase of intense sympathetic activity causing sinus tachycardia is followed by a phase of increased parasympathetic activity causing sinus bradycardia, atrioventricular block and ST segment and T wave abnormalities (Chuang et al., 1996). Kiss and Fazekas (1979) reported QT prolongation, S-T segment and T wave abnormalities with a variety of arrhythmias in 56 out of 134 patients. Repetitive ventricular tachycardia with 'torsade des pointes' phenomenon was seen in 7 patients. The tachycardia was initiated by a ventricular ectopic beat with a 'R-on-T' phenomenon. In this series, the greatest number of fatal cardiac arrhythmias were observed some days after OP exposure, when the patient's toxic clinical symptoms and signs were moderate or had resolved completely.

Luzhnikov et al. (1975) reported arrhythmias and conduction abnormalities in 18.5% of patients poisoned by OP agents whilst Ludomirsky et al. (1982) observed that 'torsade des pointes' occurred in those patients who had a prolongation of QTc greater than 0.58 s. In a retrospective study of 223 patients (Chuang et al., 1996), the ECG showed normal sinus rhythm in 50%, sinus tachycardia in 44.7%, sinus bradycardia in 3.1% and sinus arrhythmia in 0.9% of the patients. Saadeh et al. (1997) found that cardiac complications developed in 67% of patients after OP and/or carbamate poisoning.

5.3. Acute Cholinergic Syndrome and Muscle Dysfunction

The cardinal features associated with muscle are fasciculations and weakness. Fasciculations may be localised in instances where exposure has been limited to a limb or the face.

Fasciculations are considered to be due to stimulation of the presynaptic nicotinic receptors at the neuromuscular junction (Bowman *et al.*, 1986) with subsequent antidromic impulse transmission and excitation of the whole motor unit.

Electrophysiological abnormalities following OP poisoning were described by Besser *et al.* (1998a).

They were:

1. Repetitive firing following a single evoked compound muscle action potential (CMAP)
2. The decrement and decrement-increment phenomenon of the CMAP in response to repetitive nerve stimulation.

5.4. Acute Cholinergic Syndrome and Effects on Metabolism, Endocrine Function and Temperature

In a series of 104 patients studied in Rhodesia (Hayes *et al.*, 1978), 25 were febrile without evidence of infection and 48 had neutrophil leucocytosis. The blood sugar was moderately raised in 7: all showed glycosuria but ketones were absent from the urine. Low-grade fever, not related to infection was also observed in 49% of patients with OP and carbamate poisoning in Jordan (Saadeh *et al.*, 1996). Hirshberg and Lerman (1984) found fever to be a clinical problem for more than 24 h after anti-AChE exposure in 25% of the total cases.

Gordon and Rowsey (1999) suggested that mechanisms other than those involving interleukin-6 and tumour necrosis factor may be involved in OP induced fever.

In a recent case report from France (Nisse *et al.*, 1998), a blood sugar of 7.9 mmol/l and a leucocytosis of $19,100/mm^3$ was observed on admission, 30 minutes after ingestion of parathion. Kin Sang Hui (1983) from Houston reported two cases of lethal OP insecticide poisoning with diazinon where the patients had severe hyperglycaemia and severe metabolic acidosis associated with moderate hypokalaemia (serum K^+ of 2.6 MEQ/l and 2.7 MEQ/l) when first seen. These patients also had low serum magnesium levels of (0.6–0.7 mmol/l). Changes in blood glucose levels in persons occupationally exposed to OP pesticides were also reported by Owczarzy *et al.* (1982).

5.5. Changes in Hormones and Enzymes

In a prospective study of 22 patients in Turkey, Güven *et al.* (1999) observed significantly higher levels of ACTH, cortisol and prolactin during OP poisoning than after resolution of poisoning. This may have represented a pharmacological effect of OP but may also have reflected the stress of acute illness. FSH levels were significantly lower during poisoning. Sick euthyroid syndrome was detected in 7 patients.

5.6. Acute Cholinergic Phase and Pancreatitis

Following the first case of acute pancreatitis reported by Dressel *et al.* in 1979, Dagli and Shaikh (1983) reported a large series of cases of OP induced "acute pancreatitis", concluding that mild and transient pancreatitis frequently (incidence of 47% with malathion poisoning) occurred in OP poisonings. In a study of 159 patient records from Taiwan (Wui Chiang Lee *et al.*, 1998), hyperamylasemia was found in 44 of 121 patients but they considered serum lipase estimations to be a more reliable indicator of pancreatic dysfunction after OP poisoning. Elevation of serum amylase on the day of admission was predictive of subsequent respiratory failure (Matsumiya *et al.*, 1996). Persistent pancreatic involvement in malathion poisoning was recently described by Cordoba Lopez *et al.* (1999).

OPs are considered to produce a 100-fold increase in sensitivity of the human pancreas to ACh (Kandalaft *et al.*, 1991).

5.7. Other Effects of OPs which may Contribute to the Acute Cholinergic Syndrome

1. Effects on GABA, glutamate (see chapter 12) and serotonin systems. Single doses of an OP increased the number of dopamine and GABA receptors shortly after exposure (Sivam *et al.*, 1983). Leptophos affected the GABA regulated chloride channels (Gant *et al.*, 1987) and changes in the serotonergic system have been attributed to OPs (Fernando *et al.*, 1984).
2. Effects on mitochondrial enzymes. OP compounds inhibit mitochondrial enzymes, respiration and ATP generation, in addition to inducing structural changes such as matrix swelling (Carlson and Ehrich, 1999).

3. Effects on muscarinic receptors M2 and or M4. Paraoxon, malaoxon, and chlorpyrifos oxon were shown to affect second messenger systems coupled to M2 and M4 receptors (Ward and Mundy, 1996).

4. Effects on mast cells and autacoid release. Cowan *et al.* (1996) considered the possibility that the accumulation of ACh may not be the sole mechanism of OP toxicity. Soman, for example may act as a secretagogue by inducing mast cell degranulation with associated autacoid release and anaphylactoid reactions. They considered the possibility of anaphylactoid shock producing a lethal syndrome with symptoms of respiratory failure and circulatory collapse similar to the physiological sequelae observed for OP poisoning. Further, they stated that ACh can act as an agonist of autacoid release and of autacoids such as histamine augmenting soman-induced bronchospasm. Xiong and Rodgers (1997) revealed that malathion metabolites can cause rapid release of histamine from basophilic cells from a variety of origins and species.

5. Effects on nitric oxide release. Rao *et al.* (1999) observed that OP agents like malathion inhibited nitric oxide activity in the rat brain and calmodulin stimulated nitric oxide activity.

6. Interference with surface tension lowering substances, inhibition of phospholipase A2 (Bergler *et al.*, 1995; Petroianu *et al.*, 1997). The OPs were found to have a low potency for inhibition of blood clotting factors and digestive enzymes (Quistad and Casida, 2000).

7. The contribution, if any, of the reported effects on the immune system (Newcombe ,1992) to the acute cholinergic syndrome is uncertain at present.

5.8. Poisoning in Children

Presenting signs and symptoms may differ in children. Sofer *et al.* (1989) studying 25 infants and children aged three months to seven years found that the presenting signs and symptoms were mainly related to the CNS. Decreased level of consciousness including deep unresponsive coma (15 cases) and stupor (9 cases) were the most common presenting signs. In six patients coma and stupor followed an episode of generalised seizure. Fasciculations and bradycardia were uncommon on arrival to the hospital. Only 76% exhibited the classical non-reactive pupils while in four, the pupils were dilated on admission. Eventually the pupils constricted to pin point size in all patients during the first 12 hours. Sweaty cold skin was present in 52% while 10 children had warm dry skin.

Bradycardia (pulse rate 60–100 per minute) was noted on arrival in four children, while all others had either a normal heart rate or tachycardia (up to 205 beats per minute). Thirteen children had only gastro-intestinal disturbances including diarrhoea, vomiting, acute gastric dilatation and haematemesis. Hyperglycaemia was recorded in 14 (56%).

A study of 16 children intoxicated with OP (age 2–8 years) (Lifshitz *et al.*, 1999) confirmed the predominance of symptoms related to the CNS. Tear production and diaphoresis were notably absent. However, pulmonary oedema developed in 6 of these patients.

A low frequency of fasciculations following OP poisoning in children was also reported by Zwiener and Ginsburg (1988) [See chapter 9]. Nearly 25% presented with generalised tonic-clonic seizures which contrasted with the reported incidence of seizures of approximately 2.5% in adults (Hayes *et al.*, 1978; Jamil *et al.*, 1977). Zavon (1974) listed abdominal cramps, headaches, dyspnoea and weakness as the most common symptoms of intoxication in children. However, it was commented that these symptoms could not be relied upon in the very young.

Virtually all poisonings in children occurred in the home and 70% were due to ingestion of an improperly stored compound (Zwiener and Ginsburg, 1988). Following the use of OP agents to eradicate household pests (spraying, fogging), symptoms may develop within 36 h of exposure in some children. These intoxications were probably due to transdermal absorption from contaminated carpets and linen.

5.9. Duration and Outcome of Acute Cholinergic Syndrome

The muscarinic, nicotinic and central nervous system symptoms may occur in varying combinations. Most of the symptoms and clinical signs of the acute cholinergic syndrome are potentially reversible. The cholinergic syndrome usually lasts 24–48 hours and constitutes a medical emergency that requires treatment in an intensive care unit (Namba *et al.*, 1971; Hayes and Laws, 1991; Karalliedde and Senanayake, 1989).

Death during the acute cholinergic phase is due to severe bradycardia, other arrhythmias and/or respiratory depression of either central and/or peripheral origin (Wright, 1954).

A report by Mahieu *et al.* (1982) illustrates the different clinical signs and in particular the delayed and prolonged symptomatology that may occur.

After ingestion of about 30 ml of Lebaycid (equivalent to 18g fenthion), a 43-year-old man developed nausea and biliary vomiting after 20 minutes. This was followed by abundant fluid diarrhoea which persisted for about 12 h. About 22 h after ingestion atrial tachycardia, sporadic ventricular extra-systoles, hypertension (220/110 mm Hg), persistent nausea and vomiting together with sialorrhoea and bronchorrhoea were noted. The patient was still conscious and neither miosis nor fasciculations were noted. About 31 h after ingestion, generalised fasciculations and marked tracheo-bronchorrhoea associated with bronchospasm developed. These features were probably linked to the formation of active metabolites.

5.10. Mortality from OP Poisoning

A wide range of mortality figures have appeared in the literature related to adult poisoning. Virtually all of these refer to suicidal ingestion. The geographical, economic (health facilities) and cultural backgrounds of these reports vary. A uniform or accepted scale to indicate severity of poisoning has not been used. The composition of the compounds ingested (presence of impurities, solvents etc) were not always recorded. Thus comparisons are not possible. An overview is presented in Table 5.1.

5.11. Diagnosis

The diagnosis of the cholinergic syndrome in most instances is based on clinical features. Miosis in combination with fasciculations is pathognomonic of acute OP intoxication, particularly in adults. Lachrymation, salivation, bronchorrhoea and excessive sweating along with bradycardia provide supportive evidence. The OP agents possess a characteristic pungent garlic like odour which is easily recognised by clinicians in developing countries. This odour when present in the breath, vomitus or clothing is often the main diagnostic tool in these countries where in the majority of instances the agent implicated in poisoning is not known with certainty (Karalliedde, 2000).

When available, ChE assays are useful in diagnosis, evaluating the clinical course and assessing the response to oximes (Mutch et al., 1992). Inhibition of RBC AChE and butyrylcholinesterase (BuChE) may occur to differing degrees with different OPs (See appendix).

Table 5.1. Overview of the range of mortality figures related to adult poisoning

Author	Year	Number of patients	Mortality	OP agents
Surjit Singh	1980–1989		12%	
Luzhnikov *et al.*	1975	182	16%	
Hayes *et al.*	1978	105	15%	
Kiss and Fazekas	1979	168	30%	
Finkelstein	1981–1986	81	26%	
Ludomirsky	1982	15	20%	
Satoh and Hosokawa	1985–87		11.5%	
Bardin *et al.*	1987	61	16%	
Karalliedde and Senanayake	1988	92	18%	dimethoate methamidophos monocrotophos fenthion
Surjit Singh	1990	623	11%	
De Silva *et al.*	1992	45	28–29%	malathion methamidophos fenthion
Yilmazlar and Ozyurt	1992	15	17%	
Cunha *et al.*	1995	52	28.9%	
Chuang *et al.*	1996		19.6%	in patients with QTc prolongation
Chuang *et al.*	1996		4.8%	no QTc prolongation
Saadeh *et al.*	1997	46	4%	
Yamashita *et al.*	1997	130	25%	

Familiarity with OP toxicity facilitates diagnosis and assessment of severity. Following diagnosis, grading of disease severity may identify patients with serious poisoning who should receive treatment in intensive care (Bardin *et al.,* 1990). A recent report from Australia (Hollis, 1999) highlights the problems associated with diagnosis in situations where the occurrence of acute poisoning is rare.

5.12. Severity Grading of the Acute Cholinergic Phase

A clinical scale selecting five common parameters (miosis, fasciculations, respiratory depression, bradycardia and level of consciousness) validated using two consecutive series of 173 patients with OP poisoning was developed in Sri Lanka (Senanayake *et al.,* 1993).

Goswamy *et al.* (1994) used a scoring system, on a point scale of 16 using miosis, unconsciousness, fasciculations and plasma cholinesterase levels to predict ventilatory requirements.

Poison Severity Score (PSS) (Persson *et al.,* 1998) modified for OP poisoning was developed by clinicians with the International Programme on Chemical Safety in 1999 in Sao Paulo, Brazil (Haines, Personal Communication, 1999).

Bardin *et al.* (1987) retrospectively classified and graded patients on a scale of 0–3 on the basis of the initial clinical findings, blood gas values and chest radiographs, in an attempt to identify high risk patients. Patients with grade 3 intoxication (attempted suicide, stupor, PaO2 < 10kPa and an abnormal chest radiograph—two more factors present) were more likely to require ventilatory support and stayed in the Intensive Care Unit longer. The classification was further studied in 1990 (Bardin *et al.,* 1990).

5.13. Measurement of Cholinesterase Activity

ChE assays are particularly useful if pre-exposure values are known. Caution is necessary in interpreting the results as there is no uniformly accepted standard technique, and each method has its own 'normal range'. In acute poisoning, mild exposure may cause a reduction of activity to 50% of normal of BuChE, moderate exposure causing a further reduction to 20%, while severe poisoning produces values of 10% or less.

However, Bardin *et al.* (1987) who measured BuChE serially in all of their 61 consecutive patients found that estimations were not of value in predicting severity of poisoning. They considered that RBC AChE estimations were a better index of clinical poisoning and a value of 30% of normal correlated with clinical recovery with little danger of relapse. However, Cunha *et al.* (1995), following a retrospective survey of severe OP poisoning observed that BuChE recovery to above 10% of the normal value seemed to correlate with good prognosis.

BuChE measurements are more convenient because of lower cost and wider availability. However, the correlation with RBC AChE is not consistent and permanent. The measurement of RBC AChE is a more reliable manner of estimating severity of intoxication (Taitelman, 1999).

The relationship between in vivo OP toxicity and brain AChE inhibition is influenced by many factors. In general, 50–80% of nervous system AChE must be inactivated before symptoms are noted. Brain AChE activity around 10–15% of normal is associated with severe toxicity and below 10% with respiratory failure and death (Lotti, 1999). Lethal exposures in the absence of treatment have been estimated to correspond to approximately 30 to 50 times the minimal symptomatic exposure.

5.14. Recovery of Cholinesterases

The half-life of recovery of inhibited AChE in the nervous system is about 1 week in experimental animals and is believed to be the same in man (Lotti, 1999).

In an untreated patient, BuChE activity takes approximately 4–6 weeks to return to pre-exposure levels whereas RBC AChE requires 5–7 weeks. BuChE activity increases by 25–30% within the first 7–10 days which is then followed by a gradual increase. RBC AChE changes by approximately 1% per day as red cells do not have the ability to synthesise AChE and the return of levels of AChE to normal depends on formation of new red cells (Hayes and Laws, 1991; Namba *et al.*, 1971).

5.15. Measurement of Metabolites of OP in the Urine, OP Levels in the Blood

The distribution of OPs is variable. Blood half-lives are usually short, although plasma levels are, in some cases maintained for several days.

Because of the lipophilicity, high chemical reactivity and large apparent volume of distribution, it is particularly important for the clinician to appreciate that plasma levels represent a minute fraction of body burden. Further the clearance from body compartments vary substantially amongst OPs, and redistribution does occur (Lotti, 1999). Vasilic *et al.* (1999) observed that following malathion poisoning, the parent compound was detectable in the serum for only one day after poisoning.

Urinary excretion of metabolites can be used as a biomarker of exposure (COT, 1999). Most reliable data are derived from the analysis of 24 h urine collection made prior to (in workers) and after exposure. About 70% of an oral dose of 0.5 mg/kg of chlorpyrifos given to humans was recovered as metabolites in the urine within 6–7 days of dosing and this was accompanied by significant lowering of RBC AChE (Nolan *et al.*, 1984). Dermal application of a similar dose resulted in between 1–2% appearing in the urine as metabolites. The apparent elimination half-life of urinary dialkylphosphates after oral dosing of chlorpyrifos to human volunteers was 15.5 hours and after dermal dosing, the half-life was 30 hours (Griffin *et al.*, 1999). They suggested that the best time to collect urine samples for biological monitoring after dermal exposure was before the work shift the next day. Further, in their experiment, the amounts of chlorpyrifos used did not depress AChE activity but could be readily detected as urinary dialkylphosphate metabolites, indicating that the urinary assay is a more sensitive indicator of exposure. Drevenkar *et al.*, (1991) confirmed that dialkylphosphorus metabolites in the urine are a more sensitive index of absorption than cholinesterase inhibition in the serum. They suggested that both parameters should be measured because of the lack of correlation between cholinesterase inhibition and urinary metabolite concentrations. It is of interest that Richter *et al.* (1992) reported the finding of a metabolite of diazinon in the urine of symptomatic patients who resided in household which had been sprayed four and half months earlier.

Different OP compounds may produce the same metabolite (e.g. parathion-methyl and fenitrothion), thus limiting the scope of identification of an OP compound by urine analysis.

The measurement of sarin metabolites (methylphosphonic acid and isopropylmethylphosphonic acid) detected by gas chromatography after conversion to volatile derivatives was found to be a useful tool for the biological monitoring of exposure to sarin (Nakajima *et al.*, 1998). See also Chapter 15.

5.16. Carboxylesterase Levels

Carboxylesterase (CaE) is an esterase found in many mammalian tissues such as the lung, liver, kidney, brain, muscle and gonads usually as a microsomal enzyme. CaE does not react with positively charged carboxylesters such as ACh and BuChE but is involved in the metabolism of OP agents. The enzyme has broad substrate specificity and exists as several isoenzymes which creates difficulties in comparing observations obtained in different laboratories. A variety of OP compounds have been found to inhibit CaE at concentrations of 1 to 100 nM. Plasma or brain CaE activity recovers to normal levels within 24–48 h after inhibition by a single dose of sarin, soman or tabun. Clement (1989) found that the return of soman mediated lethal dose to control values occurred in the same time frame as the recovery of serum CaE activity. This correlation between the recovery of enzyme activity for CaE and soman LD 50 values contrasted with the lack of correlation observed with recovery of AChE activity which remained extensively inhibited in brain, diaphragm and erythrocytes. This work suggested that CaE activity is a better criterion of recovery from OP toxicity than is AChE activity. Lassiter *et al.* (1999) observed that foetal liver CaE inhibition was an extremely sensitive indicator of foetal chlorpyrifos exposure. Possibly serial measurements of CaE may prove to be useful in diagnosis and assessing recovery from OP intoxication.

5.17. Plasma beta-G Levels

Egasyn is an accessory protein of beta-glucuronidase (beta-G) in the liver microsomes. The egasyn-beta-glucuronidase (EG) complex was easily dissociated by administration of OPs (e.g. fenitrothion, EPN, phenthionate, bis-beta-nitrophenyl phosphate) and the resulting beta-G dissociated was released in to blood, leading to a rapid and transient increase of plasma beta-G levels with a concomitant decrease of liver microsomal beta-G level. Satoh *et al.* (1999) concluded that increase of the plasma beta-G level after OP administration is a much more sensitive biomarker than cholinesterase inhibition to acute intoxication of OPs and carbamates.

5.18. Precautions during the Acute Cholinergic Syndrome

If endotracheal intubation or general anaesthesia is required during the acute cholinergic syndrome (Karalliedde, 1999), the muscle relaxants suxamethonium and mivacurium should not be used. Further, other medications metabolised by BuChE such as esmolol and procaine should be used with caution during the cholinergic phase.

It should be noted that benzoylcholine, heroin, amethocaine and methyl prednisolone acetate too are hydrolysed by BuChE (Williams, 1985).

5.19. Sequelae of the Acute Cholinergic Syndrome

1. **Complete recovery**
2. **Death due to respiratory and/or cardiac failure**
3. **Development of the intermediate syndrome.** See Chapter 6.
4. **Development of weakness of external ocular muscles.** Tripathi and Misra (1996).
5. **Acute cholinergic phase and the neuroleptic malignant syndrome:** Ochi *et al.* (1995) reported a 60-year-old woman with schizophrenia who manifested a neuroleptic malignant-like syndrome 13 days after acute OP poisoning.
6. **Development of the delayed polyneuropathy.** (See Chapter 7). Senanayake and Karalliedde in 1987 first reported a patient who developed the cholinergic phase followed by the intermediate syndrome and later by the delayed polyneuropathy. Following methamidophos poisoning De Haro *et al.* (1999) described a similar sequence in two patients.
7. **Development of extrapyramidal manifestations: Ataxia, dystonia, rest tremor, cog-wheel rigidity, choreoathetoid movements and reversible parkinsonism.** Michotte *et al.*, (1989); Senanayake and Sanmuganathan (1995); Hsieh *et al.*, (2000); Bhatt *et al.*, (1999); Muller-Vahl *et al.*, (1999)
8. **Development of isolated recurrent laryngeal nerve palsy and vocal cord paralysis.** De Siva *et al.*, (1994); Thompson and Stocks, (1997); Aiuto *et al.*, (1993); Indhudharan, (1998a;1998b).
9. **Development of neuropsychological and behavioural effects.** (Vale, 1999). See Chapter 8.
10. **Transient diabetes insipidus:** Sidhu and Collis, (1989); Abdul-Gaffar, (1997)

5.20. Effects on Reproductive Function

a   OP poisoning during pregnancy causes pre- and postnatal death and congenital abnormalities such as vertebral deformities, limb defects, polydactyly, intestinal herniae, cleft palate and hydroureter, in experimental animals (Hayes, 1982).

b   Changes in testes, sperms and epididymis. (Contreras and Boustos–Obregon, 1996;1999; Contreras et al., 1999).

c   Increased LH levels, slightly elevated FSH levels and decreased serum testosterone levels (Padungtod et al., 1998).

d   Prevalence of sperm aneuploidy (Padungtod et al., 1999).

Other effects reported in the literature:
Reduced bone formation (Compston et al., 1999).
Ototoxicity (Ernest et al., 1995), **sphincteric involvement** (Patial et al., 1987), **Guillain—Barré like syndrome** (Adlakha et al., 1987), **Contact dermatitis** (Haenen et al., 1996), **haemorrhagic panoesophagitis** Koga et al., (1999), **renal tubular cytotoxicity** Poovala et al., (1999)

5.21. Conclusion

The acute cholinergic syndrome is a medical emergency which necessitates management in an intensive care unit. Prompt resuscitation, maintenance of vital functions, close monitoring and aggressive treatment are necessary to prevent death. The clinical presentation is varied and differs in adults and in children. Diagnosis is often clinical but serial measurements of cholinesterase activity are extremely useful in assessing severity, clinical course and treatment. Many sequelae of the acute cholinergic syndrome have been reported and it is necessary to monitor patients closely following recovery. Though most of the signs and symptoms of the acute cholinergic syndrome have been attributed to inactivation of cholinesterases, it is very likely that other hormonal and neurotransmitter disorders may contribute to the clinical scenario in a manner yet to be determined. Further knowledge of the pathogenesis of this syndrome would enable the use of more rational therapeutic procedures.

Appendix

Cholinesterase Assays in the Diagnosis of OP Intoxication.

It is useful to recall the observations of Ladell (Maynard, 1989) when interpreting the results of cholinesterase assays. He stated that:

1. The percentage depression of enzyme activity would be the same at all sites and in all tissues within the body—blood, brain, autonomic ganglia, muscles and glands if the relative concentration of cholinesterase to inhibitor was the same everywhere after poisoning which requires rapid penetration to all sites of cholinergic transmission.

2. The degree of dysfunction in a cholinergic junction is not linearly dependent upon the amount of cholinesterase present. There are considerable reserves of the enzyme at all sites and the amount required for efficient functioning is small in comparison with the total amount available. A considerable amount of inhibition can therefore take place before there is any disturbance of physiological function. Thus it is apparent that there could be no direct association between the symptomatology in anticholinesterase poisoning and the extent to which the ChE is inhibited in the blood.

As the AChE present in human erythrocytes (RBC) is the same as the enzyme present in target synapses, levels of RBC AChE are assumed to mirror the effects in the target organs.

The sensitivities of RBC AChE and plasma ChE (BuChE) to OP inhibitors differ. The plasma enzyme is inhibited preferentially by OP insecticides such as chlorpyrifos, demeton, diazinon, malathion and mipafox whilst the RBC enzyme is inhibited more by dimefox, merinphos, parathion and parathion-methyl (WHO, 1986) See chapter 15.

When reviewing results of plasma cholinesterase (BuChE) assay it is also necessary to consider the following: Also see Chapter 15.

1. The coefficient of variation for BuChE activity in samples from an individual is 8–11% (Brock, 1991).

2. BuChE activity is known to vary with age, sex and other parameters such as plasma lipids or lipoprotein fractions.

3. Males have higher BuChE activity than females—at least until the later decades of life.

4. During the first trimester of pregnancy, BuChE activity decreases to 70–80% of the pre-pregnancy level and this decrease in activity is maintained until 2–4 days after delivery. However, Garcia-Lopez and Monteoliva (1988) determining cholinesterase activity in human erythrocytes by the 'pH-stat' method in 1903 samples observed that higher AChE activity was obtained for pregnant women as compared with non-pregnant women.

5. The BuChE activity in the newborn is about 50–60% of that in healthy adults. At the age of 3–4 years the activity has increased to approximately 30% higher than the activity in young adults and activity falls to adult levels at puberty. Garcia-Lopez and Monteoliva (1988) observed significant age-related differences in AChE activity at a 99% confidence level in both men and women and that there are no significant differences in AChE activity in subjects > 10y of age.

6. In 50–75% of patients with prolonged liver disease, a substantial reduction of BuChE activity often to 50 or 25% of the initial level is seen.

7. Low levels of BuChE (30–35% of normal) may be seen in renal disease.

8. Patients with malignant tumours tend to have low BuChE activity (60–65% of normal).

9. BuChE activity falls to 20% of normal values after burns and low levels may persist for months after the trauma.

10. Low BuChE activities have been reported in patients with Crohn's disease, Dengue fever, myxoedema and tuberculosis.

11. A wide range of medications have been reported to affect BuChE levels— approximate reductions within parentheses e.g. quinidine (60–80%), corticosteroids (50%), contraceptive pill (20–30%), bambuterol (40–100%), metoclopramide (minor), cyclophosphamide (35–70%), pancuronium, vecuronium (5–15%).

12. BuChE is usually elevated in some hyperlipidaemic states and reduced in conditions where there is an acute phase response (Crook et al., 1994).

13. Malnutrition: Subjects from poor communities in Chiapas Mexico had reduced RBC AChE levels (Tinoco–Ojanguren and Halperin, 1986).
Protein and calorie malnutrition: associated with low ChE levels in mice (Cahill-Morasco et al., 1998). Subjects with protein energy malnutrition (PEM) had significantly lower values for ChE (Kumari et al., 1993).

14. Reduced RBC AChE levels in newborn and in patients with leukaemia and multiple myeloma (Wills, 1972).

15. Elevated RBC AChE levels when increased reticulocytes and young erythrocytes are present in the blood (e.g. thalassaemia major, hereditary spherocytosis) and following anti-malarial treatment.
16. Physical exercise increased total cholinesterase and BuChE levels in blood and diaphragm (Ryhanen *et al.*, 1988).
17. Houeto *et al.* (1999) reported significantly lower levels of RBC AChE in victims of residential fires.

References

Abdul–Ghaffar, N.U., Transient diabetes insipidus complicating severe suicidal malathion poisoning. *Journal of Toxicology Clinical Toxicology* 1997;**35**:221–3.

Adlakha, A., Philip, P.J., Dhar, K.L. Guillain–Barré Syndrome as a sequela of organophosphorus poisoning. *Journal of the Association of Physicians India* 1987;**35**:665–6.

Aiuto, L.A., Pavlakis, G.S., Boxer, RA. Life-threatening organophosphate-induced delayed polyneuropathy in a child after accidental chlorpyrifos ingestion. *Journal of Pediatrics* 1993;**122**:658–60.

Akbarsha, M.A., Sivasamy, P. Male reproductive toxicity of phosphamidon: histopathological changes in epididymis. *Indian Journal of Experimental Biology* 1998;**36**:34–8.

Bardin, P.G., Van Eeden, S.F., Joubert, J.R. Intensive care management of acute organophosphate poisoning. A 7 year experience in the western Cape. *South African Medical Journal* 1987;**72**:593–7.

Bardin, P.G., van Eeden, S.F. Organophosphate poisoning: grading the severity and comparing treatment between atropine and glycopyrrolate. *Critical Care Medicine* 1990;**18**:956–60.

Bergler, W., Juncker, C., Petroianu, G., *et al.* The influence of an insecticide on the function of the Eustachian tube. *Acta Otolaryngologica (Stockh)* 1995;**115**:528–31.

Besser, R., Gutmann, L., Dillmann, U., *et al.* End plate dysfunction in acute organophosphate intoxication. *Neurology* 1989;**39**:561–7.

Bhatt, M.H., Elias, M.A., Mankodi, A.K. Acute and reversible parkinsonism due to organophosphate pesticide intoxication: five cases. *Neurology* 1999;**52**:1467–71.

Bobba, R., Venkataraman, B.V., Pais, P. *et al.* Correlation between the severity of symptoms in organophosphorus poisoning and cholinesterase activity (RBC and plasma) in humans. *Indian Journal of Physiology and Pharmacology* 1996;**40**:249–52.

Bowman, W.C., Gibb, A.J., Harvey, A.L., *et al.* Prejunctional actions of cholinoreceptor agonists and antagonists and of anticholinesterase drugs. In: *New Neuromuscular Blocking Agents (Handbook of Experimental Pharmacology,* vol 79). Kharkevich, D.R. ed. Springer-Verlag; Berlin. 1986. p. 143–70.

Brock, A. Inter and intra-individual variations in plasma cholinesterase activity and substance concentration in employees of an organophosphorus insecticide factory. *British Journal of Industrial Medicine* 1991:**48**;562–7.

Burchfiel, J.L., Duffy, F.H. Organophosphate neurotoxicity: chronic effects of sarin on the electroencephalogram of monkey and man. *Neurobehavioural Toxicology Teratology* 1982:**4**:767–78.

Cahill-Morasco, R., Hoffman, R.S., Goldfrank, L.R. The effects of nutrition on plasma cholinesterase activity and cocaine toxicity in mice. *Journal of Toxicology Clinical Toxicology* 1998;**36**:667–72.

Carlson K, Ehrich M. Organophosphorus compound-induced modification of SH-SY5Y human neuroblastoma mitochondrial transmembrane potential. *Toxicology and Applied Pharmacology* 1999:**160**:33-42.

Chaudhry, R., Lall, S.B., Mishra, B. *et al.* A foodborne outbreak of organophosphate poisoning. *British Medical Journal* 1998;**317**:268–9

Chuang, F-R., Jang, S-W., Lin, J-A., *et al.* QTc prolongation indicates a poor prognosis in patients with organophosphate poisoning. *American Journal of Emergency Medicine* 1996;**14**:451–3.

Clement, J.G. Survivors of soman poisoning: recovery of the soman LD50 to control value in the presence of extensive acetylcholinesterase inhibition. *Archives of Toxicology* 1989;**63**:150-4.

Compston, J.E., Vedi, S., Stephen, A.B., *et al.* Reduced bone formation after exposure to organophosphates. *Lancet* 1999;**354**:1791–2.

Contreras, H.R., Badilla, J., Bustos-Obregon, E. Morphological disturbances of human sperm after incubation with organophosphate pesticides. *Biocell* 1999;**23**:135–41

Contreras, H.R., Bustos-Obregon, E. Effect of an organophosphorate insecticide on the testis, epididymis and preimplantational development and pregnancy outcome in mice. *International Journal of Developmental Biology* 1996;(**Suppl 1**):207 S.

Contreras, H.R., Bustos–Obregon, E. Morphological alterations in mouse testis by a single dose of malathion. *Journal of Experimental Zoology* 1999;**284**:355–9.

Cook, D.R., Stiller, R.L., Weakly, J.N., *et al.* In vitro metabolism of mivacurium chloride (BW B 1090U) and succinyl choline. *Anesthesia and Analgesia* 1989;**68**:452–6.

Cordoba Lopez, A., Bueno Alvarez–Arenas, M.I., Alzugaray Fraga, R.J., *et al.* Persistent pancreatic involvement in malathion poisoning (Spanish). *Medicina Clinica* 1999;**112**:78–9.

COT. Committee on Toxicity Report. *Organophosphates.* The Stationary Office, London. 1999.

Cowan, F.M., Shih, T.M., Lenz, D.E., *et al.* Hypothesis for synergistic toxicity of organophosphorus poisoning-induced cholinergic crisis and anaphylactoid reactions. *Journal of Applied Toxicology,* 1996;**16**:25–33.

Cunha, J., Povoa, P., Mourao, L., *et al.* Severe poisoning by organophosphate compounds. An analysis of mortality and of the value of serum cholinesterase in monitoring the clinical course. (Portuguese). *Acta Medica Portuguesa* 1995;**8**:469–75.

Dagli, A.J., Shaikh, W.A. Pancreatic involvement in malathion-anticholinesterase insecticide intoxication. A study of 75 cases. *British Journal of Clinical Practice* 1983;**37**:270–2.

De Haro, L., Arditti, J., David, J.M., *et al.* Methamidophos intoxication: immediate and late neurological toxicity; two case reports. (French). *Acta Clinica Belgica* 1999Suppl:**1**:64–7.

De Silva, H.J., Sanmuganathan, P.S., Senanayake, N. Isolated bilateral recurrent laryngeal nerve paralysis: a delayed complication of organophosphorus poisoning. *Human and Experimental Toxicology* 1994;**13**:171–3.

Dressel, T.D., Goodale, R.L., Arneson, M.A., *et al.* Pancreatitis as a complication of anticholinesterase insecticide intoxication. *Annals of Surgery* 1979;**189**:199–204.

Drevenkar, V., Radic, Z., Vasilic, Z., *et al.* Dialkylphosphorus metabolites in the urine and activities of esterases in the serum as biochemical indices for human absorption of organophosphorus pesticides. *Archives of Environmental Contamination and Toxicology* 1991;**20**:417–22.

Duffy, F.H., Burchfiel, J.L., Bartels, P.H., *et al.* Long-term effects of an organophosphate upon the human electroencephalogram. *Toxicology and Applied Pharmacology* 1979;**47**:161–76.

Ernest, K., Thomas, M., Paulose, M., *et al.* Delayed effects of exposure to organophosphorus compounds. *Indian Journal of Medical Research* 1995;**101**:81–4.

Evans, R.T. Cholinesterase phenotyping: clinical aspects and laboratory applications. *CRC Critical Reviews in Clinical Laboratory Science* 1986;**23**:35–64.

Faff, J., Rabsztyn, T., Rump, S. Investigations on the correlation between abnormalities of neuromuscular transmission due to some organophosphates and activity of acetylcholinesterase in the skeletal muscle. *Archives of Toxicology* 1973:**31**:31–8.

Fernando, J.C.R., Hoskins, B.H., Ho, I.K. A striatal serotonergic involvement in the behavioural effects of anticholinesterase organophosphates. *European Journal of Pharmacology* 1984;**98**:129–32.

Finkelstein, Y., Kushnir, A., Raikhlin–Eisenkraft, B., *et al.* Antidotal therapy of severe acute organophosphate poisoning: a multihospital study. *Neurotoxicolgy and Teratology* 1989;**11**:593–6.

Firemark, H., Barlow, C.F., Roth, L.J. The penetration of 2-PAM C14 into brain and the effect of cholinesterase inhibitors on its transport. *Journal of Pharmacology and Experimental Therapeutics* 1964;**145**:252–65.

Gaines, T.B. Acute toxicity of pesticides. *Toxicology and Applied Pharmacology* 1969;**14**:515–34.

Gant, D.B., Elderfrawi, M.E., Elderfrawi, A.T. Action of organophosphates on GABA A receptor and voltage-dependent chloride channels. *Fundamental and Applied Toxicology* 1987;**9**:698–704.

Garcia-Lopez, J.A., Monteoliva, M. Physiological changes in human erythrocyte cholinesterase as measured with the "pH-stat". *Clinical Chemistry*, 1988;**34**:2133–5.

Gordon, C.J., Rowsey, P.J. Are circulating cytokines interleukin-6 and tumour necrosis factor alpha involved in chlorpyrifos-induced fever? *Toxicology* 1999;**134**:9–17.

Goswamy R, Chaudhuri, A., Mahashur, A.A. Study of respiratory failure in organophosphate and carbamate poisoning. *Heart and Lung* 1994;**23**:466–72.

Greenaway, C., Orr, P. A foodborne outbreak causing cholinergic syndrome. *Journal of Emergency Medicine,* 1996;**14**:339–44.

Griffin, P., Mason, H., Heywood, K., *et al.* Oral and dermal absorption of chlorpyrifos: a human volunteer study. *Occupational and Environmental Medicine* 1999;**56**:10–3.

Gupta, A., Agarwal, R., Shukla, G.S. Functional impairment of blood-brain barrier following pesticide exposure during early development in rats. *Human and Experimental Toxicology* 1999;**18**:174–9.

Güven, M., Bayram, F., Ünlühızarcı, K., *et al.* Endocrine changes in patients with acute organophosphate poisoning. *Human and Experimental Toxicology* 1999;**18**:598–601.

Güven, M., Ünlühızarcı, K., Göktas, Z., *et al.* Intravenous organophosphate injection: an unusual way of poisoning. *Human and Experimental Toxicology* 1997;**16**:279–80.

Haenen, C., de Moor, A., Dooms–Goossens, A. Contact dermatitis caused by the insecticides omethoate and dimethoate. *Contact Dermatitis* 1996;**35**:54–5.

Haines, J. Personal communication. 1999.

Hata, S., Bernstein, E., Davis, L.E. Atypical ocular bobbing in acute organophosphate poisoning. *Archives of Neurology* 1986;**43**:185–6.

Hayes, M.M.M., Van Der Westhuizen, N.G., Gelfland, M. Organophosphate poisoning in Rhodesia. *South African Medical Journal* 1978;**54**:230–4.

Hayes, W.J. Jr. *Pesticides studied in man.* Baltimore: Williams and Wilkins; 1982.

Hayes, W.J. Jr, Laws, E.R. Jr. *Handbook of Pesticide Toxicology* Vols 1, 2, 3. San Diego: Academic Press; 1991.

Health and Safety Executive. Technical Developmental Survey. Exposure to Chlorpyrifos in Orchard Spraying. *Report from Health and Safety Laboratory (FOD).* HSE 1998.

Hirshberg, A., Lerman, Y. Clinical problems in organophosphate insecticide poisoning: The use of a computerised information system. *Fundamental and Applied Toxicology* 1984;**4**:S209-14.

Hollis, G.J. Organophosphate poisoning versus brain stem stroke. *Medical Journal of Australia* 1999;**170**:596–7.

Houeto, P., Borron, S.W., Baud, F.J., *et al.* Assessment of erythrocyte cholinesterase activity in victims of smoke inhalation. *Journal of Toxicology Clinical Toxicology* 1999;**37**:321–6.

Hseih, B.H., Tsai, W.J., Deng, J.F. Extrapyramidal signs related to organophosphate poisonings: 2 case reports. *EAPCCT XX International Congress Abstract 150.* 2000.

Indudharan, R., Win, M.M., Noor, A.R. Laryngeal paralysis in organophosphorus poisoning. *Journal of Laryngology and Otology* 1998a;**112**:81–2

Indudharan, R. Brief bilateral vocal cord paralysis after insecticide poisoning. *Archives of Otolaryngology Head Neck Surgery* 1998b;**124**:113.

IPCS. *Environmental Health Criteria 63. Organophosphorus Insecticides.* World Health Organisation, International Programme on Chemical Safety, Geneva. 1986.

Jamil, H., Kundi, A., Akhtar, S., *et al.* Organophosphorus insecticide poisoning - review of 53 cases. *Journal of the Pakistan Medical Association* 1977;**27**:361–3.

Johnson, P.S., Michaelis, E.K. Characterisation of organophosphate interactions at N-methyl-D-aspartate receptors in brain synaptic membranes. *Molecular Pharmacology* 1992;**41**:750–6.

Kandalaft, K., Liu, S., Manivel, C., *et al.* Organophosphate increases the sensitivity of human exocrine pancreas to acetylcholine. *Pancreas* 1991;**6**:398–403.

Karalliedde, L., Henry, J.A. Effects of organophosphates on skeletal muscle. *Human and Experimental Toxicology* 1993;**12**:289–96.

Karalliedde, L., Senanayake, N. Acute organophosphorus insecticide poisoning: a review. *Ceylon Medical Journal,* 1986;**31**:93–100.

Karalliedde, L., Senanayake, N. Acute organophosphorus insecticide poisoning in Sri Lanka. *Forensic Science International* 1988;**36**:97–100.

Karalliedde, L., Senanayake, N. Organophosphorus insecticide poisoning. *British Journal of Anaesthesia* 1989;**63**:736–50

Karalliedde, L. Organophosphorus poisoning and anaesthesia. *Anaesthesia* 1999;**54**:1073–88.

Karalliedde L. Report on retrospective study on organophosphorus insecticide poisoning in South Asia. WHO SEARO 2000. Unpublished report.

Kin Sang Hui (Hui, K.S.). Metabolic disturbances in organophosphate insecticide poisoning. *Archives of Pathology and Laboratory Medicine* 1983;**107**:154.

Kiss, Z., Fazekas, T. Arrhythmias in organophosphate poisoning. *Acta Cardiologica* 1979;**34**:323–30.

Koga, H., Yoshinaga, M., Aoyagi, K., *et al.* Hemorrhagic panoesophagitis after acute organophosphorus poisoning. *Gastrointestinal Endoscopy* 1999;**49**:642–3.

Krause, W., Homola, S. Alterations of the seminiferous epithelium and the Leydig cells of the mouse testis after the application of dichlorvos. *Bulletin of Environmental Contamination and Toxicology* 1974;**11**:429–33.

Kumari, R., Rao, Y.N., Talukdar, B., *et al.* Serum enzyme abnormalities in protein energy malnutrition. *Indian Pediatrics* 1993;**30**:469–73.

Ladell, W.S.S. The impracticability of deducing blood cholinesterase depression from clinical condition in organophosphorus poisoning. In: Maynard R.L. *A Medical Review of Chemical Warfare Agents.* 2nd Edition of CDE TP 484. 1989. p. 133–6.

Lassiter, T.L., Barone, S. Jr., Moser, V.C., *et al.* Gestational exposure to chlorpyrifos: dose response profiles for cholinesterase and carboxylesterase activity. *Toxicological Sciences* 1999;**52**:92–100.

Lifshitz, M., Shahak, E., Sofer, S. Carbamate and organophosphate poisoning in young children. *Pediatric Emergency Care* 1999;**15**:102–3.

Lotti, M. Organophosphorus compounds. In: *Experimental and Clinical Neurotoxicology* 2nd Edition Spencer, P.S., Schaumburg, H.S., Ludolph, A.C. eds. Oxford University Press, New York 2000.

Ludomirsky, A., Klein, H.O., Sarelli, P. *et al.* QT prolongation and polymorphous ("Torsade des pointes") ventricular arrhythmias associated with organophosphorus insecticide poisoning. *American Journal of Cardiology* 1982;**49**:1654–8.

Luzhnikov, E.A., Savina, A.S., Shepelev, V.M. On the pathogenesis of cardiac rhythm and conductivity disorders in cases of acute insecticide poisoning. *Kardiologia* 1975;**15**:126–9.

Mahieu, P., Hassoun, A., Van Binst, R., *et al.* Severe and prolonged poisoning by fenthion. Significance of the determination of the anticholinesterase capacity of plasma. *Journal of Toxicology-Clinical Toxicology* 1982;**19**:425–32.

Matsumiya, N., Tanaka, M., Iwai, M., *et al.* Elevated amylase is related to the development of respiratory failure in organophosphate poisoning. *Human and Experimental Toxicology* 1996;**15**:250–3.

Michotte, A., Van Dijck, I., Maes, V., *et al.* Ataxia as the only delayed neurotoxic manifestation of organophosphate insecticide poisoning. *European Neurology* 1989;**29**:23–6.

Montoya-Cabrera, M.A., Escalante-Galindo, P., Rivera-Rebolledo, J.C., *et al.* Acute methyl parathion poisoning with extrapyramidal manifestations not previously reported. (Spanish). *Gaceta Medica de Mexico* 1999;**135**:79–82.

Mortensen, M.L. Management of acute childhood poisoning by selected insecticides and herbicides. *Pediatric Clinics of North America* 1986;**33**:421–45.

Muller–Vahl, K.R., Kolbe, H., Dengler, R. Transient severe parkinsonism after acute organophosphate poisoning. *Journal of Neurology, Neurosurgery Psychiatry* 1999;**66**:253–4.

Mutch, E., Blain, P.G., Williams, F.M. Interindividual variations in enzymes controlling organophosphate toxicity in man. *Human and Experimental Toxicology* 1992;**11**:109–16.

Nakajima, T., Sasaki, K., Ozawa, H., *et al.* Urinary metabolites of sarin in a patient of the Matsumoto sarin incident. *Archives of Toxicology* 1998;**72**:601–3.

Namba, T., Nolte, C.T., Jackrel, J., *et al.* Poisoning due to organophosphate insecticides. Acute and chronic manifestations. *American Journal of Medicine* 1971;**50**:475–92.

Newcombe, D.S. Immune surveillance, organophosphorus exposure and lymphomagenesis. *Lancet* 1992:**339**:539–41.

Nisse, P., Forceville, X., Cezard, C., *et al.* Intermediate Syndrome with delayed distal polyneuropathy from ethyl parathion poisoning. *Veterinary and Human Toxicology* 1998;**40**:349–52.

Nolan, R.J., Rick, D.L., Freshour N.L., *et al.* Chlorpyrifos: pharmacokinetics in human volunteers. *Toxicology and Applied Pharmacology* 1984;**73**:8–15.

Ochi, G., Watanabe, K., Tokuoka, H., *et al.* Neuroleptic malignant-like syndrome: a complication of acute organophosphate poisoning. *Canadian Journal of Anaesthesia* 1995;**42**:1027–30.

Opawoye, A.D., Haque, T. Insecticide/organophosphorus compound poisoning in children. http://www.kfshrc.edu.sa/annals/182/97-225.html.

Owczarzy, I., Wysocki, J., Kalina, Z. Blood glucose changes in persons occupationally exposed to organophosphate pesticides. (Polish). *Polski Tygodnik Lekarski* 1982;**37**:1429–32.

Pach, J., Winnik, L., Kusmiderski, J., *et al.* The results of the brain computer tomography and clinical picture in acute cholinesterase inhibitors poisoning. *Przeglad Lekarski* 1997;**54**:677–83.

Padungtod, C., Hassold, T.J., Millie, E., *et al.* Sperm aneuploidy among Chinese pesticide factory workers: scoring by the FISH method. *American Journal of Industrial Medicine* 1999;**36**:230–8.

Padungtod, C., Lasley, B.L., Christiani, D.C., *et al.* Reproductive hormone profile among pesticide factory workers. *Journal of Occupational and Environmental Medicine* 1998;**40**:1038–47.

Pala, I., Vig, P.J.S., Desaiah, D., *et al.* In vitro effects of organophosphorus compounds on calmodulin activity. *Journal of Applied Toxicology* 1991;**11**:391–5.

Patial, R.K., Bansal, S.K., Sehgal, V.K., *et al.* Sphincteric involvement in organophosphorus poisoning. *Journal of the Association of Physicians India* 1987;**39**:492–3.

Persson, H.E., Sjoberg, G.K., Haines, J.A., *et al.* Poisoning Severity Score. Grading of Acute Poisoning. *Journal of Toxicology Clinical Toxicology* 1998;**36**:205–13.

Petroianu, G., Helfrich, U., Globig, S., *et al.* Phospholipase A_2 (PLA_2) activity in mini pigs after acute high dose iv-paraoxon (POX) intoxication. *Chemico-Biological Interactions* 1999;**119–20**:497–502.

Poovala, V.S., Huang, H., Salahudeen, A.K. Role of reactive oxygen metabolites in organophosphate-bidrin-induced renal tubular cytoxicity. *Journal of the American Society of Nephrology* 1999;**10**:1746–52.

Quistad, G.B., Casida, J.E. Sensitivity of blood clotting factors and digestive enzymes to inhibition by organophosphorus pesticides. *Journal of Biochemistry and Molecular Toxicology* 2000;**14**:51–6.

Rao, M.R., Kanji, V.K., Sekhar, V. Pesticide induced changes of nitric oxide synthase in rat brain in vitro. *Drug and Chemical Toxicology* 1999;**22**:411–20.

Relakis, K., Sifakis, S., Froudarakis, G., *et al.* Disposition of pesticides and toxicants in the human reproductive system in cases of acute poisoning. *Clinical and Experimental Obstetrics and Gynaecology* 1999;**20**:207–10.

Rengstorff, R.H. Accidental exposure to sarin: vision effects. *Archives of Toxicology,* 1985;**56**:201–3.

Richter E.D., Kowalski, M., Leventhal A., *et al.* Illness and excretion of organophosphate metabolites four months after household pest extermination. *Archives of Environmental Health* 1992;**47**:135–8.

Rocha, E.S., Santos, M.D., Chebabo, S.R., *et al.* Low concentrations of the organophosphate VX affect spontaneous and evoked transmitter release from hippocampal neurons: toxicological relevance of cholinesterase-independent actions. *Toxicology and Applied Pharmacology* 1999;**159**:31–40.

Rodgers, K., Xiong, S. Effect of acute administration of malathion by oral and dermal routes on serum histamine levels. *International Journal of Immunopharmacology* 1997;**19**:437–41.

Rodgers, K.E., Grayson, M.H., Ware, C.F. Inhibition of cytotoxic T lymphocyte and natural killer cell-mediated lysis by O,S,S-trimethyl phosphorodithioate is at an early post recognition step. *Journal of Immunology* 1988;**140**:564–70.

Rodgers, K.E., Leung, N., Ware, C.F., *et al.* Lack of immunosuppressive effects of acute and sub acute administration of malathion. *Pesticide Biochemical Physiology* 1986;**25**:358–64.

Ryhanen, R., Kajovaara, M., Harri, M., *et al.* Physical exercise affects cholinesterases and organophosphate response. *General Pharmacology* 1988;**19**:815–8.

Saadeh, A.M., al–Ali, M.K., Farsakh, N.A., *et al.* Clinical and socio-demographic features of acute carbamate and organophosphate poisoning: a study of 70 adult patients in north Jordan. *Journal of Toxicology Clinical Toxicology* 1996;**34**:45–51.

Saadeh, A.M., Farsakh, N.A., al–Ali, M.K. Cardiac manifestations of acute carbamate and organophosphate poisoning. *Heart* 1997;**77**:461–4.

Satoh, T., Hosokawa, M. Organophosphates and their impact on the global environment. *Neurotoxicology* 2000;**21**:223–7.

Satoh, T., Suzuki, S., Kawai, N., *et al.* Toxicological significance in the cleavage of esterase-beta-glucuronidase complex in liver microsomes by organophosphorus compounds. *Chemico-Biological Interactions* 1999;**119-120**:471–8.

Savage, E.P., Keefe, T.J., Mounce, L.M., *et al.* Chronic neurologic sequelae of acute organophosphorus pesticide poisoning. *Archives of Environmental Health* 1998;**43**:38–45.

Senanayake, N., de Silva, H.J., Karalliedde, L. A scale to assess severity on organophosphorus intoxication: POP Scale. *Human and Experimental Toxicology* 1993;**12**:297–9.

Senanayake, N., Karalliedde, L. Neurotoxic effects of organophosphorus insecticides: an intermediate syndrome. *New England Journal of Medicine* 1987;**316**:761–3.

Senanayake, N., Sanmuganathan, P.S. Extrapyramidal manifestations complicating organophosphorus insecticide poisoning. *Human and Experimental Toxicology,* 1995;**14**:600–4.

Senanayake, N. Organophosphorus insecticide poisoning. *Ceylon Medical Journal,* 1998;**43**:22–9.

Serrano, N., Fedriani, J. Fenthion suicide poisoning by subcutaneous injection. *Intensive Care Medicine* 1997;**23**:129.

Sidhu, K.S., Collisi, M.B.   A case of an accidental exposure to a veterinary insecticide product formulation. *Veterinary and Human Toxicology* 1989;**31**:63–4.

Singh, S., Sharma, B.K., Wahi, P.L., *et al.* Spectrum of acute poisoning in adults- 10 year experience. *Journal of the Association of Physicians of India* 1984;**32**:561–3.

Singh, S., Wig, N., Chaudhry, D., *et al.* Changing pattern of acute poisoning in adults: experience of a large northwest Indian Hospital. *Journal of the Association of Physicians of India,* 1997;**45**, 194–7.

Sivam, S.P., Norris, J.C., Kim, D.K., *et al.*   Effect of acute and chronic cholinesterase inhibition with diisopropylfluorophosphate on muscarinic, dopamine and GABA receptors of the rat striatum. *Journal of Neurochemistry* 1983;**40**:1414–22.

Sofer, S., Tal, A., Shahak, E.   Carbamate and organophosphate poisoning in early childhood. *Pediatric Emergency Care* 1989;**5**:222–5.

Stewart, W.C., Anderson, E.A.   Effect of a cholinesterase inhibitor when injected in to the medulla of the rabbit. *Journal of Pharmacology and Experimental Therapeutics* 1968;**162**:309–18.

Stewart, W.C.   The effects of sarin and atropine on the respiratory center and neuromuscular junctions of the rat. *Canadian Journal of Biochemistry Physiology* 1959;**37**:361.

Taitelman, N.I.   Affinity of organophosphate insecticides to acetylcholinesterase compared to plasma cholinesterase. *NACCT Abstracts.* Abstract No 194. 1999.

Thompson, J.W., Stocks, R.M.   Brief bilateral vocal cord paralysis after insecticide poisoning: a new variant of toxicity. *Archives of Otolaryngology Head and Neck Surgery* 1997;**123**:93–6.

Tielemans, E., van Kooij, R., Velde, E.R., *et al.* Pesticide exposure and decreased fertilisation rates in vitro. *Lancet* 1999;**354**:484–5.

Tinoco–Ojanguren, R., Halperin, D.C.   Poverty, production and health: inhibition of erythrocyte cholinesterase via occupational exposure to organophosphate insecticides in Chiapas, Mexico. *Archives of Environmental Health* 1998;**53**:29–35.

Tripathi, A.K., Misra, U.K.   Ophthalmoplegia in dimethoate poisoning. *Journal of Physicians India* 1996;**44**:225.

Vale, J.A.   Are there long-term sequelae from a single acute organophosphorus insecticide exposure? *Proceedings of European Society of Toxicology* 1999. p. 367.

Van Bao, T., Szabo, I., Ruzicska, P., *et al.* Chromosome aberrations in patients suffering acute organic phosphate insecticide poisoning. *Humangenetik* 1974;**24**:33–57.

Vasilic, Z., Stengl, B., Drevenkar, V. Dimethylphosphorus metabolites in serum and urine of persons poisoned by malathion or thiometon. *Chemico-Biological Interaction* 1999;**119-120**:479–87.

Wadia, R.S., Sadagopan, C., Amin, R.B., *et al.* Neurological manifestations of organophosphorus insecticide poisoning. *Journal of Neurology, Neurosurgery and Psychiatry* 1974;**37**:841–7.

Ward, T.R., Mundy, W.R. Organophosphorus compounds preferentially affect second messenger systems coupled to M2/M4 receptors in rat frontal cortex. *Brain Research Bulletin* 1996;**39**:49–55.

Whorton, M.D., Obrinsky, D.L. Persistence of symptoms after mild to moderate acute organophosphate poisoning among 19 farm field workers. *Journal of Toxicology and Environmental Health* 1983;**11**:347–54.

Williams, F.M. Clinical significance of esterases. *Clinical Pharmacokinetics* 1985;**10**:392–403.

Wills, J.H. The measurement and significance of changes in the cholinesterase activities of erythrocytes and plasma in man and animals. *CRC Critical Reviews in Toxicology* 1972;**1**:153–202.

Wright, P.G. An analysis of the central and peripheral components of respiratory failure produced by anticholinesterase poisoning in the rabbit. *Journal of Physiology* 1954;**126**:52.

Wui–Chiang, Lee, Chen–Chang, Yang., Jou–Fang, Deng. *et al.* The clinical significance of hyperamylasemia in organophosphate poisoning. *Journal of Toxicology Clinical Toxicology* 1998;**36**:673–81.

Xiong, S., Rodgers, K. Effects of malathion metabolites on degranulation of and mediator release by human and rat basophilic cells. *Journal of Toxicology and Environmental Health* 1997;**51**:159–75.

Yamashita, M., Yamashita, M., Tanaka, J., *et al.* Human mortality in organophosphate poisonings. *Veterinary and Human Toxicology* 1997;**39**:84–5.

Yilmazlar, A., Ozyurt, G. Brain involvement in organophosphate poisoning. *Environmental Research* 1997;**74**:104–9.

Zavon, M.R. Poisoning from pesticides: diagnosis and treatment. *Pediatrics* 1974;**54**:332–6.

Zoppellari, R., Borron, S.W., Chieregato, A., *et al.* Isofenphos poisoning: prolonged intoxication after intramuscular injection. *Journal of Toxicology Clinical Toxicology* 1997;**35**:401–4.

Zwiener, R.J., Ginsburg, M. Organophosphate and carbamate poisoning in infants and children. *Pediatrics* 1988;**81**:121–6.

CHAPTER 6

The Intermediate Syndrome

Jan L. De Bleecker

6.1. Introduction

In 1987, Senanayake and Karalliedde in a landmark *New England Journal of Medicine* paper reported 10 patients who developed facial, proximal limb and respiratory muscle weakness (Senanayake and Karalliedde, 1987). Because this occurs in the interval between the acute cholinergic crisis and the possible development of a delayed motor neuropathy called OP-induced delayed polyneuropathy, they termed this new entity the "Intermediate Syndrome" (IMS). The acute cholinergic crisis is due to inhibition of carboxylic esterases, of which acetylcholinesterase (AChE) is clinically the most important (Grob, 1963), and the delayed neuropathy has been linked to inhibition of a separate esterase termed the neuropathy target esterase (Abou-Donia and Lapadula, 1990; Johnson, 1975). The pathogenesis of the IMS was unclear and the question arose whether or not the IMS bore a separate structure-activity relationship (Marrs, 1993; De Bleecker *et al.*, 1992).

6.2. Original Description

Senanayake and Karalliedde observed 10 patients of Asian origin who were admitted with a well-defined cholinergic crisis. Following treatment with atropine and oximes in conventional doses, the initial outcome was favourable, but the patients went on to develop an IMS usually 1 to 4 days after the cholinergic poisoning (Senanayake and Karalliedde, 1987). The most threatening clinical symptom was the occurrence of sudden respiratory distress, often requiring re-intubation and positive-pressure ventilation. Various degrees of weakness of muscles innervated by several cranial nerves were present in 8 patients. All subjects had weakness of neck flexors and of proximal limb muscles. In all but 1 patient, the tendon reflexes were absent or markedly decreased. There was no sensory impairment. Transient dystonic movements appeared in 2 fenthion-poisoned victims.

Two patients died on the third and fifth hospital day from respiratory failure, whereas 1 patient died on the fifteenth day because of a technical failure.

There was no distinct pattern in the development of the symptoms, but their regression followed a characteristic order in the 7 survivors. Cranial nerve palsies, palatal, facial, and external ocular, in that order—were the first to recover. Then followed improvement of respiratory function and proximal limb muscle strength, and neck flexion was the last to recover. The time to recovery ranged from 5 to 18 days. One methamidophos-poisoned patient developed delayed neuropathy.

In 9 subjects, the causative OP was identified: 4 fenthion, 2 dimethoate, 2 monocrotophos, and 1 methamidophos. Standard biochemistry and cerebrospinal fluid examination were normal. Cholinesterase assays were not available.

Electromyography (EMG) showed normal motor and sensory nerve conduction velocities and normal needle myography. Tetanic stimulation of the abductor pollicis brevis muscle 24 to 48 h after the onset of the IMS showed a marked fade at 20 and 50 Hz. A train of 4 stimuli at 2 Hz produced no changes in the amplitude of the compound muscle action potential (CMAP).

Treatment was mainly symptomatic. Atropine did not seem to influence the course of the IMS. No definite mechanism of the IMS was identified, but the authors wondered whether the necrotising myopathy induced by acute OP poisoning in patients (Tattersall, 1990; De Reuck and Willems, 1975; Wecker et al., 1986) and experimental animals (Ariëns et al., 1969; Dettbarn, 1984; Inns et al., 1990; De Bleecker et al., 1991; De Bleecker et al., 1991;1992;1998) might underlie the selective muscle weakness.

6.3. Previous Reports

Several patients reported before the recognition of the IMS by Senanayake and Karalliedde can retrospectively be related to this syndrome.

The largest cohort was presented by Wadia et al. (1974) in diazinon poisoning. These authors divided the signs and symptoms into Type I (those present on admission) and Type II (those appearing 24 h after onset of poisoning). Type I signs included impaired consciousness and fasciculations, and were responsive to atropine therapy. Type II signs were very much like the IMS and included proximal limb weakness, areflexia, and cranial nerve palsies, and were not influenced by atropine. Some Type I patients developed Type II signs after an initial recovery.

Thirty-six of 200 consecutive patients developed Type II signs, and 15 died from respiratory paralysis.

In 1966, Clarmann and Geldmacher-von Mallinkdrodt successfully managed a fenthion-poisoned patient with relapse of respiratory paralysis a few hours after initial improvement. Atropine and oxime administration finally appeared successful in this patient. The oxime used was obidoxime (Toxogonin®). In another fenthion-poisoned victim, sudden respiratory insufficiency necessitating artificial ventilation occurred 72 h after ingestion (Dean et al., 1967). This patient at the same time was restless, sweating, salivating, and had profuse fasciculations. He had considerable strength in all limbs and could lift his trunk from the bed. Combined atropine and oxime (PAM) treatment was successful in rapidly controlling the muscarinic signs; it took 7 days however, before spontaneous breathing returned. The authors mentioned the disproportion between respiratory (intercostal, bulbar and diaphragm muscles) and non-respiratory muscle strength as the most striking feature in their patient. A Belgian group (Mahieu et al., 1982) reported severe relapses of an initial cholinergic crisis 31 h, 72 h, 7, 12, 13 and 16 days after ingestion of fenthion, despite atropine (not on day 2 and 3) and oxime administration. Biochemical investigations disclosed that disappearance or reappearance of cholinergic signs coincided with the initial decrease and subsequent increase of free cholinesterase inhibitor in serum. In all those cases of fenthion poisoning, the initial cholinergic symptoms started within 0.5 h after oral ingestion and were moderately intense.

Relapse of cholinergic symptoms and unconsciousness has also been reported following dimethoate intoxication (Molphy and Rathus, 1964). A tractor driver with subacute dicrotophos poisoning probably through both skin contact and inhalation recovered from a moderate cholinergic crisis after atropine and pralidoxime treatment. He further improved when atropine dosage was tapered, but on the seventh day after the last exposure, he relapsed with prominent respiratory paralysis. Response to drug treatment, if any, was not mentioned. The ultimate outcome was favourable (Perron and Johnson, 1969).

Gadoth and Fisher (1978) reported a victim of malathion ingestion who 20 h after a mild and apparently well-treated cholinergic crisis, needed urgent re-intubation, with vomiting, muscle cramps, and diarrhoea at the same time. A progressive paresis emerged, and after 50 h, a neurological evaluation revealed complete respiratory paralysis, bilateral ptosis, myosis, orbicularis oculi muscle fasciculations and external ophthalmoplegia. Deep tendon reflexes were absent. Repeated doses of atropine and obidoxime gave no improvement. The ultimate outcome was favourable.

6.4. Further Characterisation of the Syndrome: Author's Observations

6.4.1. Experimental Animal Studies

Our group compared in Wistar rats, the acutely toxic OP paraoxon with fenthion; one of the agents frequently involved in the human IMS. The clinical course was related to the development of muscle fibre necrosis, histochemically assessed AChE activity at the neuromuscular junction, biochemically assessed brain AChE activity, and electromyographic studies including repetitive nerve stimulation at various frequencies.

Marked differences in the clinical course of the cholinergic crisis were noted between paraoxon and fenthion poisoning, regardless of the route of administration (De Bleecker *et al.*, 1994). Paraoxon provoked an acute, severe and short-lasting cholinergic crisis lasting less than 24 h. In contrast, fenthion poisoning produced a gradual increase of cholinergic signs lasting several days. All surviving animals were symptom-free after 1 week. Fasciculations peaked within the first days of fenthion poisoning, and gradually decreased and ultimately disappeared when the rats got weaker. Single poisoning with these 2 OPs turned out to be a good model to compare acute and chronic types of poisoning in animals, but most clinical signs relevant to the human IMS cannot be ascertained in rodents.

Histochemically determined endplate AChE and spectrophotometrically determined brain AChE activity closely paralleled each other. In paraoxon poisoning, AChE inhibition was severe between 1 and 3 h after subcutaneous injection and gradually recovered within 24 h. In fenthion-poisoned animals, a slowly progressive decline in AChE activity occurred with maximal inhibition after 8 days. At that time, most animals had no more weakness or fasciculations.

The necrotising myopathy began shortly after the initiation of the cholinergic crisis with both OPs and involved a maximal number of muscle fibres after 24 to 48 h. The necrotising myopathy did not get worse by a further decline in AChE activity in fenthion-poisoned animals. It appeared to be a monophasic event related to the initial decline in endplate AChE activity. The severity of the myopathy was similar in paraoxon- and fenthion-poisoned rats with similar degrees of fasciculations.

Repetitive activity after single motor nerve stimulation and decrement after repetitive nerve stimulation were the major EMG findings in either type of poisoning (Fig. 6.1.) (Besser *et al.*, 1989a, 1989b, 1992; Van Dijk *et al.*, 1996; De Bleecker *et al.*, 1994; Singh *et al.*, 1998).

Repetitive activity is defined as at least one negative deflection occurring immediately after the initial biphasic compound muscle action potential (for review see (Bowman *et al.* 1986)) (Fig. 6.1.A-B).

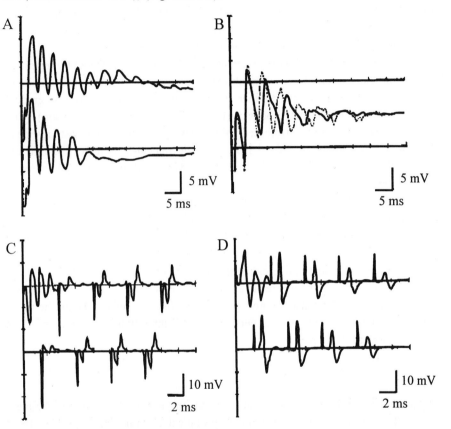

Figure 6.1. Electromyographic findings in OP-poisoned rats.

<u>A:</u> Response to two subsequent stimuli at 2 Hz administered 2.5 h after subcutaneous injection of paraoxon. Note prominent repetitive activity after the first stimulus (upper line). After the second stimulus, the repetitive activity is less marked. The initial compound muscle action potential (CMAP) amplitudes are normal. <u>B:</u> Response to two subsequent nerve stimuli at 3 Hz administered 2.5 h after subcutaneous paraoxon poisoning. Repetitive action potentials at the second stimulus (full line) are less frequent, are delayed and have less steep slopes. Note slightly decreased CMAP amplitude at the second response. <u>C:</u> Decrement-increment phenomenon in response to 50 Hz repetitive nerve stimulation 3 h after subcutaneous paraoxon injection. The odd responses are displayed on top, the even at the bottom.

The second response has the smallest amplitude, with gradual but incomplete recovery in the subsequent responses. Note that the marked repetitive activity at the first response is entirely abrogated at the second response and does not recur. The sharp initial deflection preceding each CMAP represents the stimulation artefact. D: Decrement phenomenon in response to 50 Hzrepetitive nerve stimulation 9 days after subcutaneous injection of fenthion. Gradual decrease in amplitude and area towards the ninth response. The repetitive activity disappears completely at the second response.

Compound muscle action potential amplitude decrements provoked by repetitive nerve stimulation occurred only in weak rats with severe endplate AChE inhibition. The smallest amplitude occurred either at the second response followed by gradual increase in the subsequent responses (decrement-increment phenomenon) (Fig. 6.1.C), or the amplitude decreased progressively towards the last response (decrement phenomenon) (Fig. 6.1.D). The decrement-increment phenomenon preceded the decrement phenomenon and occurred at a slightly less severe degree of AChE inhibition.

Conclusions from the animal studies were that:

1.   The AChE inhibition by fenthion is much prolonged.
2.   The necrotising myopathy is determined by the initial decline in endplate AChE activity, and is not further aggravated by continued inhibition.
3.   Decrement-increment and decrement responses on EMG are related to severe AChE inhibition and appeared at a slightly different extent of AChE inhibition.

The data argued against the monophasic necrotising myopathy being the cause of the IMS, and were suggestive of persistent AChE inhibition being involved. This hypothesis was tested in patients.

6.4.2. Observations in Patients

Consecutive OP-poisoned patients admitted to our institution were prospectively studied. The study included a standard neurological examination at frequent fixed time intervals, serum cholinesterase and erythrocyte AChE activity, urinary OP metabolite excretion and EMG with repetitive nerve stimulation. Some patients underwent a muscle biopsy. Eight out of 19 patients developed clinical signs and symptoms of the IMS. In some, short relapses of muscarinic symptoms were superimposed on the IMS. No clinical, electromyographic, biochemical or other differences were noted between patients with or without "symptom-free interval", or those with or without short relapses of muscarinic signs and symptoms. OPs such as fenthion (n=1), dimethoate (n=1) (De Bleecker et al., 1992) and methyl-parathion (n=5) (De Bleecker et al., 1992a) apparently carried a higher risk.

However, we also noted a prolonged IMS in a parathion-poisoned man with severe renal and hepatic failure, indicating that the IMS is not restricted to a few OP agents (De Bleecker *et al.*, 1992b). Table 6.1. lists the OPs frequently involved in IMS (cases cited in this chapter). Prospective studies on the relative incidence of IMS with certain OP agents are needed to avoid a number of biases inherent to case reports.

The clinical signs of the IMS were weakness in the territory of multiple cranial nerves (diplopia, dysphagia, facial diplegia), sudden respiratory distress necessitating re-intubation, neck and proximal limb muscle weakness, and depression of the deep tendon reflexes. Fasciculations were not part of the IMS but coincided with the appearance of muscarinic signs. The duration of the IMS varied from a few days to several weeks. The outcome was good. No patients developed clinical or EMG features of delayed polyneuropathy (De Bleecker *et al.*, 1993).

All patients had severe AChE inhibition during the entire period of the IMS. Metabolite excretion was also prolonged. Consecutive EMG findings in the evolution of the IMS were: decrement, decrement-increment, increment, and finally normal repetitive nerve stimulation studies. The EMG normalised before the last neurological symptom i.e. fatigable external ocular muscle weakness had disappeared (De Bleecker *et al.*, 1993).

In the 4 patients who underwent muscle biopsy, a few necrotic muscle fibres were noted, but these were too sparse to explain severe muscle weakness and were no more frequent in IMS than in non-IMS patients.

We concluded from the prospective patient study that:

1. The IMS is not rare, and although it is more likely to occur with certain OP agents, it is not restricted to these agents. Toxicokinetic factors such as high lipid-solubility of certain OPs (Davies *et al.*, 1975), but also impaired systemic functions (cardiovascular, hepatic, renal) (Berrosian *et al.*, 1995) with prolongation of OP metabolism and excretion, can probably all contribute to the development of an IMS (Table 6.1.1).

2. The syndrome invariably coincides with prolonged AChE inhibition and is not due to muscle fibre necrosis. No separate structure-activity relationship is involved.

3. When viewed together, the clinical and EMG features are best explained by combined pre- and post-synaptic impairment of neuromuscular transmission (De Wilde *et al.*, 1991) (see also 6.X.X).

4. The IMS is not related to incipient delayed neuropathy.

Table 6.1. Causative OPs in Intermediate Syndrome

Total number of cases:	43 + 36
Fenthion	11
Dimethoate – omethoate	6-5
Parathion	8
Parathion-methyl	5
Malathion	2
Monocrotophos - dicrotophos	2-1
Methamidophos	1
Dichlorvos – trichlorfon	1 + 1
Diazinon (16)	36

6.5. Comparison with other Human Diseases with Impaired Neuromuscular Transmission

The clinical, electromyographic, electrophysiological, microelectrophysiological and morphological features of a number of acquired or congenital human disorders of neuromuscular transmission have been well characterised.

Comparison of the IMS with some of these syndromes is helpful in interpreting the observations made in IMS patients. Besides practical problems involved in studies of endplate-rich human intercostal muscle biopsies, the changing dynamics of the endplate AChE inhibition in the course of OP poisonings make the IMS more difficult to study than more frequent or stable disorders.

Table 6.2 summarises the main clinical and EMG characteristics of some disorders of neuromuscular transmission. Myasthenia gravis is an autoimmune disorder with post-synaptic impairment of neuromuscular transmission due to complement deposition at the ACh receptor sites. In the Lambert-Eaton myasthenic syndrome, antibodies against the pre-synaptic voltage-sensitive calcium channels cause reduced release of ACh quanta from the motor nerve terminal. In botulinum toxin poisoning, the ACh release from the nerve terminal is reduced by impaired fusion of pre-synaptic vesicles with the pre-synaptic membrane.

The distribution of the weakness and the obvious fatigability of some muscle groups in the IMS are very similar to myasthenia gravis. Areflexia or hyporeflexia, on the other hand, is more typical of pre-synaptic disorders. Likewise, the EMG findings of the IMS are a combination of those observed in pre-and post-synaptic disorders of neuromuscular transmission.

In some IMS patients with severe weakness, persistent decrements at low stimulation frequencies were found, just like in severe myasthenia gravis. In most patients, a decrement-increment phenomenon with the smallest amplitude at the second stimulus occurred at intermediate or high frequency- stimulation only. This is more like in pre-synaptic disorders. However, reduced amplitude of the CMAP after a single nerve stimulus, the most typical and constant EMG feature of the Lambert-Eaton myasthenic syndrome, was never noted. The decrement-increment phenomenon, with the smallest amplitude at the second muscle action potential, turns out to be rather typical of the IMS.

Taken together, the data in IMS are compatible with a combined pre- and post-synaptic disturbance of neuromuscular transmission, presumably to a different proportion during the evolution of the IMS.

A congenital myasthenic syndrome with synaptic AChE deficiency, resulting from a mutation in the collagenic tail subunit of asymmetric AChE, has been described by Engel et al. and others (Ohno et al., 1998). Clinically these patients are much like IMS patients. They have persistent fatigable weakness of external ocular, facial, palatal, masticatory, neck, and proximal limb muscles, and depressed deep tendon reflexes. EMG shows repetitive compound muscle action potentials after single nerve stimulation, and decrements at slow and rapid rates of repetitive nerve stimulation.

Detailed microelectrophysiological and morphological studies have revealed combined pre- and post-synaptic abnormalities of neuromuscular transmission (Table 6.2.).

6.6. Later Reports

In the years following the initial description, the IMS has been diagnosed increasingly due to heightened awareness. He et al. (1998) found IMS in 21 of 272 cases (7.7%). The causative OPs were parathion, omethoate, dimethoate, diclorvos and some pesticide mixtures. Persisting blood AChE inhibition was a constant finding and decrements were noted in weak patients on 20 or 30 Hz repetitive nerve stimulation.

The fatality rate was 19%. Choi and Quinonez (1998) reported a case of IMS in malathion poisoning. Karademir et al. (1990) observed IMS in a young female poisoned by trichlorfon and the carbamate proxyfur, and in a fenthion-poisoned female, both with complete recovery. Two pregnant fenthion-poisoned women were successfully managed by Karalliedde et al. (1988).

Table 6.2. Main characteristics of some human disorders of neuromuscular transmission

	Myasthenia gravis	Lambert-Eaton myasthenic syndrome	Botulinum toxin poisoning	Intermediate Syndrome	Congenital AChE deficiency
Site of defect	Post-synaptic	Pre-synaptic	Pre-synaptic	Pre- and post-synaptic	Pre- and post-synaptic
Clinical findings	Fatigable	Fatigable	Fatigable, descending	Fatigable	Fatigable
Distribution of muscle weakness	Extraocular bulbar, facial, respiratory, proximal limb	Proximal limb	Extraocular head and neck, trunk and proximal limb	Extraocular bulbar, facial, neck, respiratory, proximal limb	Extraocular bulbar, facial, neck, proximal limb
Tendon reflexes	Normal	Decreased	Decreased	Decreased	Decreased
Response to AChE inhibitors	Yes	Poor or absent	Absent	Absent or adverse	Absent
Electromyography					
CMAP amplitude	Normal	Small	Some small	Normal	Normal
Repetitive activity	No	No	No	Yes	Yes
Repetitive nerve stimulation	Decrement at low frequency	Increment at high frequency	Increment at high frequency	Decrement at low frequency; increment at intermediate/high frequency	Decrement at low and high frequency

An acute poisoning in a 44-year-old female who ingested 50ml of parathion concentrate (25g) was described by Nisse *et al.* (1999). She was admitted 30 minutes after ingestion of OP agent and was treated with a continuous infusion of atropine and 400mg of pralidoxime methyl sulphate 4 hourly, a gastric lavage, oral administration of paraffin oil along with endotracheal intubation and mechanical ventilation. On day 3, consciousness was normal and treatment was discontinued. On day 4, deep hypotonic coma occurred with absence of muscle reflexes, bilateral ptosis and apnoea. Atropine and pralidoxime (200mg/4 hourly) was recommenced. A distal polyneuropathy developed on day 23. Assisted ventilation was required for 35 days. The first group of muscles to recover were those innervated by cranial nerves. On day 28, patient regained consciousness and on day 40 she returned to normal.

A 33-year-old female ingested an unknown quantity of malathion in a suicide attempt. Cholinergic signs consistent with severe OP intoxication developed and were treated within 6 hours of ingestion with intravenous atropine and continuous infusion of pralidoxime (400mg/h). Prolonged depression of plasma and red cell cholinesterases were documented. Despite the presence of plasma pralidoxime concentrations in excess of 4 µg/ml, the patient developed profound motor paralysis on the third day after apparent recovery (moving all extremities with strong hand grip) from the acute cholinergic crisis. Weakness persisted until hospital day 8 when weaning parameters appeared favourable (Sudakin *et al.*, 2000).

Other investigators undertook *in vivo* electrodiagnostic studies in experimental animals (Dongren *et al.*, 1999) and in man (Baker and Sedgwick, 1996; Singh *et al.*, 1998).

Baker and Sedgwick (1986) performed an elegant study using single fibre EMG, a more sensitive technique than repetitive motor nerve stimulation to detect subtle changes in neuromuscular transmission. In sarin-poisoned healthy volunteers, they found small changes in single fibre EMG at 3 hours and 3 days after exposure to a small dose of sarin sufficient to cause a reduction of red blood cell AChE of 60%. These people had no clinical neuromuscular signs or symptoms. They and others (Norman, 1990) considered that a non-depolarising block underlies the IMS, and concluded from their studies in volunteers that reversible sub-clinical changes indicating a non-depolarising block could be found to a variable extent in all study persons and probably, also in patients.

Inter-individual differences in the safety factor of neuromuscular transmission; the degree and duration of endplate AChE inhibition; and conformational changes of the acetylcholine (ACh) receptors in the post-synaptic membrane due to the precedent cholinergic crisis may explain why not all OP-poisoned patients with a similar severity of intoxication develop the IMS. Based on observations in a fenthion-poisoned IMS patient, the same group proposed down regulation of post-synaptic acetylcholine receptors as a possible explanation for the clinical and electrophysiological abnormalities in that patient (Sedgwick and Senanayake, 1997). Different affinity of different OPs for nicotinic versus muscarinic cholinesterases or selective distribution of some OPs to muscle have also been proposed (Benson et al., 1992).

A study by Dongren et al. (1999) in dimethoate-poisoned rats confirmed the higher sensitivity of single fibre EMG over repetitive nerve stimulation to detect subtle changes in neuromuscular transmission after OP poisoning.

Two recent reports are of particular interest as they associate IMS despite early oxime therapy.

6.7. Diagnostic Criteria

On the basis of our personal observations and the cases reported from experienced centers all over the world we propose the following diagnostic guidelines:

1. Persistent acquired inhibition of red blood cell AChE through OP or possibly carbamate poisoning.
2. Fatigable weakness of the extraocular, bulbar, facial, respiratory, neck flexor, and proximal limb muscles. The weakness occurs 1–4 days after a cholinergic crisis, with or without symptom-free interval.
   Short relapses of muscarinic signs and symptoms do not exclude the diagnosis.
3. Absent or depressed deep tendon reflexes without other identifiable cause (e.g. pre-existent polyneuropathy).
4. EMG abnormalities indicating pre- or post-synaptic impairment of neuromuscular transmission are not constant. Decrement studies may reveal decrement, decrement-increment or abnormal increment. Single fibre EMG is likely to be more sensitive, but further prospective studies are required to see if single fibre EMG changes are constant and/or specific.

6.8. Future Studies

The clinical recognition of the IMS is no longer problematic for most medical workers in the field, and considerable progress towards the elucidation of the underlying mechanisms has been made in the past 10 years. A number of pertinent questions remain unanswered. Most importantly, why do not all patients with a similar degree of anticholinesterase poisoning develop IMS? Which are the precise pre- and post-synaptic factors that reduce the safety factor of neuromuscular transmission? Do these factors change over time? Does post-synaptic membrane damage with decreased numbers or altered conformation of post-synaptic ACh receptors play a role? What are the microelectrophysiological characteristics of neuromuscular transmission in IMS patients?

Possible tools to solve these questions include studies in chronically poisoned rodents, with detailed morphological and electrophysiological studies on repeated muscle biopsies in the same animal. The morphological studies should include estimations of the number of ACh receptor sites by quantitative electron microscopy and immunocytochemistry at the light and electron microscopic level, as well as the measurement of the number of ^{125}I-labelled alpha-bungarotoxin binding sites. EMG studies, including decrement studies at various frequencies of stimulation and single fibre EMG, should be complemented and correlated with *in vitro* electrophysiology studies on the same biopsy tissue. The latter should combine conventional microelectrode studies to determine miniature endplate potential (MEPP), miniature endplate current (MEPC), and evoked quantal release, with noise analysis and preferably also single-channel patch-clamp recordings. Identical studies could be done on endplate-rich intercostal muscle biopsies of IMS patients. Ethical and practical considerations then come into play.

The precise incidence of the IMS, and the relative incidence of IMS with different OP agents are unknown. All studies are case reports or suffer from a number of other biases. Prospective studies are needed to avoid a number of biases inherent to case reports.

Finally, the possible role of therapeutic interventions is unclear. Is the IMS an artefact of insufficient oxime therapy, as suggested by Benson *et al.* (1992). Should early, continuous high-dose oxime administration be the standard ? (Besser *et al.*, 1995; Willems *et al.,* 1992; Tush and Anstead, 1997; Thiermann *et al.,* 1999)

References

Abou-Donia M.B., Lapadula D.M. Mechanisms of organophosphorous ester-induced delayed neurotoxicity: type I and type II. *Annual Review of Phamacology and Toxicology* 1990;**30**:405–40.

Ariëns A.T., Meeter E., Wolthuis O.L., *et al.* Reversible necrosis at the end-plate region in striated muscles of the rat poisoned with cholinesterase inhibitors. *Experimentia* 1969;**25**:57–9.

Baker, D., Sedgwick M.E. Single fibre electromyographic changes in man after organophosphate exposure. *Human and Experimental Toxicology* 1996;**15**:369–75.

Benson, B., Tolo, D., McIntire, M. Is the intermediate symdrome in organophosphate poisoning the result of insufficient oxime therapy. *Journal of Toxicology Clinical Toxicology* 1992;**30**:347–9.

Berrosian, A., Balla, M., Kafiri, G., *et al.* Multiple systems organ failure from organophosphate poisoning. *Journal of Toxicology Clinical Toxicology* 1995;**33**:257–60.

Besser, R, Weilemann, L.S., Gutmann, L. Efficacy of obidoxime in human organophosphorous poisoning: determination by neuromuscular transmission studies. *Muscle Nerve* 1995;**18**:15–22.

Besser, R., Gutmann, L., Dillmann, U., *et al.* End-plate dysfunction in acute organophosphate intoxication. *Neurology* 1989a;**39**:561–7.

Besser, R., Gutmann, L., Weilemann L.S. Inactivation of end-plate acetylcholinesterase during the course of organophosphate intoxications. *Archives of Toxicology* 1989b;**63**:412–5.

Besser, R., Vogt, T., Gutmann, L., *et al.* Impaired neuromuscular transmission during partial inhibition of acetylcholinesterase: the role of stimulus induced antidromic backfiring in the generation of the decrement increment phenomenon. *Muscle Nerve* 1992;**15**:1072–80.

Bowman W. C., Gibb A. S., Harvey A. C., *et al.* New neuromuscular blocking agents. In: *Handbook of Experimental Pharmacology.* Kharkevich D.A., ed. Springer–Verlag; Berlin, Heidelberg, New York. 1986. p. 141–70

Choi, P-L., Quinonez, L., Cook, D.J., *et al.* The use of glycopyrrolate in a case of intermediate syndrome following acute organophosphate poisoning *Canadian Journal of Anaesthesia* 1998;**45**:337–40.

Clarmann, M., Geldmacher-von Mallinckrodt, M. Über eine erfolgreich behandelte akute orale Vergiftung durch Fenthion und desson Nachweis in Mageninhalt und Harn. *Archiv Für Toxikologie* 1966;**22**:2–11.

Davies, J. E. *et al.* Human pesticide poisonings by a fat-soluble organophosphate insecticide. *Archives of Environmental Health* 1975;**30**:608–13.

De Bleecker, J.L., De Reuck, J.L., Willems, J.L. Neurological aspects of organophosphate poisoning. *Clinical Neurology Neurosurgery* 1992;**94**:93–103.

De Bleecker, J.L., Vogelaers, D., Ceuterick, C. et al. Intermediate syndrome due to prolonged parathion poisoning. *Acta Neurologica Scandinavica* 1992b;**86**:421–4.

De Bleecker, J.L., Lison. D., Van Den Abeele, K. et al. Acute and subacute organophosphate poisoning in the rat. *Neurotoxicology* 1994;**15**:341–8.

De Bleecker, J.L., Meire, V.I., Pappens, S. Quinidine prevents paraoxon-induced necrotizing myopathy in rats. *Neurotoxicology* 1998;**19**:833–8.

De Bleecker, J.L., Van Den Abeele, K.G., De Reuck, J.L. Variable involvement of rat skeletal muscles in paraoxon-induced necrotizing myopathy. *Research Commununications in Chemical Pathology and Pharmacology* 1992a;**75**:309–22.

De Bleecker, J.L., Van Den Abeele, K.G., De Reuck, J.L. Electromyography in relation to end-plate acetylcholinesterase in rats poisoned by different organophosphates. *Neurotoxicology* 1994;**15**:331–40.

De Bleecker, J.L., Van Den Neucker, K., Colardyn, F. Intermediate syndrome in organophosphorous poisoning: a prospective study. *Critical Care Medicine* 1993;**21**:1706–11.

De Bleecker, J.L., Van Den Neucker, K., Willems, J.L. The intermediate syndrome in organophosphate poisoning: presentation of a case and review of the literature. *Journal of Toxicology Clinical Toxicology* 1992;**30**:321–9.

De Bleecker, J.L., Willems, J., De Reuck, J.L. et al. Histological and histochemical study of paraoxon-induced myopathy in the rat. *Acta Neurologica Belgica* 1991;**91**:255–70.

De Bleecker, J.L., Willems, J., Van Den Neucker, K., *et al.* Prolonged toxicity with intermediate syndrome after combined parathion and methyl-parathion poisoning. *Journal of Toxicology Clinical Toxicology* 1992a;**30**:333–45.

De Reuck J.L., Willems J.L. Acute parathion poisoning: myopathic changes in the diaphragm. *Journal of Neurology* 1975;**208**:309–14.

De Wilde, V., Vogelaers, D., Colardyn, F., *et al.* Post-synaptic neuromuscular dysfunction in organophosphate induced neuromuscular syndrome. *Klinische Wochenschrift* 1991;**69**:177–83.

Dean G., Coxon, J., Brereton, D. Poisoning by an organophosphorous compound; a case report. *South African Medical Journal* 1967;**41**:1017–9.

Dettbarn, W-D. Pesticide induced muscle necrosis: mechanisms and prevention. *Fundamental and Applied Toxicology* 1984;**4**:518–26.

Dongren Y., Tao L., Fengsheng H. Electroneurophysiological studies in rats of acute dimethoate poisoning. *Toxicology Letters* 1999;**107**:249–54.

Engel, A.G., Lambert E. H., Gomez M. R. A new myasthenic syndrome with end-plate acetylcholinesterase deficiency, small nerve terminals, and reduced acetylcholine release. *Annals of Neurology* 1977;**1**:315–30.

Gadoth, N., Fisher, A. Late onset of neuromuscular block in organophosphorous poisoning. *Annals of Internal Medicine* 1978;**88**:654–5.

Grob D. Anticholinesterase intoxication in man and its treatment. In: *Cholinesterases and Anticholinesterase Agents.* Koelle, G.B. ed. Springer–Verlag; Berlin: (Gottingen, Heidelberg, 1963). p. 989–1027.

He, F., Xu, H., Qin, F., *et al.* Intermediate myasthenia syndrome following acute organophosphate poisoning-an analysis of 21 cases. *Human and Experimental Toxicology* 1998;**17**:4045.

Inns, R.H., Tuckwell, N.J., Bright, J.E., *et al.* Histochemical demonstration of calcium accumulation in muscle fibres after experimental organophosphate poisoning. *Human and Experimental Toxicology* 1990;**9**:245–50.

Johnson, M.K. The delayed neuropathy caused by some organophosphorous esters: mechanism and challenge. *Critical Reviews of Toxicology* 1975;**3**:289–316.

Karademir M., Ertürk F., Koçak R. Two cases of organophosphate poisoning with development of intermediate syndrome. *Human and Experimental Toxicology* 1990;**9**:187–9.

Karalliedde, L., Senanayake, N., Ariaratnam, A. Acute organophosphorous insecticde poisoning during pregnancy. *Human Toxicology* 1988;**7**:363–4.

Mahieu, P., Hassoun, A., Van Binst, R., *et al.* Severe and prolonged poisoning by fenthion: significance of the determination of the anticholinesterase capacity of plasma. *Journal of Toxicology Clinical Toxicology* 1982;**19**:425–32.

Marrs, T.C. Organophosphate poisoning. *Pharmacology and Therapeutics* 1993;**58**:51–66

Molphy, R., Rathus, E.M. Organic phosphorous. *Medical Journal of Australia* 1964;**2**:337–40.

Nisse, P., Forceville, X., Cezard, C., *et al.* Intermediate syndrome with delayed distal polyneuropathy from ethyl parathion poisoning. *Veterinary and Human Toxicology* 1998;**40**:349–51

Norman J. In: *A textbook of Anaesthesia.* Aitkenhead A.R., Smith, G. eds.:Churchill Livingstone; London 1990. p. 211–24

Ohno, K., Brengman, J.M., Tsujino, A., *et al.* Human end-plate acetylcholinesterase deficiency caused by mutations in the collagen-like tail subunit (Col Q) of the asymmetric enzyme. *Proceedings National Academy of Sciences* 1998;**95**:9654–9.

Perron, R., Johnson, B.B. Insecticide poisoning. *New England Journal of Medicine* 1969;**281**:274–5.

Sedgwick, M.F., Senanayake, N. Pathophysiology of the intermediate syndrome of organophosphorous poisoning. *Journal of Neurology, Neurosurgery and Psychiatry* 1997;**62**:201–2.

Senanayake, N., Karalliedde, L. Neurotoxic effects of organophosphorous insecticides: an intermediate syndrome. *New England Journal of Medicine* 1987;**316**:761–3.

Singh, G., Mahanjan, R., Whig, J. The importance of electrodiagnostic studies in acute organophosphate poisoning. *Journal of Neurological Science* 1998;**157**:191–200.

Sudakin, D.L., Mullins, M.E., Horowitz, B.Z., *et al.* Intermediate syndrome after malathion ingestion despite continuous infusion of pralidoxime. *Journal of Toxicology Clinical Toxicology* 2000;**38**:47–50

Tattersall, J.E.H. Effects of organophosphorous anticholinesterases on nicotinic receptor ion channels at adult mouse end-plates. *British Journal of Pharmacology* 1990;**101**:349–57

Thiermann, H., Szinicz, L., Eyer, F. Modern strategies in therapy of organophosphate poisoning. *Toxicology Letters* 1999;**107**:233–9.

Tush, G., Anstead, M. Pralidoxime continuous infusion in the treatment of organophosphate poisoning. *Annals of Pharmacotherapy* 1997;**31**:441–4.

Van Dijk, J.G., Lammers, G.J., Wintzen, A.R., *et al.* Repetition CMAPs: mechanisms of neural and synaptic genesis. *Muscle Nerve* 1996;**19**:1127–33.

Wadia, R.S., Sadagopan, C., Amin, R.B., *et al.* Neurological manifestations of organophosphate insecticide poisoning. *Journal of Neurology, Neurosurgery and Psychiatry* 1974;**37**:841–7.

Wecker, L., Mrak, R.E., Dettbarn, W. Evidence of necrosis in human intercostal muscle following inhalation of an organophosphate insecticide. *Fundamental and Applied Toxicology* 1986;**6**:172–4.

Willems, J.L., Langenberg J.P., Verstraete A.G., *et al.* Plasma concentrations of pralidoxime methylsulphate in organophosphorous poisoned patients. *Archives of Toxicology* 1992;**66**:260–6.

CHAPTER 7

Organophosphorus-Induced Delayed Polyneuropathy

Nimal Senanayake

7.1. Introduction

The earliest reports of paralysis due to organophosphorus (OP) intoxication were in the late 1880s, when patients with tuberculosis were treated with phospho-creosote, a mixture of esters derived from phosphoric acid and coal-tar phenols (Lorot, 1899). Awareness of this condition became widespread after the massive epidemic in the United States in the 1930s, during the days of the prohibition. The poisoning was caused by the consumption of a popular substitute for alcohol called *Ginger jake.* This ginger extract was diluted with *Lindol,* which consisted mainly of tri-orthocresyl phosphate (TOCP), drunk neat or used to flavour illicitly distilled liquors (Smith *et al.,* 1930). As many as 20,000 people were paralysed (Kidd and Langworthy, 1933).

Several more outbreaks of neuropathy were reported in the 1930s and 1940s from other parts of the world. An abortifacient known as *Apiol,* which contained TOCP, affected 60 European women (Cavanagh, 1964a). In South Africa, about 60 people developed paralysis after using contaminated cooking oil, which had been stored in drums previously used for storing lubricating oil containing TOCP (Sampson, 1942). In a unit of the Swiss army, 80 men were affected when machine-gun oil accidentally contaminated cooking oil (Cavanagh, 1964a).

Three men working at a TOCP manufacturing plant developed paralysis following exposure to toxic vapour (Hunter *et al.,* 1944). Two outbreaks occurred in the 1950s, one affecting 11 South Africans who drank contaminated water from a drum taken from a paint factory where it had been used to store TOCP (Susser and Stein, 1957), and the other involving some 10,000 people in Morocco who consumed cooking oil adulterated with jet-airplane lubricating oil (Smith and Spalding, 1959). More recent outbreaks include those reported from India (Vora, 1962; Mehta, 1975) and elsewhere (Inoue *et al.,* 1988).

TOCP and TCP are widely used industrial chemicals found in organic solvents a lubricating oils. In all these epidemics, the exposure had been by way contamination food, edible oils, drinks or water.

During 1977–78, we investigated an epidemic of acute polyneuropathy, whi occurred in the central tea plantation area of Sri Lanka, affecting 20 Tamil girls menarche. The toxic agent was tri-cresyl phosphate (TCP), found as a contaminant gingili oil, the contamination presumably having occurred during transport of the oil containers previously used for storing mineral oils. Gingili (jinjili, ginelly) oil, which an extract of the seeds from a kind of sesame plant, is a cooking oil used commonly the Tamils. Because of its presumed nutritive value, the raw oil is given in lar quantities to girls as a special diet during the immediate post-menarche period. Th strange custom was responsible for the selective affliction of the adolescent Tamil gir in this epidemic (Senanayake and Jeyaratnam, 1981; Senanayake, 1981).

OP insecticides (OPI) producing polyneuropathy and paralysis had bee documented from 1950 to 1980 in occasional patients exposed to mipafox, leptopho trichlorfon (Chlorophos or Dipterex), and trichloronate (Phytosol) (Bidstrup *et al.* 195 Hierons and Johnson, 1978; Jedrzejowsksa *et al.,* 1980). In 1982, we reported isolated cases of polyneuropathy seen over 3 years in Sri Lanka, following exposure methamidophos (Senanayake and Johnson, 1982). Since then, more case have bee reported from Sri Lanka (Senanayake, 1985; 1990) and elsewhere (Shiraishi *et al.,* 198 Vasilescu *et al.,* 1984; Wadia *et al.,* 1985; Csik *et al.,* 1986; Capodicasa *et al.,* 199 Komori *et al.,* 1991).

Polyneuropathy has now been recognised as a distinct manifestation of toxicity both non-insecticidal and some insecticidal OP, and named organophosphorus-induc delayed polyneuropathy or neuropathy (OPIDP or OPIDN) (Lotti *et al.,* 1984).

7.2. Epidemiology

Quantitative data about the frequency of OPIDP after OP poisoning are not readi available. In China, where methamidophos is responsible for half of pestici intoxications and fatality, a follow up study of 104 patients has identified 14 cases OPIDP, giving a frequency of 13.5%.

The risk of OPIDP was associated with the severity of intoxication. All cases of OPIDP recovered in one and half year without permanent disability. No association was found between the frequency of OPIDP and age, sex, or treatment with dexamethasone during the acute phase of poisoning (Sun *et al.*, 1998).

7.3. Clinical features

Symptoms of OPIDP begin about 1 to 3 weeks after acute exposure, and after a more uncertain interval following chronic exposure. The delay between exposure and onset of symptoms depends, in part, on the dose and the nature of the exposure. The neuropathy due to OPIDP generally manifests after a delay following the acute cholinergic symptoms. In the case of TOCP or TCP, there is no distinct acute cholinergic phase, but the patient may experience some gastrointestinal distress with nausea, vomiting, and diarrhoea, lasting a few hours to a few days, shortly after ingestion of the poison. Cramping muscle pain in the legs is the usual initial complaint of OPIDP, sometimes followed by numbness and paraesthesiae in the distal parts of the limbs. Acute weakness of the feet and legs then occurs, followed by weakness of the hands and forearms. Sensory loss develops sometimes, initially in the feet and then in the hands, but it is often mild or inconspicuous.

Physical examination shows a predominantly motor polyneuropathy, with flaccid weakness of distal muscles, especially in the legs. This is of variable severity, but most patients develop foot- and wrist-drop. The weakness is usually symmetrical, but we have noticed asymmetrical weakness, the dominant hand being worse affected.

The reason for the asymmetry has not been established, but a likely explanation is that muscular exercise at the onset of the neuropathy aggravates the subsequent muscle weakness. After a few weeks, the affected parts may show muscle wasting and deformities, such as wasting of small muscles and clawing of hands. The tendon reflexes are reduced or lost, absent ankle reflex being a constant feature. Objective sensory impairment is usually slight or absent, and when present, is of glove-and-stocking distribution, characteristic of polyneuropathy.

Mild pyramidal signs may be found after a few weeks, manifesting as mild spasticity of legs and exaggerated knee reflexes. With time, the pyramidal and other central nervous system signs become more evident. The degree of pyramidal involvement may determine the ultimate prognosis for functional recovery.

Electrophysiological tests reveal partial denervation of the affected muscles, with increased insertional activity, abnormal spontaneous activity (fibrillation potentials and positive sharp waves), and a reduced interference pattern. Large polyphasic motor unit potentials may also be found after a few weeks. The compound muscle action potentials to supramaximal stimulation of motor nerves are reduced in amplitude, and the terminal motor latencies are delayed. The maximal motor conduction velocity is usually normal or only slightly reduced.

Exclusively sensory neuropathy in eight patients after repeated unquantified exposures to chlorpyrifos spray, which did not cause clear-cut cholinergic symptoms has recently been reported (Kaplan, 1993). Moretto and Lotti (1998) have questioned whether OP poisoning was responsible for these cases. They studied 11 patients after acute OP poisoning among which two were poisoned with chlorpyrifos. Three patients developed OPIDP, including one poisoned by chlorpyrifos. A mild sensory component was associated with a severe motor component in two of the three cases, the other was an exclusively motor polyneuropathy. Pure sensory neuropathy was never seen after either single or repeated acute OP poisoning.

7.4. Diagnosis

The diagnosis is basically clinical. Measurement of serum or red cell cholinesterase activity is unlikely to be of help even in the case of compounds which are active inhibitors of this enzyme, because the enzyme activity could have recovered by the time the neuropathy develops.

Acute, distal, purely or predominantly motor polyneuropathy following recent exposure to a neurotoxic OP compound is diagnostic of OPIDP. When the exposure to OP is denied or unavailable, an inexperienced clinician may confuse the condition for acute infective polyneuritis or Guillain–Barré syndrome (GBS).

But, the weakness of limbs in GBS is more generalised or more proximal in contrast the very focal, distal weakness in OPIDP. Other features of GBS, such as unilateral bilateral facial weakness, bulbar involvement and respiratory paralysis are absent in PIDP.

The intermediate syndrome described by us is a state of muscle paralysis, which has much earlier onset following OP poisoning, but it is unlikely to cause confusion in agnosis because the clinical features of the two conditions are very distinct (Table 7.1.) enanayake and Karalliedde, 1987).

Table 7.1. Comparison of OPIDP with the intermediate syndrome

Variable	Intermediate Syndrome	Delayed Neuropathy
me of onset, after isoning	1–4 Days	2–3 Wk
tes of weakness		
Limb muscles	Proximal	Distal
Neck muscles	+	-
Cranial nerves	+	-
Respiratory muscles	+	-
ectromyogram	Tetanic fade	Denervation
ecovery, from time of onset	4–18 Days	6–12 Mo
rganophosphorous agents commonly involved	Fenthion Dimethoate Monocrotophos	Methamidophos Trichlorphon Leptophos

eproduced with the permission of Senanayake N, Karalliedde L. (1987) and the publishers. Neurotoxic ects of organophosphate insecticides: an intermediate syndrome. N Engl J Med 316:761–3)

5. Treatment

ysiotherapy, passive in the initial stages and active subsequently, is the cornerstone of eatment.

There is no specific drug for the treatment or the prevention of OPIDP. Several adrenocortical steroids, calcium-channel blockers, and gangliosides have been used in animal experiments and clinical studies as potential therapeutic agents, but no convincing benefits have been established.

7.6. Prognosis

Recovery from OPIDP is considered poor, mainly because of central long-tract involvement. Eleven survivors of the Ginger Jake epidemic, at a 47-year follow-up, still showed the spasticity and abnormal reflexes of an upper motor neuron syndrome (Morgan and Penovich, 1978). In the Moroccan outbreak, only 10% of the patients recovered completely (Smith and Spalding, 1959). Our experience, however, is rather different. All the patients in the gingili oil outbreak, seen one year after poisoning, were asymptomatic, despite complete paralysis of some of the muscle groups during the early phase. The young age of the patients, the difference in the chemical structure of the cresyl phosphate, and the duration of initial intoxication, in addition to the relatively mild pyramidal tract involvement, probably contributed to the favourable outcome (Senanayake, 1981). Patients who developed polyneuropathy after OPIDP poisoning, in our experience, have also made a good functional recovery at review 1 to 2 years after poisoning.

7.7. Recurrent Laryngeal Palsy

Recurrent laryngeal nerve (RLN) paralysis due to OPs has been described in animals. In Sri Lanka, we observed three patients who, 25 to 35 days after poisoning, developed isolated bilateral RLN palsy (de Silva et al., 1994). After successful treatment of the acute cholinergic crisis with atropine and pralidoxime, all three of them developed IMS requiring endotracheal intubation and intermittent positive pressure ventilation. They recovered, and two of them left hospital asymptomatic, 3 and 4 days after extubation. The other patient remained in hospital for the treatment of pressure-sores. But, none of them had difficulty in breathing or hoarseness at this stage.

Fourteen to 26 days after extubation (25 to 35 days after ingesting OP), the patients eveloped symptoms suggestive of laryngeal dysfunction. Two of them presented with tridor, and the other developed aphonia. Laryngoscopy showed bilateral vocal cord aralysis in all three of them. The cords were fully adducted in the two patients with stridor, nd partially adducted in the other patient. There were no local lesions in the larynx. The ervous system was otherwise normal, in particular, there was no clinical or lectropysiological evidence of polyneuropathy.

One of the two patients who developed stridor became cyanosed requiring racheostomy. The other two received conservative treatment. All three patients recovered 4 ɔ 15 weeks after the onset of the laryngeal symptoms.

The OPs, which caused poisoning in these patients—chlorpyriphos, parathion and ɪethamidophos, are known to have delayed neurotoxic properties in man. The delay of 25 ɔ 35 days from the poisoning to the onset of the laryngeal symptoms corresponds with the ɪme delay to develop OPIDP. As such, we believe that the mechanism of delayed RLN ɪalsy in our patients was similar to that of OPIDP.

ˈ.8. Neuropathology

ꓱeuropathological data of OPIDP come mainly from animal studies. The disease has ɪeen reproduced in a number of species, the hen (female of *Gallus gallus domesticus*), lassically, being the species of choice. Generally, the young of a species is resistant to ingle, but not repeated, doses of neurotoxic OPs (Johnson and Barnes, 1970). Adult rats ɪnd guinea pigs are also affected only by repeated dosing.

The morphological pattern of OPIDP consists of symmetrical, distal axonal ꓲegeneration of ascending and descending nerve tracts located both in the central and ɪeripheral nervous systems. Primarily, long, large diameter fibres are affected ꓚavanagh, 1954 and 1964a; Bischoff, 1967 and 1970; Prineas, 1969). In the peripheral ꓲervous system, the longer nerve fibres to the hindlimbs undergo axonal degeneration ɪefore the shorter fibres to the forelimbs. Concurrently, the long spinal cord tracts, such ᴸs the dorsal columns, the corticospinal pathways, and the spinocerebellar tracts, show ꓲistal axonal degeneration. The degenerative change appears to move in a retrograde ꓲanner, the neuronal damage increasing in severity from proximal to distal.

The vulnerability of nerve fibres is directly related to axonal length and diameter large-diameter and long fibres being more susceptible than small and short fibres. Thi pathological process was earlier referred to as the "dying back" phenomenon (Cavanagh 1964b and 1979), but now the preferred term is central-peripheral distal axonopathy.

7.9. Pathogenesis

The pathogenesis of OPIDP is independent of the ability of OPs to inhibit acety cholinesterase (AChE), but related to a different enzyme system in the nervous tissu called the neuropathy target esterase (NTE) (formerly, neurotoxic esterase). The identification of NTE and subsequent studies of molecular changes induced b; neuropathic OPs date back to the 1960s (Johnson, 1969a, 1969b and 1970). Since then NTE has been and is still being monitored routinely to assess neuropathic potential o OPs as well as to perform mechanistic studies on OPIDP. The concept of NTE has also been challenged (Abou-Donia, 1981; Carrington, 1989), but most objections have bee considered to have little validity (Johnson, 1990).

Measurement of NTE activity soon after dosing enables a quantitative assessment o the neuropathic potential of OPs. The grading of NTE and AChE inhibition after OPs together with clinical and neuropathological evaluation, allows a more precis assessment of OPIDP.

Following the detection of NTE in lymphatic tissues, initially in the hen, th measurement of NTE in circulating lymphocytes has been employed for monitorin; OPIDP. Lymphocytic NTE has also been characterised in human lymphocytes an platelets. NTE inhibition in lymphatic and neural tissues has been found to correspond even though a good correlation is evident only 24 hr after dosing. Lymphocytic NTE ha been employed as a biomonitor of OPIDP in man, after acute poisoning and also durin; occupational exposures. A better understanding of the pathogenesis of OPIDP wil enable the more precise use of these tests, and perhaps the discovery of others (Lott 1992).

Certain esterase inhibitors (OPs, organophosphinates, sulfonyl halides, carbamate and thiocarbamates) exacerbate the clinical and morphological expression of toxic an traumatic axonopathies, and this phenomenon is referred to as "promotion".

This is believed to interfere with mechanisms of compensation or repair of the ͺes. The target of promotion is unknown, but there are indications that it might be ͺlar and/or linked to NTE. OPIDP is the model axonopathy used to characterise ͺnotion. Identification and characterisation of the target of promotion might be ͺful in understanding the mechanism(s) of compensation and repair of the peripheral ͺous system (Moretto, 2000).

ͺendix

proposed mechanism of pathogenesis is a two-step process: progressive inhibition of ͺ by neuropathic OPs (certain phosphates, phosphonates, and phosphoramidates) and ͺng of the phosphorylated enzyme. Ageing involves the loss of an alkyl or aryl group in ͺcovalently bound moiety of the inhibited NTE, leaving a negatively charged group. ͺen more than 70% of NTE is modified by this process, neuropathy develops a few ͺks later. Other chemicals (some carbamates, phosphinates and sulfonyl halides) ͺducing an inhibited NTE, which is incapable of ageing, were thought to be not ͺropathic. When given before a challenging dose of a neuropathic OP, they protect ͺnals from neuropathy. The ability to form ageable inhibited NTE was thought to ͺerentiate between neuropathic and protective inhibitors of NTE. Less NTE inhibition ͺained by protective inhibitors (30–40%) before challenging doses of neuropathic OPs ͺelated with protection from OPIDP (Johnson, 1990; Lotti, 1992).

Clinical outcomes correlate with these changes in spinal cord and peripheral nerve ͺ (Lotti *et al.,* 1987; Moretto *et al.,* 1989). Recent evidence indicates that ageing ͺ not always be essential in causing neuropathy. Mipafox and methamidophos as well ͺertain classic protective inhibitors such as carbamate and sulfonyl fluoride form an ͺibited NTE, which apparently does not age and yet produces neuropathy. It has now ͺn proposed that all NTE inhibitors may have the potential to cause neuropathy (Lotti ͺ*l.,* 1993).

In analogy with pharmacological models of drug-receptor interactions, NTE inhibitors ͺht have variable intrinsic activities to initiate neuropathy once attached to the protein. ͺng neuropathic chemicals require about 70% inhibition of NTE, others 80–90%, and the ͺ potent almost 100%.

Protection from OPIDP by the least neuropathic inhibitors can be explained by their weak intrinsic activity. Occupying recognition sites on NTE, they prevent the binding of more neuropathic compounds. Methamidophos represents a particular example because it is protective at lower doses and neuropathic at high doses (Lotti et al., 1993).

Because of the structural similarity to TOCP, concern has been raised about the neuropathic potential of triaryl phosphates, which have been widely used in commerce for over 30 years as flame retardents in fluids and plastics. Johnson (1975a and 1975b) found that certain structural features are required for a triaryl phosphate to react with NTE in manner to induce OPIDP.

Animal studies fail to demonstrate a potential to elicit OPIDP by products, such as triphenyl phosphate and butylated triaryl phosphates, after a single dose. Studies on the mixed isopropyl phenyl phopshates indicate that, while some are neurotoxic, they are much less potent than TCP and TOCP in the induction of OPIDP. Most commercial isopropylated triaryl phosphates lack the potential to induce acute OPIDP using a limit dose of 2000mg/kg. Recent advances in the synthesis of commercial TCP have resulted in products with reduced neurotoxic potential. These data are indicative of the safety of these aviation lubricants at levels currently employed (Weiner et al., 1999)

Little is known about the cascade of biochemical and physiological events, which follow NTE inhibition and precede the clinical and morphological expression of OPIDP. Retrograde axonal transport is selectively affected, but the relationship between effect on NTE, reduction of retrograde axonal transport, accumulation of NTE in distal parts of nerves, and expression of OPIDP is unknown (Lotti, 1992).

NTE is an integral membrane protein present in all neurons and in some non-neural-cell types of vertebrates. Recent data indicate that NTE is involved in a cell-signalling pathway controlling interactions between neurons and accessory glial cells in the developing nervous system. NTE has serine esterase activity. It efficiently catalyses the hydrolysis of phenyl valerate in vitro, but its physiological substrate is unknown. NTE comprises at least two functional domains: an N-terminal putative regulatory domain and a C-terminal effector domain which contains the esterase activity and is, in part, conserved in proteins found in bacteria, yeast, nematodes and insects. NTE's esterase activity appears to be largely redundant in adult vertebrates, but OPs which react with NTE in vivo initiate unknown events which lead, after a delay of 1–3 weeks, to a neuropathy with degeneration of long axons.

These neuropathic OPs leave a negatively charged group covalently attached to the active-site serine residue, and it is suggested that this may cause a toxic gain of function in NTE (Glynn, 1999).

References

Abou-Donia, M.B. Organophosphorus ester-induced delayed neurotoxicity. *Annual Review of Pharmacology and Toxicology* 1981;**21**:511–48.

Bidstrup P.L., Bonnell J.A., Beckett A.G. Paralysis following poisoning by a new organic phosphorus insecticide (mipafox). *British Medical Journal* 1953;**i**:1068–72.

Bischoff, A. The ultrastncture of tri-ortho-cresyl phosphate poisoning; I. Studies on myelin and axonal alterations in the sciatic nerve. *Acta Neuropathologica* 1967;**9**:158.

Bischoff, A. The ultrastructure of tri-ortho-cresyl phosphate poisoning in the chicken; II. Studies on spinal cord alterations. *Acta Neuropathologica* 1970;**15**:142.

Capodicasa, E., Scapellato, M.L., Moretto, A., *et al.* Chlorpyrifos-induced delayed polyneuropathy, *Archives of Toxicology* 1991;**65**:150.

Carrington, C.D. Prophylaxis and the mechanism for the initiation of organophosphorus compound-induced delayed neurotoxieity. *Archives of Toxicology* 1989;**63**:165–72.

Cavanagh, J.B. The toxic effect of tri-ortho-cresyl phosphate on the nervous system. *Journal of Neurology, Neurosurgery and Psychiatry* 1954;**17**:163.

Cavanagh, J.B. Peripheral nerve changes in *ortho*-cresyl phosphate poisoning in the cat. *Journal of Pathology and Bacteriology* 1964;**87**:365.

Cavanagh, J.B. The significance of the "dying back" process in experimental and human neurological disease. *International Review of Experimental Pathology* 1964;**3**:219–67.

Cavanagh, J.B. The "dying back" process: a common denominator in many naturally occurring and toxic neuropathies. *Archives of Pathology and Laboratory Medicines* 1979;**103**:659–64

Csik, V., Motika, D., Marosi, G.Y. Delayed neuropathy after trichlorfon intoxication, *Journal Neurology, Neurosurgery and Psychiatry* 1986;**49**:222.

de Silva, H.J., Sanmuganathan, P.S., Senanayake, N. Isolated bilateral recurrent laryngeal nerve paralysis: a delayed complication of organophosphorus poisoning. *Human and Experimental Toxicology* 1994;**13**:171–3

Glynn, P. Neuropathy target esterase. *Biochemical Journal* 1999;**344**:625–31

Hierons, R., Johnson, M.K. Clinical and toxicological investigations of a case of delayed neurophathy in man after acute poisoning by an organophosphorus pesticide. *Archives of Toxicology* 1978;**40**:279–84.

Hunter, D., Perry, K.M.A., Evan, R.B. Toxic polyneuritis arising during manufacture of tricresyl phosphate. *British Journal of Industrial Medicine* 1944;**1**:227.

Inoue, N., Fujishiro, K., Mori, K., *et al.* Triorthocresyl phosphate poisoning—a review of human cases. *Sangyo Ika Daigaku Zasshi* 1988;**10**:433–42

Jedrzejowsksa, H., Rowinska-Marcinska, K., Hoppe, B. Neuropathy due to phytosol (Agritox): Report of a case. *Acta Neuropathologica* 1980;**49**:163–8.

Johnson, M.K., Barnes, J.M. Age and the sensitivity of chicks to the delayed neurotoxic effects of some organophosphorus compounds. *Biochemical Pharmacology* 1970;**19**:3045.

Johnson, M.K. A phosphorylation site in brain and the delayed neurotoxic effect of some organophosphorous compounds. *Biochemical Journal* 1969a;**111**:487–95

Johnson, M.K. The delayed neurotoxic effect of some organophosphorus compounds. *Biochemical Journal* 1969b;**114**:711–7

Johnson, M.K. Organophosphorus and other inhibitors of brain "neurotoxic esterase" and the development of delayed neuropathy in hens, *Biochemical Journal* 1970;**120**:523–31

Johnson, M.K. Organophosphorus esters causing delayed neurotoxic effects. *Archives of Toxicology* 1975a;**34**:259–88

Johnson, M.K. The delayed neuropathy caused by some organophosphorus esters: mechanism and challenge. *CRC Critical Reviews in Toxicology* 1975b;**3**:289

Johnson, M.K. Organophosphates and delayed neuropathy—Is NTE alive and well? *Toxicology and Applied. Pharmacology* 1990;102:385–99.

Kaplan, J.G., Kessler, J., Rosenberg, N., *et al.* Sensory neuropathy associated with Dursban (chlorpyrifos) exposure. *Neurology* 1993;**43**:2139–6

Kidd, J.O., Langworthy, O.R. Paralysis following the ingestion of Jamaica Ginger Extract adulterated with tri-ortho-cresyl phosphate. *Johns Hopkins Medical Journal* 1933;**52**:39.

Komori, T., Yamane, K., Nagayama, T., *et al*. [A case of delayed myeloneuropathy due to malathion intoxication]. *No to Shinkei Brain and Nerve*. 1991;**43**:969–74

Lorot, C. Les combinaisons de la creosote dans le traitement de la tuberculose pulmonaire, Thesis, Paris, 1899, cited by D. Hunter. In: *Industrial Toxicology*, Clarendon Press, Oxford; 1944

Lotti, M., Becker, C.E., Aminoff, M.J. Organophosphate polyneuropathy: pathogenesis and prevention. *Neurology* (Cleveland) 1984;**34**:658–62

Lotti, M., Moretto, A., Capodicasa, E., *et al*. Interactions between neuropathy target esterase and its inhibitors and the development of polyneuropathy. *Toxicology and Applied Pharmacology* 1993;122:165–71

Lotti, M., Caroldi, S., Moretto, A., *et al*. Central-peripheral delayed neuropathy caused by diisopropyl phosphorofluoridate(DFP): Segregation of peripheral nerve and spinal cord effects using biochemical, clinical and morphological criteria. *Toxicology and Applied Pharmacology* 1987;**88**:87–96.

Lotti, M. The pathogenesis of organophosphate polyneuropathy. *Critical Reviews in Toxicology* 1992;**21**:465–87.

Mehta, R.S., Dixit, I.P., Khakharia, S.J. Toxic neuropathy in Raipur due to triorthocresylphosphate (TOCP). *Journal of the Association of Physicians of India* 1975;**23**:133–8.

Moretto, A., Lotti, M. Poisoning by organophopshorus insecticides and sensory neuropathy. *Journal Neurology, Neurosurgery and Psychiatry* 1998;64(4):463–8

Moretto, A. Promoters and promotion of axonopathies. *Toxicology Letters* 2000;**112**:17–21

Moretto, A., Lotti, M., Spencer, P.S. *In vivo* and *in vitro* regional differential sensitivity of neuropathy target esterase to di-*n*-butyl-2,2 dichlorovinyl phosphate. *Archives of Toxicology* 1989;**63**:469–73.

Morgan, J.P., Penovich, P. Jamaica Ginger paralysis. *Archives of Neurology* 1978;**35**:530.

Prineas, J. The pathogenesis of dying-back polyneuropathies. Part 1. An ultrastructural study of experimental triorthocresyl phosphate intoxication in the cat. *Journal of Neuropathology and Experimental Neurology* 1969;**28**:571

Sampson, B.F. The strange Durban epidemic of 1937. *South African Medical Journal* 1942;**16**:1- 3

Senanayake, N. Tri-cresyl phosphate neuropathy in Sri Lanka: a clinical and neurophysiological study with a three year follow up. *Journal of Neurology, Neurosurgery and Psychiatry* 1981;**44**:775–80

Senanayake, N. Polyneuropathy following insecticide poisoning: a clinical and electrophysiological study. *Proceedings of the XIIIth World Congress of Neurology* 1985;**232 (Suppl.)**:203

Senanayake, N. Toxic polyneuropathies. *Ceylon Medical Journal* 1990;**35**:45–55

Senanayake, N. and Jeyaratnam, J. Toxic polyneuropathy due to gingili oil contaminated with tri-cresyl phosphate affecting adolescent girls in Sri Lanka *Lancet* 1981; i:88–89

Senanayake, N., Johnson, M.K. Acute polyneuropathy after poisoning by a new organophosphate insecticide. *New England Journal of Medicine* 1982;**306**:155–57

Senanayake, N., Karalliedde, L. Neurotoxic effects of organophosphate insecticides: an intermediate syndrome. *New England Journal of Medicine* 1987;**316**:761–3

Shiraishi, S., Inoue, N., Murai, Y., *et al*. Dipterex (trichlorfon) poisoning. Clinical and pathological studies in human and monkeys. *Sangyo Ika Daigaku Zashi* 1983:5:125–32.

Smith, H.V., Spalding, J.M.K. Outbreak of paralysis in Morocco due to ortho-cresyl phosphate. *Lancet* 1959;**ii**:1019–21

Smith, M.I., Elvove, E., Valaer, P.J., *et al*. Pharmacological and chemical studies of the cause of so-called ginger paralysis. *US Public Health Reports* 1930;**45**:1703

Sun, D.H., Zhou, H.D., Xue, S.Z. Epidemiologic survey on organophosphate-induced delayed polyneuropathy (OPIDP) among patients recovered from methamidophos poisoning. *Medicina del Lavoro* 1998;**89(Suppl** 2):S123–8.

Susser, M., Stein, Z. An outbreak of tri-ortho-cresyl phosphate (T.O.C.P.) poisoning in Durban. *British Journal of Industrial Medicine* 1957;**14**:111–20

Vasilescu, C., Alexianu, M., Dan, A. Delayed neuropathy after organophosphorus insecticide (Dipterex) poisoning: a clinical, electrophysiological and nerve biopsy study, *Journal of. Neurology,. Neurosurgery and. Psychiatry* 1984;**47**:543.

'ora, D.D., Dastur, D.K., Braganca, B.M., *et al.* Toxic polyneuritis in Bombay due to ortho-cresyl-phosphate poisoning. *Journal of Neurology, Neurosurgery and Psychiatry* 1962;**25**:234–42

Wadia, R.S., Shinde, S.N., Vaidya, S. Delayed neurotoxicity after an episode of poisoning with dichlorvos. *Neurology* (India) 1985;**33**:247

Weiner, M.L., Jortner, B.S. Organophosphate-induced delayed neurotoxicity of triarylphosphates. *Neurotoxicology* 1999;**20**:653–73.

CHAPTER 8

The Effects of Organophosphates on Neuropsychiatric and Psychological Functioning

Malcolm Lader

8.1. Introduction

Organophosphates (OPs) have widespread effects in the body. They pass easily into the brain so that central nervous system effects are quite marked, especially during acute exposure. Both acute and chronic exposure have been claimed to result in a variety of effects and these will be discussed in detail in this chapter. One difficulty preparing the information is that there are major methodological considerations to be taken into account, particularly with respect to the "softness" of psychiatric data, diagnosis and assessment.

The OPs are extensively used as pesticides in spraying crops and in dipping sheep. They act by inhibiting the enzyme cholinesterase, thereby enabling the accumulation of acetylcholine (ACh) in the synaptic cleft and neuromuscular junction. This prolongs the effects of ACh, an important neurotransmitter in the CNS, and gives rise to a multiplicity of symptoms, a wide range of toxic effects are readily induced with acute overdose. More controversial is the claim that continued or even intermittent low dose exposure can give rise to permanent changes in the CNS with associated psychiatric and neuropsychological deficits. Much public controversy has attended the use of sheep dips and other compounds. In some countries, the use of these dips is compulsory to protect sheep from a range of ectoparasites. Consequently any apparent toxicity can be blamed on the official agencies and the governments. As a result the link between exposure to OP pesticides and putative neurological and psychiatric damage has become an important scientific, political, and medico-legal issue (Dyer, 1997).

Another area in which these compounds are available is as so-called "nerve gases". These have been used in war on only limited occasions, but terrorist organisations have access to, and have used, these compounds, as in Japan. Many countries have tested these substances on human volunteers with particular reference to the effectiveness of possible protective measures such as the carbamates.

Claims have been made that these volunteers have suffered in a rather similar way to sheep dippers.

Before evaluating the fairly extensive literature on this topic, a critique of the techniques used to assess possible damage in those exposed to these substances will be presented. In particular, the limitations and vagaries of psychiatric diagnosis are emphasised. Furthermore, the implications of the difficulty of obtaining adequate control groups in most of these descriptive and epidemiological studies will be addressed.

8.2. Methodological Considerations

Another problem with the OPs, is that of developing an accurate index of exposure. These considerations, with respect to the central nervous system, are the same as those with other systems in the body and are dealt with elsewhere. An index of exposure might be developed by analysing hair samples (Tsatsakis et al., 1998). This technique has proven successful with respect to illicit drugs such as heroin. In many of the studies, to be outlined later, reports of psychiatric and psychological disturbances are often quite inadequate, frequently to the point of being uninformative or actually misleading. Phrases purporting to be diagnostic are dotted around in the literature, such as "anxiety and depression", "memory disturbance", and "CNS effects". Even allowing for the changes in psychiatric diagnoses over the past 30 years, many obsolescent diagnoses are still used such as "cerebral decline", "neurasthenia" and "neurotic symptoms". The use of standardised diagnostic instruments in these studies has only come about in the last few years. However, it is fair to point out that this only happened in mainstream psychiatry itself relatively recently. The use of diagnostic categories is helpful but does not of course address the issue of whether the OP compounds are associated with a characteristic syndrome or disorder, which has not yet been identified and categorised. Consequently, a symptomatic history may be necessary and that is more difficult to standardise. Nevertheless, it can be accomplished and personnel can be trained to administer standardised instruments to rate symptoms. The use of such interviewing techniques are not for the inexpert. For example, in the assessment of new therapeutic agents, proper training sessions, assessment of test, and re-test reliability, etc. are insisted on by the drug regulatory authorities. A similar level of rigour is necessary to assess people claiming deleterious effects from OP insecticide and other exposure.

The first step in such a proceeding should be a fairly open-ended interview in which as many symptoms as possible are carefully elicited by asking "neutral" questions. The use of trained interviewers is essential but these can be nursing staff or psychologists of fairly junior level, providing adequate training is given. Following the amassment of a whole range of symptoms, they should be factored in some standard way to develop a cluster of core symptoms, which may reasonably relate to that condition. A rating scale can then be drawn up listing these various core symptoms or syndromes with ratings of a) severity, b) chronicity and c) interference with functional activities at work, in the home, and in social relationships. Unfortunately, the characterisation of any such syndrome has not been attempted in any rigorous or systematic way. Various other approaches have been tried and will be dealt with later.

A further complication is the plethora of symptoms complained of by those exposed to these chemicals. Because of this, a wide range of symptoms have to be assessed and it is manifestly impossible to have just one discipline in medicine involved in this task. Nevertheless, with proper training a comprehensive battery of questions dealing with a variety of symptoms could be utilised.

The psychiatric sequelae to OPs and similar compounds can occur at the symptomatic, the syndromal or the disorder level. At the lowest level, many symptoms are exaggerations of the normal, giving rise to issues relating to the style of reporting of individuals, their proneness to developing physical symptoms and their reactions to stress. For example, anxiety is a ubiquitous emotion experienced by everyone. Many people know that they respond to stresses in their lives with anxiety, together with a range of physical symptoms such as palpitations and bowel upsets. However, they do not seek medical attention for these symptoms. Others, with perhaps less insight, become concerned at their physical symptoms and seek medical advice for what is still within normal physiological limits. Accordingly, some index of the "illness style" of the individual is also an useful part of the assessment.

Even neuropsychological testing with its apparent objectivity can give rise to problems. The tests used have usually been developed in another context; for example, traditional 10 tests have been criticised because of the heavy cultural bias which they contain. Other tests have been developed to address specific areas of brain damage and while they appear to be more relevant, they might miss a unique pattern of decrement in performance associated with OP exposure. A further complicating factor is the interaction of any psychiatric symptoms, such as anxiety and depression, with the test performance.

These symptoms are well-known to lower motivation, cause distraction and lessen attention and concentration. This in itself can give rise to impaired test performance almost across the whole range of testing. It is therefore important that independent measures of common symptoms of this type be obtained at the time of testing. The most careful neuropsychological experts routinely incorporate such tests into their battery. Careful double-blind assessments are essential (Mearns *et al.*, 1994).

The bodily symptoms induced by the OP insecticides can be primary or secondary. The primary symptoms are directly induced, for example, sweating or anorexia whereas secondary symptoms accompany central emotional states, for example, sweating as a symptom of indirectly produced anxiety or loss of appetite with the onset of a depressive disorder. Again, careful questioning is necessary to sort out the type of symptom pattern.

At the next level, the syndromal level, a recognisable constellation of symptoms and signs is encountered. For example, in acute poisoning, the syndrome of "delirium" is characterised by clouding of consciousness, disorientation in time and space, anxiety and agitation, and frightening visual hallucinations. A complicating factor is that there is usually partial or complete amnesia for the episode so retrospective questioning of the victim is of limited usefulness. Other syndromes which can be induced on a more chronic basis often comprise memory disturbances which can be subtle and localised. For example, it may affect short-term learning such as remembering a telephone number but not long-term recollection of childhood events. The memory deficits may be fairly circumscribed or part of a much wider dementia. The dementia itself may be intellectual, but also include many elements of emotional changes such as disinhibition in personality and irritability. The syndrome can merge into more obvious neurological conditions such as aphasia, apraxia, and agnosia. Executive functioning may be affected and this can result in difficulties in every day living.

Finally, at the disorder level, a range of conditions have been recognised much earlier. These are complex and relate to substance use. They are listed in Table 8.1. Note, however, that not all of these are encountered or claimed after OP exposure.

The range of neuropsychological tests is quite extensive. Examples of these are set out in Table 8.2., together with the psychological function which tests are believed to sample. This is a highly technical area and it is essential in studies that specialised neuropsychological not just psychological advice is obtained.

The use of neuropsychological tests has been reviewed several times. In these overviews, the use of behavioural measures was reviewed (Weiss, 1988).

Table 8.1. Mental and behavioural disorders due to psychoactive substance use Source: ICD-10, WHO, 1992, pp.70–71.

Acute Intoxication	Harmful Use
Uncomplicated	Dependence syndrome
With trauma or other bodily injury	Currently abstinent
With other medical complications	Currently abstinent, but in a protected
With delirium	environment
With perceptual distortions	Currently on a clinically supervised
With coma	maintenance or replacement regime
With convulsions	(controlled dependence)
Pathological intoxication	Currently using the substance (active
	dependence)
	Continuous use
	Episodic use (dipsomania)
Withdrawal state	Psychotic disorder
Uncomplicated	Schizophrenia-like
With complications	Predominantly delusional
Withdrawal state with delirium	Predominantly hallucinatory
Without convulsions	Predominantly polymorphic
With convulsions	Predominantly depressive symptoms
	Predominantly manic symptoms
Mixed	Other
Amnesic syndrome	Unspecified mental and behavioural
Residual and late-onset psychotic	disorder
disorder	
Flashbacks	
Personality or behaviour disorder	
Residual affective disorder	
Dementia	
Other persisting cognitive	
impairment	
Late-onset psychotic disorder	

The nature of any relationship between behavioural indices and the underlying neuropsychological pathology gives rise to problems in interpretation of the results.

An International Workshop was held in the UK in 1996 (Stephens and Barker, 1998). The review of this meeting suggested that there were various steps in establishing the effects of chemicals on neurobehavioural tests.

The factors which could potentially confirm or modify the tests were numerous and are reproduced in Table 8.3.

The first step is to establish that a neurobehavioural effect has been shown after taking into account all the factors that potentially confound or modify the results. The second step is the interpretation of the data. The nature and severity of the effects and whether these were of clinical significance are important issues. The importance of taking an epidemiological view was emphasised. Thus, a substance which caused a minor impairment in a very large group of individuals might have a more profound implications for society than a compound which caused major impairment in only a few of those exposed.

The use of control groups is a very difficult problem. There is ample evidence that farmers, the bulk of those exposed to OP insecticides, are themselves in many countries or parts of the UK, subject to a high rate of psychiatric disability. A large-scale study carried out with the funding of the Department of Health in the UK used an in-depth investigation of a sample of farmers who had died by suicide (Hawton *et al.*, 1998) and included interviews with relatives and other informants and an examination of coroners and medical records. In addition, a random sample of 1000 farmers was sent a postal questionnaire survey to identify the types of problems which farmers face. The most common methods used for suicide were firearms and hanging. The use of firearms reflects the easy access of farmers to guns. Self-poisoning was less frequent in male suicides than in the general population but more than half of the self-poisoning involved agricultural or horticultural chemicals and pharmaceutical preparations. Over half of the farmers who committed suicide gave signals of a clear prior intention. Another important factor was lack of social support. Sheep farmers did not seem to be more likely to commit suicide than other farmers. In farmers who died by suicide, mental disorder was present in about 4 out of 5, where good information could be obtained. Most suffered from clinical depression of severe or moderate intensity.

About a third of these farmers were receiving antidepressants but others had not been seen by either their General Practitioner or the local psychiatric services. Occupational and financial problems were very common, being present in about two thirds of working farmers, in this study. Thus, tenant farmers were worried about the loss of living accommodation on impending retirement.

Table 8.2. Examples of neuropsychological tests for use in neurotoxicology examinations

Intellectual ability	Memory
Wechsler Adult Intelligence Scale-Revised (WAIS-R) Vocabulary Subtest of the WAIR-R Raven's Progressive Matrices Shipley Institute of Living Scale	Wechsler Memory Scale-Revised (WMS-R)
Language	Verbal memory
Peabody Picture Vocabulary Test-Revised (PPVT-R) Boston Naming Test Wide Range Achievement Test Revised (WRAT-R); Reading and spelling Subtests Boston Diagnostic Aphasia Examination (BDAE) Western Aphasia Battery (WAB)	Ray Auditory Verbal Learning Test (RAVLT) Logical Memory passages of the WMS-R California Verbal Learning Test (CVLT) System
Manual dexterity/motor	Nonverbal memory
Finger Tapping Test Purdue Pegboard Grooved Pegboard	Visual Reproduction Subtest of the WMS-R Rey—Ostemeth Complex Figure Test Symbol Digit Paired Associate
Visuoperception/visuoconstruction	Computerised batteries
Judgement of Line Orientation Hooper Visual Organisation Test Block Design of the WAIS-R Rey—Osterrieth Complex Figure Test (copy)	Neurobehavioural Evaluation System (NES-2) Milan Automated Neuropsychological
Executive psychomotor functions	Psychological functioning
Wisconsin Card Sorting Test Stroop Category Test Digit Symbol Subtest of the WAIS-R Symbol Digit Modalities Test Trail Making Test Reaction Time Continuous Performance Test	Mood Minnesota Multiphasic Personality Inventory-2 (MMPI-2) Symptom Checklist (SCL-90-R Profile of Mood States (POMS) Center for Epidemiologic Studies Depression Scale (CES-D) (MANS-WHQ) Automated Neuropsychological
Learning Test	Assessment Metrics (ANAM)

Table 8.3. Factors that potentially confound or modify

Stable factors	Varying factors
Age (date of birth)	Alcohol (recent use)
Sex	Caffeine (recent use)
Socioeconomic group or occupation	Nicotine (recent use)
First language	Medicines or drugs (recent use)
Preferred hand	Paints, glues or pesticides (recent use)
Caffeine (habitual use)	Near visual acuity
Computer experience (automated tests only	Upper body injury restricting movement
Alcohol (habitual use)	Recent cold or flu
Nicotine (habitual use)	Stress
Medicines or drugs (habitual use)	Arousal (and fatigue), sleep last night
Head injury causing unconsciousness for >1 h	Screen luminance (automated tests only)
Diabetic	Time of day
Epileptic	Time of year
Other nervous system disease	
Paints, glues or pesticides (habitual use)	
Alcohol or drug addiction problem	
Level of physical activity at work	

A particular enquiry was made into the use of OPs. In the sample of sheep farmers who committed suicide, the history of sheep dip use was more frequent than in other sheep farmers but this was not to a statistically significant extent. However, the proportions of all working farmers describing adverse effects attributing to OPs were similar in the suicides and the control group. Just over half of sheep farmers responding to the questionnaire used OP sheep dips and about a third said they had been drenched or soaked in them at some time. About 16% of sheep farmers thought that their health had been affected by OPs. In the postal survey, about three-quarters of farmers responded and were worried about their finances and nearly a quarter indicated that they had definite financial problems. Farmers with small farms and those with mixed operations appeared to be most vulnerable to financial and other problems. Similar data have been obtained in other studies (e.g. Gunderson *et al.*, 1993). The need to alert GPs in rural areas has been emphasised (Malmberg *et al.*, 1999).

These types of findings emphasise the need for caution in interpreting studies in farmers using OP insecticides in which they appear to have a high rate of suicide (Parrón et al., 1996).

It is against this background of an above average rate of mental illness, irrespective of exposure to OP insecticides, that the various studies of long-term effects of these compounds need to be evaluated. Thus, predisposition to psychiatric disorders may be an important factor in the induction of reactions to environmental toxins. Not only should current psychiatric status be assessed but a detailed previous psychiatric history and assessment of psychological, occupational and interpersonal functioning is essential in assessing reactions to environmental insults. Often on detailed questioning of people alleging deleterious effects of OP insecticides, a history is obtained of similar symptoms occurring spontaneously, chronically or sporadically, prior to the exposure. Ascribing causation may be very difficult in view of the multiplicity of factors. On a more theoretical basis, it is possible that polymorphisms in factors such as drug metabolism may render some individuals particularly susceptible to CNS damage. Similar polymorphisms are already suspected of influencing susceptibility to recognised psychiatric disorders.

8.3. Acute Exposure to OP Insecticides

The acute toxic effects of exposure to OP insecticides are well known, the first symptoms are chiefly psychological with tension, anxiety, restlessness, emotional lability with fluctuations in depression and elation. Insomnia is a cardinal feature with excessive dreaming. Other non-specific symptoms include drowsiness, headache, dizziness, tremor. Some of these symptoms such as headache may be quite marked and distressing to the sufferer. With both subjective complaints and on formal assessment, disturbances of attention concentration, and memory have been reported. Depression, social withdrawal and demoralisation can occur but less frequently than does anxiety.

These acute effects have been known since the introduction of the pesticides (Kraybill, 1969). An early study comprised observations on people exposed to the OP insecticides (Holmes and Gaon, 1956). They described over 400 cases of exposure to the insecticide over 5 years. Their results with respect to the CNS are shown in Table 8.4. The 449 cases of poisoning are classified according to the reduction in the cholinesterase activity of the red blood cells.

It can be seen that the commonest symptom is headache except in the most extreme exposure where dreams and poor sleep become more prevalent.

Some of the symptoms such as increased perspiration and dizziness show a clear effect increasing with the cholinesterase inhibition. The syndrome was treated with maintenance of adequate respiration and large doses of atropine. Some persistent symptoms occurred in more severe exposures and in those with multiple exposures. These included forgetfulness, irritability and confused thinking.

A similar study was carried out more recently and involved 190 OP poisoning cases admitted to hospital in Ahmedabad, India (Agarwal, 1993). Physical symptoms included nausea, constriction of the pupil, excessive salivation and blurred vision. The commonest CNS manifestations were giddiness (94%), headache (84%), and disturbance of consciousness (44%). In 5–6% of cases decrements in alertness and memory, increased irritability, memory deficit, lethargy and lack of energy were observed. Overall, about 90% of the cases recovered completely, 6% died and 4% were lost to observation. Neuropsychological testing was employed in one of the earlier studies (Durham et al., 1965). They used various tests of "mental alertness", including complex reaction time and paced vigilance tests. A group of crop sprayers with varying degrees of exposure were tested and compared with a group of controls who had no history of exposure. Although immediately after exposure testing revealed decrements in performance, these did not persist beyond the short-term. No dose-effect relationships were found between the acute testing decrements and the estimates of exposure.

In 23 workers exposed to OP pesticides, abnormalities of memory, signal processing, vigilance, semantic performance and proprioceptive feedback were evaluated (Rodnitzky et al., 1975). No deficits were detected in the exposed workers, compared with unexposed individuals.

The authors concluded that higher CNS functions are relatively resistant to the acute effects of OPs. In a smaller study using 99 pest control workers tested before and after their work shift, no unequivocal decrements in performance were detected (Maizlish et al., 1987). However, the exposure to the OP, diazinon, was at a fairly low level.

A recent study was designed to measure the exposure of a group of farmers to OP insecticide and sheep dip and to record the incidence of any symptoms after exposure (Rees, 1996). The study was prospective and involved; a) working methods assessed by questionnaire; b) absorption of OP pesticide by measuring indicators such as cholinesterase levels; c) symptoms recorded by questionnaire at the same time as the biological monitoring.

Table 8.4. Exposure to anticholinesterase agents
Shows the incidence of symptoms in a group of anticholinesterase poisoning. These are grouped according to the percent reduction in red cell cholinesterase. This serves as an index of the severity of the exposure (Holmes and Gaon, 1956).

System involved and Signs and Symptoms	RBC ChE Reduction 0–10% % of 169 Cases	RBC ChE Reduction 10–25% % of 153 Cases	RBC ChE Reduction 25–40% % of 78 Cases	RBC ChE Reduction 40–60% % of 33 Cases	RBC ChE Reduction over 60% % of 16 Cases
Headache	43.2	45.7	61.5	75.7	68.7
Dreams, poor sleep	33.1	27.4	33.3	54.5	75.0
Fatigability	34.3	31.4	32.0	33.3	31.3
Nervous and Irritable mood changes	23.7	24.2	38.5	39.4	37.5
Increased perspiration	13.0	17.6	29.5	30.3	62.5
Dizziness	11.2	11.8	15.4	30.3	31.3
Tremor and twitch, fasciculation	3.5	3.3	6.4	3.0	25.0
Paraesthesia and cold	5.9	6.5	11.5	21.2	25.0

The study took place in a sheep farming area in Wales and involved 38 men. Twenty-four of these completed the study. Inadequate handling of the pesticide with significant contamination occurred and 2 subjects had significant depression of RBC cholinesterase after dipping. However, this did not seem to be at a level usually associated with toxicity. Other subjects had no significant change in cholinesterase concentrations but many reported new symptoms during the 24 hours at the end of dipping. Many of these symptoms are known to occur with poisoning with OP substances and most have a pharmacological rationale. These include urinary frequency, diarrhoea, insomnia, headache, wheezing and tremor. Accordingly, although in this limited study farmers did not seem to have specific OP toxicity (despite using inadequate handling precautions), the characteristic symptoms were still found.

8.4. Chronic Effects of Acute Exposure to OP Substances

Delayed effects of OP exposure have been described. Symptoms begin about 1–3 weeks after the acute exposure and resemble those of the acute exposure itself. However, psychiatric symptoms have not been described other than those which are a reflection of the physical symptoms such as pain, numbness and limb weakness. In one study of 229 Egyptian pesticide workers (Soliman et al., 1993), reduced tactile sensitivity was detected but there was no impairment on either the Blocked Design or the Santa Ana Dexterity Test.

Tabershaw and Cooper (1966) studied a group of 235 individuals who had been reported by their doctors as having been poisoned by OP insecticides during the 1960s. At follow up 3 or 4 years later, three-quarters of the poisoned individuals were located and half were examined. Of 114 individuals regarded as having had definite OP poisoning, 6 were graded as having had severe poisoning, 54 moderate and 54 mild. Of the 114, 43 had complaints which persisted for more than 6 months after poisoning, and 33 still had complaints. Among the CNS complaints, 7 individuals had headaches but not with any clear pattern. No individual had any episode which could be regarded as psychotic. Many of them developed intolerance to the odour of pesticide preparations. Thus, it appears that subjective complaints are not necessarily consistent and do not form a pattern.

Savage and his colleagues (1998) compared 100 individuals who had a history of acute exposure to OPs with 100 carefully matched individuals who had not been poisoned. A wide range of tests was used including a physical examination with neurological evaluations, EEG recordings and various neuropsychological and personality tests. The last battery comprised the Wechsler Adult Intelligent Scale (WAIS) and the expanded Halstead—Reitan battery, and 3 sub-tests from the Peabody individual achievement tests (reading recognition, reading comprehension and spelling). An objective personality test, the Minnesota Multiphasic Personality Inventory (MMPI) was also given in order to determine whether exposure to pesticides exaggerated pre-existing tendencies towards psychiatric disturbances. In addition, each study participant and a close relative or spouse independently completed questionnaires rating the participants' functioning with respect to memory, communication skills, academic skills, sensory and motor abilities, various cognitive and intellectual abilities, and emotional status. The results from the 100 matched pairs indicated that the groups did not differ with respect to special sense function or the EEG. However, those previously exposed to OPs performed worse than the controls on 4 out of 5 summary measures.

Deficits were found with respect to widely differing abilities such as intellectual functioning, academic skills, flexibility of thinking and simple motor skills. The conclusion was that the most likely possible source of neuropsychological impairment was the exposure to the OP poisoning. However, close analysis of the data shows that pre-morbid intelligence, as assessed by verbal IQ, was significantly higher in the controls; however, it was not used as a covariate in analysing the other variables. Accordingly, the differences might have been pre-existing ones which had shown up by chance. A retrospective study of agricultural workers in Nicaragua compared 36 men who had been definitely exposed to OPs with episodes of poisoning with men who although possibly exposed to OP use, had not had documented episodes of poisoning (Rosenstock *et al.,* 1990, 1991). To test these workers, a standard battery of neuropsychological tests developed under the aegis of the WHO was used. Differences were found in the digit span, digit vigilance, Benton visual retention, digit symbol, sequencing (trails A), problem solving (block design), pursuit aiming, and dexterity tests. As above, the poisoned groups had lower vocabulary scores than the non-poisoned group. This was included in the analysis of the other variables and only lessened the contrast between the groups to a minor degree. No psychiatric symptoms were reported in the paper.

Another such study (Ames *et al.,* 1995), compared 45 agricultural pesticide applicators with a known previous history of cholinesterase inhibition (falling short, however, of clear toxicity) with 90 such workers who had no previous history of this type. Of a range of psychomotor, cognitive and mood measures, only one test differed between the groups. In fact, there was actually better performance on the serial digit test in those with a prior history of cholinesterase inhibition! The authors concluded by signifying their reassurance that by preventing acute OP poisoning as a result intervening before frank signs of toxicity are manifest, chronic sequelae may be obviated.

After reviewing the data pertaining to the long-term sequelae of acute poisoning, the Committee on Toxicity of Chemicals in Food, Consumer Products and the Environment (1999) concluded that:

a) Neuropsychological abnormality can occur as a complication of acute OP poisoning. Sustained attention and "mental agility" were most affected whereas long-term memory was unaffected.

b) No form conclusions were drawn concerning psychiatric illness as a sequel to acute OP poisoning.

8.5. Chronic Exposure to OP Substances

This topic is the most controversial of all. It has long been claimed that low and apparently subclinical but repeated exposure to OP substances can result in permanent damage to various systems of the body including the nerves, muscles, and the CNS. However, even the neurological effects of chronic exposure to low OP levels are difficult to detect (Beach *et al.*, 1996). Psychiatric abnormalities after chronic exposure have long been believed to be a problem. As far back as 1961, Gershon and Shaw reported on 16 cases in Australia in whom psychiatric problems following chronic exposure to OP pesticides were claimed. Of these, 11 had actually experienced acute episodes of schizophrenic and depressive type symptoms as well as more chronic problems. The psychological symptoms included severe impairment of memory and difficulty in concentration. However, on follow-up, 12 months later, almost all had reverted to normal. The concern raised by this study prompted an epidemiological study, also in Australia, which evaluated the incidence of psychiatric admissions in Victoria (Stoller *et al.*, 1965). A crude measure of possible exposure was used, namely sales of OP pesticides. No relationship of psychiatric admissions was found to this parameter. However, patients who did develop milder OP symptoms, not warranting admission to hospital, would be missed totally in this study.

In another early study, Dille and Smith (1964) studied 2 crop-spraying pilots who developed psychiatric symptoms such as depression, phobia and acute anxiety. In their account they state that it was routine practice for pilots at that time to take atropine to suppress the acute symptoms of exposure in order that they could continue working. A study by Davignon and her co-workers (1965) compared 441 apple growers who had been exposed to OP insecticides with 170 people living in the same environment but not exposed and 162 other controls. No psychiatric differences were found although some soft neurological signs were claimed. Another study dating from 1960s is that of Durham *et al.* (1965). Various tests of "mental alertness" were used and a variety of subjects were studied. These included crop-spraying pilots and cases of suspected OP poisoning. The authors state "there were no cases in which mental effect was noted in the complete absence of physical signs or symptoms of illness". They concluded that the OP compounds "may affect mental illness if absorbed in amounts great enough to cause clinical signs of symptoms of systemic illness".

A study in Spain involved 44 green house workers with high exposure to OP insecticides (Alvarez *et al.*, 1993).

Although a half claimed to have symptoms after using these agents, no significant decrease in cholinesterase activity was observed.

Another, essentially negative study was reported by Fiedler and her co-workers (1997). Fifty-seven male fruit farmers with a history of exposure to OP insecticides were compared with 4 age-matched cranberry/blueberry growers and hardware store owners (unexposed). The exposed subjects had slower reaction times. However, a range of other tests were negative, raising the possibility of a chance finding. The authors concluded that: "Long-term use of organophosphates without evidence of an acute poisoning episode appears to produce, at most, subtle changes in neuropsychological performance".

An index of chronic exposure levels to OPs was developed and used to divide 59 male workers in high and low exposure groups (Korsak and Sato, 1977). The outcome measures included tests from a neuropsychological test battery and EEG records analysed by computer methods (power spectra). Plasma cholinesterase estimates were also made. Impairment was detected in the trail making test and the Bender Visual Motor Gestalt test with respect to the high vs. low exposure groups. Some EEG differences were also detected. The authors concluded that the part of the brain particularly vulnerable to OPs was the left frontal lobe.

All this work was reviewed by Eyer (1995). He concluded that it is possible that neuropsychological and psychiatric effects can occur after OP poisoning. However, he concluded, "The available data do not indicate that asymptomatic exposure to organophosphates is connected with an increasing risk of delayed or permanent neuropsychopathological effects". In other words, in his opinion, definite episodes of poisoning in the past or continuing to occur are necessary in order to demonstrate psychiatric and neuropsychological deficits.

A series of toxicology studies have come out of the Institute of Occupational Health at the University of Birmingham. In 1995 a detailed study was published looking at the relationship between chronic and acute exposure effects to OPs (Stephens et al., 1995). The subjects comprised 146 sheep farmers exposed to OP during sheep dipping and 143 non-exposed quarry workers. The General Health Questionnaire developed by Goldberg was used to assess "vulnerability to psychiatric disorder". A battery of 8 neuropsychological tests was also used. Exposed subjects were 1.5 times more likely to reach criteria for "caseness" on the GHQ (p=0.035). In addition, the farmers performed significantly worse than controls on tests of sustained attention and speed of information processing. There were numerous intergroup differences, which were pre-existing, but co-varying these out still left performance differences.

A limitation of the study was that time-of-day and place-of-test effects may have acted differently on the two groups as the farmers were visited at home in the evening and the quarrymen tested during the day at work. Nevertheless, this study raised concerns about the effects of chronic exposure.

The data were analysed further (Stephens *et al.*, 1996). In their evaluation, acute exposure effects were assessed prospectively using a purpose-built symptom questionnaire. Furthermore, urine was analysed for chemical levels of OP to confirm recent exposure. Quite sophisticated statistical techniques were used to assess relationships between reported symptom levels and chronic neuropsychological effects. However, no such relationship was found. The authors concluded that chronic effects of OP exposure which they detected appeared to occur independently of symptoms that might immediately follow acute OP exposure. They raise the warning that individuals might experience chronic effects without knowing that they had been exposed to dangerous levels because the acute exposure had not resulted in any discernible subjective or objective effects.

Very recently, a large-scale complex study has been reported from the Institute of Occupational Medicine in Edinburgh. The study took place in 3 phases. The first phase was conducted in the summer of 1996 in order to develop a way of quantifying the uptake of OPs based on simple task, procedural and behavioural aspects of sheep dipping (Sewell *et al.*, 1999). The study involved 1-day surveys of 20 dipping sessions at farms located mostly in the Scottish borders. The survey comprised observation and recording of activities performed by various individuals and included frequency, extent of and time of contact with the dip concentrate and the dip wash (actual dip which the sheep pass through); the amount of protective clothing worn; hand washing, smoking and eating habits, and other significant incidents. Sheep dippers also provided urine samples before and after the day of dipping. Metabolites of diazinon were measured to enable an estimate of the uptake to be made. Finally, a questionnaire on exposure to sheep dip and other pesticides during the 72 hours prior to the visit was completed. This study found that the most important source of exposure to OPs was contact with concentrated dip that occurred almost always on the hands and usually when the farmer was handling the concentrate container during the preparation and repeated replenishment of the dipping bath. Levels of urinary metabolite increased with increased handling of the concentrate containers. This increase was usually confined to the one person at the farm responsible for handling the concentrate. A mathematical model was developed to give an estimate of the uptake.

The refined uptake model was used to develop a questionnaire for retrospective exposure assessment to be used in the second part of the study.

This second phase comprised a cross-sectional comparison of exposure to sheep dip OPs and its relation to complaints suggestive of chronic peripheral neuropathy (Pilkington *et al.*, 1999a). It was based on two areas of the UK, Hereford and Worcester in England, and the border area of Scotland. A group of pig and chicken farmers and farm workers not exposed to OPs was used as the first control group. The second control group were ceramic workers in a factory. Farms were identified from a sampling frame and then contact was made with the farm owner. Retrospective exposure information was obtained for the period of common usage of OPs (1970 onwards) using the questionnaire developed during the first phase of the study, as outlined above. Aspects of the work history were later summarised into various indices of cumulative exposure and a combined index was obtained based on the uptake model outlined above.

Neurological assessments combined a symptom questionnaire with a series of quantitative sensory tests. The symptom questionnaire was a standardised one and the sensory tests were two automated tests for thermal sensation (hot and cold) and another for vibration sensation. They were given by a trained technician on site using portable equipment. However, rather a high incidence of positive testing on the sensory test raised questions about possible false positives, especially as many of the control group also showed abnormalities on these tests.

The study group eventually comprised 612 farmers with sheep dipping experience (SD farmers), 53 farmers with no sheep dip experience (NSD) and 107 ceramics workers. Among the SD farmers cumulative exposure was found to be highly skewed. Most subjects experienced fewer than 100 days dipped, although a few individuals had taken part in over 1000 dipping days. In all groups, autonomic symptoms were more prevalent than sensory or motor symptoms. The crude prevalence was highest amongst SD farmers (19%) followed by NSD farmers (11%) and ceramics workers (5%). However, the symptom prevalence was associated with age and was much higher in English than in Scottish farmers. Adjusting for age and country, the prevalence of symptoms among SD farmers was high compared to ceramics workers (Odds Ratio 4.3), but was similar to NSD farmers (OR=1.3). Age was also found to be positively related to all three sensory thresholds.

Associations were found between symptom score and various indices of cumulative exposure to OPs and suggested that at least some of the reported symptoms were due to exposure to sheep dip chemicals. The critical exposure factors seemed to be working with the concentrate in that markedly higher rates of reported symptoms were noted amongst those who have at some time been the principal concentrate handlers. "There was no evidence that cumulative exposure was associated with impairment of measured sensory thresholds". It thus appeared that if there was any relationship, it was confined to dippers who had handled the concentrate.

The third phase of the study is that most relevant to the present chapter (Pilkington et al., 1999b). In phase 3 a subset of subjects involved in the phase 2 field study were invited to participate in clinical studies at the Institute of Neurological Sciences (INS) in Glasgow. Seventy-nine subjects attended these assessments but all were sheep farmers. The study attempted to relate any abnormalities with the finding in the field study of "no", "possible" and "probable/definite" categories of impairment in the field study. The symptom questionnaire was repeated and the same range of sensory tests was performed. Additional tests included nerve conduction and electromyography. A battery of neuropsychological tests was performed to assess general intelligence, psychomotor function, attention, memory, mood and affect.

A third of 72 subjects had confirmation of their neuropathy by neurological signs or nerve conduction abnormality. Only one of the 15 subjects from the known neuropathy group had neurological abnormalities as compared with about a third of those having possible neuropathy and a half of those with probable/definite neuropathy.

Subjects classified as being probable/definite cases of neuropathy had poorer self-reported general mental health and experienced greater self-reported anxiety and depression than other subjects with less likely neuropathy. The neuropsychological tests did not however show any consistent results. There was some evidence perhaps of slower processing time amongst probable/definite cases of neuropathy but there was no clear evidence of an overall slowing of processing time. There was no evidence of any differences in memory capability.

These studies have been subject to very careful scrutiny. The main finding is that English farmers are more likely to be symptomatic than Scottish farmers by a factor of almost 2. The estimate of neuropathy was mainly on subjective grounds as the sensory test seemed overly sensitive and were probably giving many false positives. The phase 3 was within-group comparison, relating to the degree of subjective neuropathy in the field. As such, it does not provide independent estimates of either exposure or objective damage. The neuropsychological tests were almost uniformly uninformative, not distinguishing between the groups in any consistent way. The study therefore raises more questions than it answers.

The Committee on Toxicity of Chemicals in Food, Consumer Products and the Environment (1999) concluded that with chronic low-level exposure:

a)   The evidence, on balance, did not show any clinically significant effects on performance in neuropsychological tests.

b)   The psychiatric evidence was insufficient to draw useful conclusions but exposure to OP sheep dips was not a major factor in the excess suicide mortality among British farmers.

8.6. Organophosphate Nerve Agents

These comprise a rather diverse group of rapidly acting cholinesterase inhibitors (for review see Marrs and Maynard, 1994). There are few data concerning accidental poisoning with OP nerve agents but there are some experimental studies mainly involving primates. One study involved 77 workers with one or more definite exposures to sarin, but not within the previous year (Duffy *et al.,* 1979). Both clinical and computer abnormalities followed these exposures. The controls were 38 workers from the same factory in whom there was no history of such exposure. A collection of sophisticated EEG analyses was used including all night EEG and spectral analysis of the records. Some differences between the groups were found both during waking and sleeping and were interpreted to reflect long-term sequelae. The variables which showed differences included beta activity, increased delta and beta slowing, decreased alpha and increased rapid eye movement sleep in the exposed population.

A large case series of acute sarin poisonings eventuated as a result of the terrorist attack in the subway in Tokyo (Okamura *et al.,* 1996). Of these cases, 0.6% showed severe poisoning and 17% moderate poisoning. In a third of all cases an acute stress reaction requiring antidepressant therapy supervened. In 4 of 111 cases of severe or moderate poisoning this was succeeded by a post-traumatic stress disorder noted at a 3-month follow-up examination. However, these psychiatric symptoms must be presumed to be a reaction to the stress rather than to the direct poisoning.

In the experimental studies single or repeated doses of sarin or dieldrin were administered to small groups of rhesus monkeys (Burchfiel *et al.,* 1976). EEG changes were induced which persisted for a year. However, the single large dose of the OP induced convulsions which may have accounted for the later changes in the EEG.

8.7. Conclusions and Summary

The OPs have complex effects on the body, including the brain. Methodological issues are complex both with respect to the provision of well-matched controls and to choice of valid, reliable and sensitive psychiatric and neuropsychological measures. Physical symptoms following acute exposure to OPs are usually accompanied by a range of psychological symptoms such as anxiety, insomnia and emotional instability. Depression may ensue. The chronic effects of acute exposure are less well-defined but it is probably that long-lasting sequelae may follow proven exposure to toxic levels of OPs. The most controversial issue relates to possible psychiatric and neuropsychological impairments following repeated exposure to OP substances, with or without transient symptomatic episodes following each exposure. This is the usual pattern in sheep farmers who dip sheep on an annual basis. Some negative studies have been reported. Other studies suggesting differences between OP users and OP non-users have been criticised for lack of carefully selected controls or on methodological grounds. Many other factors including previous psychiatric and medical history, previous personality, familiarity with psychological tests, level of education and media publicity may vitiate the interpretation of data. No firm conclusions are yet possible regarding chronic effects of low exposure of OPs.

References

Agarwal, S.B.   A clinical, biochemical, neurobehavioral and sociopsychological study of 190 patients admitted to hospital as a result of acute organophosphorus poisoning. *Environmental Research* 1993;**62**:63–70.

Alvarez, E., Aurrekoetxea, J., Santa Manna, L., *et al.*   Exposure to organophosphorus plaguicides in greenhouse workers in the Basque Country (Spain). *Medicine Ojinica* 1993;**101**:681–3.

Ames, R. G., Steenland, K., Jenkins, B., *et al.*   Chronic neurologic sequelae to cholinesterase inhibition among agricultural pesticide applicators. *Archives of Environmental Health* 1995;**50**:440–3.

Amr, M.M., Halim, Z.S., Mousse, S.S.   Psychiatric disorders among Egyptian pesticide applicators and formulators. *Environmental Research* 1997;**73**:193–9.

Beach, J.R., Spurgeon, A., Stephens, F., *et al.*   Abnormalities on neurological examination among sheep farmers exposed to organophosphorous pesticides. *Occupational and Environmental Medicine* 1996;**53**:520–5.

Blain, Prof P.G. The long-term neurotoxicity of anticholinesterases. Report of a DSAC Working Party, Ministry of Defence. Personal Communication. 1999.

Bolla, K.I.   Neuropsychological evaluation for detecting alterations in the central nervous system after chemical exposure. *Regulatory Toxicology and Pharmacology* 1996;**24**:548–51.

Burchfiel, J.L., Duffy, F.H., Sim, V.M.   Persistent effects of sarin and dieldrin upon the primate electroencephalogram. *Toxicology and Applied Pharmacology* 1976;**35**:365–79.

Committee on Toxicity of Chemicals in Food, Consumer Products and the Environment. Organophosphates. Department of Health. London. 1999

Davignon, L.F., St-Pierre, J., Charest, G., *et al.*   A study of the chronic effects of insecticides in man. *Journal of the Canadian Medical Association* 1965;**92**:597–602.

Dille, J.F., Smith, P.W.   Central nervous system effects of chronic exposure to organophosphate insecticides. *Aerospace Medicine* 1964;**6**:475–8.

Duffy, F.H., Burchfiel, J.L., Bartels, P.H., *et al.*   Long-term effects of an organophosphate upon the human electroencephalogram. *Toxicology and Applied Pharmacology* 1979;**47**:161–76.

Durham, W.F., Wolfe, H.R., Quinby, G.E.   Organophosphorus insecticides and mental alertness. *Archives of Environmental Health* 1965;**10**:55–66.

Dyer, C. Organophosphates do cause long term damage. *British Medical Journal* 1997;**315**:1113.

Eyer, P. Neuropsychopathological changes by organophosphorus compounds—a review. *Human and Experimental Toxicology* 1995;**14**:857–64.

Fieder, N., Kipen, H., Kelly-McNeil, K., *et al.* Long-term use of organophosphates and neuropsychological performance. *American Journal of Industrial Medicine* 1997;**32**:487–96.

Gershon, S., Shaw, F.H. Psychiatric sequelae of chronic exposure to organophosphorus insecticides. *Lancet* 1961;i:1371–4.

Gunderson, P., Donner, D., Nashold, R., *et al.* The epidemiology of suicide among farmer residents or workers in five north-central states. *American Journal of Preventative Medicine* 1993;**9**:26–32.

Hawton, K., Simkin, S., Malmberg, A., *et al.* Suicide and stress in farmers. Department of Health funded research: London. The Stationery Office. 1998.

Holmes, J.H., Gaon, M.D. Observations on acute and multiple exposure to anticholinesterase agents. *Transactions of the American Clinical Chemistry Association* 1956;**68**:86–103.

Korsak, R.J., Sato, M.M. Effects of chronic organophosphate pesticide exposure on the central nervous system. *Clinical Toxicology* 1977;**11**:83–95.

Kraybill, H.F. Biological effects of pesticide in mammalian systems. *Annals of the New York Academy of Sciences* 1969;**160**:1–422.

Maizish, N., Schenker, M., Weisskopf, C., *et al.* A behavioral evaluation of pest control workers with short-term, low-level exposure to the organophosphate diazinon. *American Journal of Industrial Medicine* 1987;**12**:153–72.

Malmberg, A., Simkin, S., Hawton, K. Suicide in farmers. *British Journal of Psychiatry* 1999;**175**:103–5.

Marrs, T.C., Maynard, R.L. Neurotoxicity of chemical warfare agents. *Handbook of Clinical Neurology* 1994;**20**:223–38.

Mearns, J., Dunn, J., Lees-Haley, P.R. Psychological effects of organophosphate pesticides; a review and call for research by psychologists. *Journal of Clinical Psychology* 1994;**50**:286–94.

Okumara, I., Takasu, N., Ishimatsu, S., *et al.* Report on 640 victims of the Tokyo subway sarin attack. *Annals of Emergency Medicine* 1993;**28**:129–35.

Parron, T., Hernandez, A.F., Villanueva, E. Increased risk of suicide with exposure to pesticides in an intensive agricultural area. A 12-year retrospective study. *Forensic Science International* 1996;**79**:53–63.

Pilkington, A., Buchanan, D., Jamal, G.A., *et al.* Epidemiological study of the relationships between exposure to organophosphate pesticides and indices of chronic peripheral neuropathy, and neuropsychological abnormalities in sheep farmers and dippers. Phase 2. Cross-sectional exposure-response study of sheep dippers. Institute of Occupational Medicine, Edinburgh, and Institute of Neurological Sciences, Glasgow, Report no TMI99I02b. 1999a.

Pilkington, A., Jamal, C.A., Cilham, R., *et al.* Epidemiological study of the relationships between exposure to organophosphate pesticides and indices of chronic peripheral neuropathy, and neuropsychological abnormalities in sheep farmers and dippers. Phase 3. Clinical Neurological, Neurophysiological Study. Institute of Occupational Medicine, Edinburgh, and Institute of Neurological Sciences, Glasgow, Report no TM/99102c. 1999b.

Rees, H. Exposure to sheep dip and the incidence of acute symptoms in a group of Welsh sheep farmers. *Occupational and Environmental Medicine* 1996;**53**:258–63.

Rodnitzky, R.L., Levin, H.S., Mick, D.L. Occupational exposure to organophosphate pesticides. *Archives of Environmental Health* 1975;**30**:98–103.

Rosenstock, L., Daniell, W., Barnhart, S., *et al.* Chronic neuropsychological sequelae of occupational exposure to organophosphate insecticides. *American Journal of Industrial Medicine* 1990;**18**:321–5.

Rosenstock, L., Keifer, M., Daniell, W.E., *et al.,* and the Pesticide Health Effects Study Group. Chronic central nervous system effects of acute organophosphate pesticide intoxication. *Lancet* 1991;**338**:223–7.

Savage, E.P., Keefe, I.J., Mounce, L.M., *et al.* Chronic neurological sequelae of acute organophosphate pesticide poisoning. *Archives of Environmental Health* 1988;**43**:38–45.

Sewell, C., Pilkington, A., Buchanan, D., *et al.* Epidemiological study of the relationships between exposure to organophosphate pesticides and indices of chronic peripheral neuropathy, and neuropsychological abnormalities in sheep farmers and dippers. Phase 1. Development and Validation of an organophosphate Uptake Model for Sheep Dippers. Institute of Occupational Medicine, Edinburgh, and Institute of Neurological Sciences, Glasgow; Report no TMI99I02a. 1999.

Soliman, S.A., Svendsgaard, I.D., Otto, D., *et al.* Biochemical and neurobehavioural assessment of neurotoxicity in workers occupationally exposed to organophosphorus pesticides. *Proceedings of the International Conference on Peripheral Nerve Toxicity* 1993;29–32.

Stephens, R., Barker, P. Role of human neurobehavioural tests in regulatory activity on chemicals. *Occupational and Environmental Medicine* 1998;**55**:210–4.

Stephens, R., Spurgeon, A., Berry, H. Organophosphates: the relationship between chronic and acute exposure effects. *Neurotoxicology and Teratology* 1996;**18**:449–53.

Stephens, R., Spurgeon, A., Calvert, I.A., *et al.* Neuropsychological effects of long term exposure to organophosphates in sheep dip. *Lancet* 1995;**345**:1135–9.

Stoller, A., Krupinski, J., Christophers, A.J., *et al.* Organophosphorus insecticides and major mental illness. *Lancet* 1965;**i**:1387–8.

Tabershaw, I.R., Cooper, C.W. Sequelae of acute organic phosphate poisoning. *Journal of Occupational Medicine* 1966;**8**:5–20.

Tsatsakis, A.M., Tutudaki, M.I., Tzatzarakis, B.S., *et al.* Pesticide deposition in hair: preliminary results of a model study of methomyl incorporation into rabbit hair. *Veterinary and Human Toxicology* 1998;**40**:200–3.

Weiss, B. Behaviour as an early indicator of pesticide toxicity. *Toxicology and Industrial Health*, 1988;**4**:351–9.

World Heath Organization. The ICD-10 Classification of Mental and Behavioural Disorders. Diagnostic criteria for research. Geneva; WHO. 1993.

CHAPTER 9

Effects of Organophosphates on the Neuromuscular Junction and Muscle

Stanley Feldman

1. Introduction

is probable that when primitive life form emerged from the primordial swamp into the tmosphere it found a hostile environment, relatively rich in ammonia, carbon dioxide nd carbon monoxide. It is likely that it was these circumstances that were responsible or the development of the variety of amino acids that became the building blocks of our enes, of DNA and proteins and for the formation of the earliest mechanism for the oordination of multicellular animals utilising a simple chemical substance formed from mmonia, carbon and oxygen—acetylcholine (ACh). Cholinergic mechanisms exist videly in the animal kingdom, in invertebrates as well as in advanced mammals and 1an where they have become the most ubiquitous transmitter substance playing a major ole in regulating human physiology. Its wide spread importance as a transmitter ubstance causes it to influence endocrine and exocrine secretions, cardiac function, the ut and its secretions, muscle power by which we move and the function of the brain. It s hardly surprising that drugs and poisons that interfere with ACh, either its production r its release have widespread and dangerous consequences for the body. Indeed there is vidence that the cholinergic system is so fundamental to bodily function that various nechanisms have developed to protect it from the effects of false transmitters, hemically similar to ACh. It is for this reason that the organophosphate (OP) poisons vhich, by preventing the normal destruction of the transmitter, are so lethal and why heir effects are so widespread.

The formation of the motor nerves and skeletal muscle is a relatively late hyllogentic development. The cholinergic transmission system involved in ommunicating a signal from the motor nerve to the muscle it innervates is therefore nore sophisticated and complex than most other, more primitive, cholinergic nechanisms.

It involves a series of checks and balances that we are only now beginning to full appreciate. As a result of this new information it is now possible to hazard informe guesses as to the many apparent paradoxes seen after poisoning with OPs. However i would be wrong to believe that we have definitive answers to explain all the symptom associated with OP poisoning or that we fully understood the effects of long terr administration.

9.2. Neuromuscular Transmission

In order to breathe, to walk, to talk or to move in any way, we have to initiate a train o nerve impulses in the brain, in the form of micro-currents, which travel down a moto nerve. When the electrical currents reach the swollen end of the motor nerve, as it lies o the muscle, enveloped by a tent like membrane to form the neuromuscular junction, i has to cross a minute gap, the synaptic cleft, in order to excite the muscle and cause it t contract. By itself the current would be insufficient to achieve this end but by releasing chemical transmitter, ACh, which diffuses across the synapse it amplifies its effect (De Castillo and Katz, 1954). This is the basis of neuromuscular transmission (Ginsberg an Jenkinson, 1976). Failure of any part of this process results in apparent muscl weakness or paralysis. The most vulnerable link in this chain of events is the mechanisn for the formation and release of ACh and the activation of the receptor sites on th muscle. It is this process that is most readily affected by drugs and poisons. In order t understand how the OP compounds produce their effects it is essential to understand th current knowledge of the mechanisms involved in normal neuromuscular conduction.

9.3. Depolarisation

A bilipid membrane surrounds the cells that make up our body and separates the flui inside surrounding the intracellular structures from those outside. The composition especially of the salt and proteins contained in the cells differs greatly from that in th extracellular fluid and plasma.

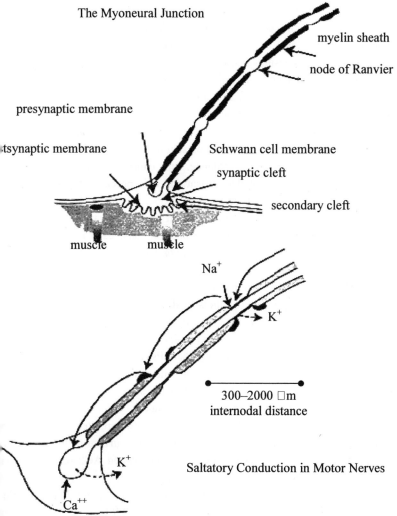

Figure 9.1. The myoneural junction and saltatory conduction of nerve impulses from one node of Ranvier to the next.

The membrane is leaky and has a selective permeability for the small hydra[t] potassium ions which is not shared by that for larger ions of sodium. As a result, [t] high concentration of sodium that exists outside the cell, is not found inside Potassium accumulates in the cell in order to compensate for the potential io[n] imbalance caused by the lack of sodium. However, because of the effect of [t] concentration gradient for potassium that this produces, it reaches equilibrium befor[e] achieves electrical balance. This ionic imbalance produces the resting transmembra[ne] potential that is characteristic of excitable tissues (Ginsberg and Jenkinson, 197[6]. When ACh receptors at the neuromuscular junction are stimulated they cause [t] opening of discrete pores in the membrane, the so called sodium channels. As a res[ult] the differential permeability of sodium and potassium is temporarily lost and sodi[um] ions enter the cell to correct the ionic imbalance. This causes the local potential acr[oss] the membrane to fall; the process of depolarisation. This process of depolarisation fundamental to neuromuscular transmission.

As an impulse travels down the motor nerve it causes a wave of depolarisati[on] associated with increased local permeability to sodium ions, each of which carrie[s] minute positive charge. The movement spreads over the surface membrane, skippi[ng] from one node of Ranvier to the next (the nodes of Ranvier are produced by perio[dic] breaks in the insulating myelin sheath), when it arrives at the nerve ending, [the] presynaptic site, it causes opening of channels in the membrane allowing an influx calcium ions (Birks, 1963). Although various drugs have been shown to influence [the] rate or duration of the channel opening (such as amino-pyridine) (Marshall, Parsons a[nd] Paul, 1976), this has not been demonstrated with the OPs (Fig. 9.1.).

The effect of the inflow of calcium ions into the nerve terminal is to cause [a] sudden release of contents of some 50 packets of ACh stored in readiness within [the] nerve terminal. Each packet, or quanta, contains about 8000 molecules of A[Ch] (McIntosh, 1963). This sudden rush of ACh diffuses across the minute gap that separa[tes] the nerve from the muscle to reach special receptors on the surface of the muscle ([the] post synaptic membrane) where it reacts with highly developed ACh recognition si[tes] within the receptors. Each receptor guards a sodium channel.

When the receptor is activated the central pore dilates making it permeable sodium ions (see Appendix 9.1) (Ginsberg and Jenkinson, 1976). If sufficient chann[els] open simultaneously the minute current from each summates.

If this reaches a critical threshold it will trigger off a propagated wave of
ɔolarisation in the muscle membrane, the action potential, resulting in contraction of
t muscle fibre (Feldman, 1996). For a muscle to contract this process must occur in
ny fibres simultaneously. If only a few fibres reach threshold depolarisation and
ɔond, then it presents as muscle weakness.

Normal muscle activity depends upon a rapid series of nerve stimuli at between 10
i 50 Hz. Lesser rates of stimulation produce a single, unphysiological, twitch
ɔonse. In order to respond to each stimulation of a rapid series it is evident that a
chanism must exist to increase the rate of ACh production and release so as to meet
increase in demand. It is the recognition of the existence of a complex feed back
tem that has allowed us to understand how this takes place (Bowman and Webb,
76). Some of the ACh released acts upon receptors presynaptically on the nerve
minal (Gibb et al., 1984; Bowman et al., 1984; Bowman et al., 1990). These receptors
fer from those on the post synaptic membrane and more closely resemble those found
the CNS. Stimulation of these receptors cause calcium pores to open in zone of the
synaptic membrane resulting in the contents of the ACh vesicles being discharged
ɔ the synaptic cleft (Bennett et al., 1992). Calcium ions also cause an increase in size
the pool of ACh immediately available for release. It does this by reacting with the
minal serine on the filament of synapsin 1 holding the reserve vesicles to microtubular
uctures in the axoplasm (Fig. 9.2.).

At the same time it speeds up the active process involved in packaging ACh
ɔlecules against their concentration gradient into the ACh vesicle ready for release
arshall et al., 1976) (Fig. 9.3.). This process, which is depressed by parathion and
ɑlathion, is calmodulin dependent and requires energy. (For a fuller description see
pendix 9.2. and 9.3.). (Fig. 9.2.). Without this presynaptic feed back mechanism
uromuscular transmission is depressed and in extreme cases it is blocked, causing
ralysis (Bowman et al., 1990; Standaert, 1964; Standaert, 1986). It is characteristic of
s kind of block that it will affect a train of stimuli or tetanic stimuli causing a
ɔgressive depression in the response (train of four or tetanic fade) whilst it is less
ely to affect the response to a single stimulus. It also prevents the normal overshoot
llowing tetanic stimulation, post tetanic potentiation (Standaert, 1964). As these
ects are the result of a failure to release sufficient ACh they are reversed, to a variable
tent, by anticholinesterases.

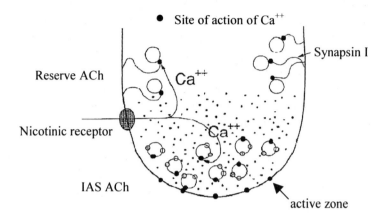

Figure 9.2. Calcium affects both the mobilisation and the release of acetylcholine in the motor nerve.

ACh is emptied from its vesicles into the synaptic cleft at active sites on **t** presynaptic membrane as the result of the interaction of specialised sites on the A**c** vesicle; synaptotagmin and docking protein in the nerve membrane. This process **i** calcium dependent (Clementi and Meldolesi, 1990). The active sites on the nerve **a** opposite the highest density of cholinergic receptors which is found on the shoulders **o** longitudinal clefts at the end plate on the muscle (the secondary clefts). As th**e** transverse the synaptic cleft they are minimally exposed to the molecules of long tai**l** cholinesterase which are found in high concentration in the meshes of the basem**e** membrane filling the cleft. However, once ACh leaves the receptor site it is immediat**e** exposed to the enzyme-acetylcholinesterase, and is hydrolysed in a fraction of a seco**n** Under usual quiet activity it is the same small fraction of the total vesicular populati**o** of the nerve terminal that participates in this process. These few (about 20% of the to**t** number of vesicles) are constantly emptying their contents into the synaptic cleft a**n** being refilled from newly formed ACh in the cytoplasm. With most transmitters **t** production of an excess or the failure of it to be destroyed leads to a down regulation **o** its rate of production. Although up regulation has been occasionally described followi**n** depression of motor nerve activity it is unusual (Martyn *et al.,* 1992).

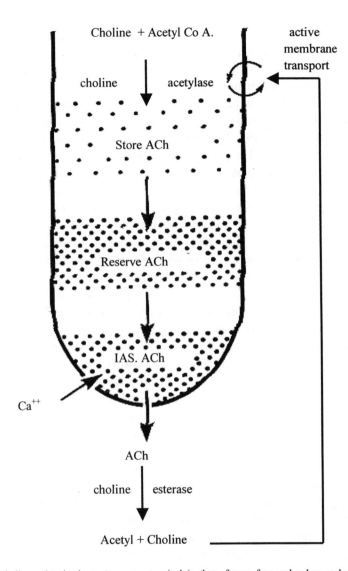

Figure 9.3. Acetylcholine exists in the motor nerve terminal in three forms; free molecules; packaged molecules that are tethered and as IAS, the immediately available store of vesicles

In the case of ACh as a neuromuscular transmitter other mechanisms come into p
to restrict its production and release. This involves presynaptic cholinergic recept
and a complex feed back mechanism (Bowman, 1990; Bowman *et al.,* 1984).

Relatively little is known about these presynaptic receptors except that they differ
certain functions from those on the muscle. They are blocked, to a lesser extent th
post synaptic receptors, by curare like agents although the effect is more rapid and la
longer (Feldman, 1996; Hubbard *et al.,* 1969). They are rapidly desensitised. A;
result after prolonged or excessive stimulation they appear to become refractory (Rik
1975). Following prolonged bombardment by ACh or ACh like drugs, they m
become desensitised for long periods causing muscle weakness or paralysis due to 1
loss of the important feed back mechanism (Bowman, 1984; Riker, 1966).

The OPs act by preventing the normal rapid destruction of ACh
acetylcholinesterase. This causes a prolonged accumulation of excess ACh at 1
neuromuscular junction. Our present concept of the effects caused by the continu
action of an excess of ACh is to some extent conjectural and depend upon observatic
in experimental conditions using relatively stable drugs, ACh agonists, that act like AC

Our understanding of the different pre and post synaptic effects are due largely
studies using incomplete and complex blockers of these receptors, like the methonii
compounds. These drugs are structurally like 2 molecules of ACh with a chain
methyl groups separating them. The more methyl groups the greater the separation of 1
2 ACh moieties. They were studied extensively in the 1950s by Burns, Paton a
Zaimis (Burns and Paton, 1951; Zaimis and Head, 1976; Paton and Zaimis, 1994; Pat
and Zaimis, 1952). They concluded that if the chain was short (5 or 6 methyl groups'
acted on neural ganglia, i.e. had a presynaptic effect, if it were longer i.e. if it had
methyl groups - decamethonium, it acted at post synaptic sites causing neuromuscu
block (Paton and Zaimis, 1994; Paton and Zaimis, 1952). They showed that it c
indeed cause a small short lived ACh like effect on the muscle end plate which th
termed 'depolarisation block' by analogy to the type of block which can be caused by
cathodal current applied to the muscle membrane (Burns and Paton, 1951). The effect
such a current is to antagonise the resting transmembrane potential causi
depolarisation. This view held sway for many years and depolarising neuromuscu
block became part of anaesthetic literature. As ACh and the methonium compoui
decamethonium, both have a similar effect at the post synaptic membrane, it was he
that OP poisons caused a decamethonium like action at this site.

As a result it has been suggested that they produce muscle weakness and paralysis a depolarising block. It is now realised that although depolarisation occurs this is y part of the story.

From the outset Zaimis had difficulty in explaining why in certain animals ›olarising agents caused tonic contractions whilst in others it caused flaccid paralysis ‹imis, 1953; Zaimis, 1976). She had difficulty in explaining why in humans, ›ecially those with myasthenia gravis, prolonged action by these drugs caused a form paralysis that outlasted the drugs presence in the blood stream by hours or days ›urchill Davidson and Richardson, 1952) and why this secondary, or phase II effect ›uld be in part reversible by giving an anticholinesterase.

The problem was compounded when Katz and Thesleff (1975) demonstrated that ‹ only was the degree of depolarisation produced by these drugs less than that monstrated by Jenerick and Gerrard (1953) to be required to produce cathodal block ‹ that the post synaptic events were far shorter than the duration of the block.

They attributed the block to desensitisation of the receptor. In 1966, Riker and later ‹lindo (1971) demonstrated that ACh affected not only post synaptic receptors but also : motor nerve terminal. This was followed by an accumulation of evidence that the ‹thonium compounds, muscle relaxants, the anticholineserases and ACh itself have portant presynaptic actions (Standaert and Adams 1965, Otsaka et al. 1962, Bowman 80, Wessler 1992). Their actions cause stimulation of the feed back mechanism in ‹v doses for relatively short periods but induce a refractory block, or desensitisation, .er prolonged exposure (Roberts and Wilson 1968).

We now have the theoretical basis for the paradox of why anticholinesterases like Ps, drugs that increase the availability of transmitter, should produce a block of uromuscular conduction and why that block might continue, or may only occur, long ‹er the drug has disappeared from the blood stream, why when it does so it might spond, at least partially, to a further dose of anticholinesterase. An interesting analogy seen in the treatment of myasthenia gravis by long term anticholinesterase therapy ‹eter and Cherian, 2000). It has been observed that increasing refractoriness to the drug ›velops in these patients which can result in a severe form of paralysis. This can be ‹ated by stopping the therapy and ventilating the patient artificially.

9.4. Neuromuscular Effects of the Organophosphates

The effect produced by an OP on the neuromuscular transmission depends upon the ty
of drug involved, the dose and the route by which it is administered. With some dru
such as parathion, the effect of the poison is delayed in the body whilst metabo
conversion takes place replacing the sulphur atom with oxygen. As this occ
progressively over the 24 hours following ingestion, the onset of the drug eff
develops slowly. Other poisons, such as the nerve gases, act with alarming rapid
following inhalation. Pharmacokinetic considerations render the oral route the slowe
as the drug is subjected to a first pass effect in the liver following absorption from t
gut, an effect that would be increased by lipophillicity. Many factors affect the rate
which the drug enters the blood stream and the rapidity with which inactivation
acetylcholinesterase occurs.   Against this must be set the rate of reactivation a
regeneration of the enzyme.

In this context the inactivation of plasma, or pseudocholinesterase (BuChE)
unimportant except in so far as it provides a physiological flypaper or 'sink' to mop
some of the drug and to offer protection against low doses of anticholinesterases
drugs of low potency (see Chapter 2). It is more important, however, in relation
anaesthesia. (see Chapter 5).

9.5. Acute Organophosphate Poisoning (Haddad, 1990; Karalliedde, 1999)

The acute symptoms caused by the actions of OP poisons upon the heart, circulatic
salivary glands and gut predominate, although even at this stage, with mild to moder
poisoning, muscle fasciculation and cramps may occur. Provided atropine has prevent
cardiovascular collapse, overwhelming intoxication produces some degree of musc
paralysis in between 30 and 50% of patients suffering from acute intoxication. This
frequently most pronounced in the muscles of respiration and in those supporting t
airway. This presents as increasing respiratory embarrassment made worse l
bronchoconstriction and bronchorhea which often accompany it. In about a third of a
cases admitted to hospital a flaccid paralysis requiring ventilatory support develo
within 12 hours. The duration of the paralysis varies but is generally in the order of 2-
days (see Chapter 5).

The cause of the muscle fasciculations, twitching and possibly the cramps which are nmonly seen after OP intoxication and also occur following administration of agonist gs, such as suxamethonium, have been variously ascribed to uncoordinated muscle ·e contraction, muscle fibre damage and action on muscle spindles which are involved maintaining the tone of postural muscles (Karalliedde, 1999; Brodsky and renworth, 1980). Whilst these effects are possible the present view is that they are the ult of antidromic and orthodromic firing of motor nerves resulting from stimulation of synaptic receptors (Katamura et al., 1981; Goldstein et al., 1987). This effect has n clearly demonstrated in animal by Standaert and Adams (1965) and would fit the dings of Besser et al. (1991) of repetitive after discharge found in the compound ion potentials of affected muscles.

The onset of muscle paralysis is usually attributed to the occurrence of depolarising ck (Peter and Cherain, 2000). Whilst some degree of depolarisation undoubtedly urs it would be anticipated that the effect would be insufficient to produce the longed paralysis observed in these patients. Prolonged drug induced depolarising ck of neuromuscular conduction has never been convincingly demonstrated. It would account for the neurophysiological findings, such as fade at rapid stimulation rates, orted in those few cases where it has been studied in the acute state. Depolarisation been assumed to be the cause of the paralysis by analogy with the block that was ieved to be caused by the methonium compounds, a theory that is now challenged iker, 1966; Galindo, 1971; Standaert and Adams, 1965; Otsaka et al., 1962; Bowman, 80; Wessler, 1992; Feldman and Hood, 1994). Before we can safely ascribe the block a specific post synaptic depolarising mechanism further studies of patients with the ite syndrome are required. It is likely that these studies would reveal initial polarisation (phase I block) rapidly giving way to a predominantly desensitisation ck (phase II). It is possible that an element of channel block may also be involved e Appendix 1) and that like neostigmine, a potent short acting anticholinesterase, the ·s may act directly on ion channels in the presynaptic membrane (Braga et al., 1993). is quite possible for both a pre and post synaptic mechanism to be occur nultaneously as a complex interdependence exists between the two effects.

9.6.   The Intermediate Syndrome (see Chapter 6) (Wadia *et al.*, 1974; Senanayake ε Karalliedde, 1987, De Bleeker 1995)

This syndrome has been reported in between 8 and 50% of intoxications treated hospital. It can occur up to 4 days following exposure to the poison when the level acetylcholineserase is usually recovering towards normality. It presents as respirate paralysis and the weakness often involves the cranial or bulbar nerves. Most patie respond to ventilatory support and recovery of full muscle power usually occurs. So cases have demonstrated a disproportionate weakness of the respiratory muscles wh compared to those of the limbs—Senanayake and Karalliedde (1987) and De Blee (1995) described the presence of the tetanic fade, a lack of post-tetanic potentiation a well maintained twitch response in these patients.

These are the neuromuscular characteristics of presynaptic block. Others ha described a low voltage response which could result either from pre or post synap block (He *et al.*, 1998). Some studies have found EMG evidence of an axonal def compatible with a prejunctional deficit (Baker and Sedgwick, 1996). This could be ι result of a depression of phosphodiesterase activity causing neuro-degenerative-chang affecting ACh synthesis. Although more evidence would allow a definitive expositi of the cause of this syndrome, its late occurrence, the presence of tetanic fade ι maintained twitch response and its predilection for muscles in which the mechanisms acetylcholine production are most consistently stretched, would suggest a ma presynaptic component in this type of neuromuscular block. This conclusion does ι exclude the possibility of other mechanisms such as a neuro-degenerative processes al being involved.

As long ago as 1969, Ariens and co workers described a necrotising myopathy that followed the administration of parathion to rats. This observation has been repeated by Fenichel et al (1974) who demonstrated that it was due to the effect on the muscle of excess ACh. It was prevented by treatment with hemicholinium, a drug that prevents choline transport into the nerve, reducing the rate of ACh synthesis and by section of the nerve supplying the muscle. It could be replicated by administering guanidine: a substance known to increase ACh production and prevented by tubocurarine and alpha bungarotoxin, both of which prevent the reaction of ACh with the receptor on the muscle (Fenichel et al 1972). The OP induced myopathy can be prevented if 2-PAM is given to experimental animals in a dose sufficient to reactivate cholinesterase within 10-20 minutes of poisoning with paraoxon (Dettbarn 1984). It has been observed that the muscles principally affected in this syndrome are the postural muscles and the muscles associated with respiration. These muscles are subject to continuous activity and therefore are most likely to produce an excess of ACh following OP poisoning.

It would appear that the muscle necrosis caused by OP poisons is a consequence of excessive stimulation of the post-synaptic cholinoceptor by ACh. There is evidence that this is associated with the release of calcium ions from the sarcoplasmic reticulum and its accumulation in toxic concentrations in the cytosol. In experiments using prostigmine, a pharmacologically similar drug to the OP anticholinesterases, Leonard and Saltpeter (1972) demonstrated that chelating agents reduced the severity of the myopathy. Other workers (Csillik and Savay 1963) had demonstrated that there is accumulation of calcium in the muscle fibres adjacent to the end plate, following cholinesterase administration.

9.7. Delayed Neuropathy (OPIDP)

The symptoms of this syndrome differ from those of the Acute and Intermediate Syndromes, they occur later and they are seldom reversible. Recovery, if it occurs at all, takes many months or years.

It is associated with pathological degenerative changes in the nerve and mus
producing loss of function. The part played by neuromuscular events in this syndrome
conjectural as the symptoms only appear after a delay of days or weeks follow
exposure to the poison. In some cases it follows as long as three weeks after a ma
exposure to OPs. It is characterised by progressive muscle weakness often associa
with some sensory loss (Moretto and Lotti, 1998). It often occurs in patients who ha
not been exposed to high doses of poison or to one of the more potent OPs.
occasionally occurs in patients who have developed the Intermediate Syndrome.

Studies carried out in these patients suggest that, in the less seriously affect
individuals, the defect initially starts in the nerve and that this causes secondary chang
in the muscle. In those exposed to more toxic concentrations of poison, nee
degeneration is overshadowed by focal necrosis of the muscle itself. Most of t
evidence, as to the manner in which the pathological changes observed in patie
develop, has come from experiments in rodents.

A condition has been described in mouse muscle, exposed to prolong
anticholinesterase activity, in which activation of some of the cholinoceptors on the pe
synaptic membrane fail to release the calcium ions necessary to initiate mus
contraction. The occurrence of this has been attributed to the blocking action of the O
upon neuropathy target esterase which is essential for normal neural function (Kimura
al., 1995; Johnson and Lauwerys, 1969). The resulting defect causes a demyelinati
degeneration of the nerve and of its associated Schwann cell. This produces a conditi
similar to that seen in the 'die back' neuropathies (Drachman et al., 1969). Although t
exact mechanism by which this causes muscle weakness remains unclear it is possit
that it could be the result of the loss of the trophic function of the motor nerve upon t
neuromuscular end plate. It is now recognised that the focal anatomy of the end-pl
depends upon the trophic effect of continuing motor nerve activity mediated throu
peptides, such as the Calcitonin Gene Related Peptide (CGRP). If the motor nerve fa
to secrete these peptides then the discrete architecture of the post synaptic end plate
lost resulting in changes characteristic of denervation. This includes loss of the foc
structure of the muscle end plate and a diffuse spread of immature cholinoceptors ov
the surface of the muscle. Associated degenerative changes develop in the muscle fib
in the region of the end plate. In experimental models these changes are reversible.

It seems likely that most of the long term effects of the OPIDP syndrome are due
more serious and less readily reversible changes.

It would appear that the OPIDP syndrome is caused by a mixture of the effects of ᶜenerative changes, which are predominantly neural in the milder cases and which ᵖgress to more permanent and debilitating muscle necrosis, in those more severely ᵉcted.

3. Other Possible Neuromuscular Effects

many different situations where anticholinesterases have been administered for ᵖlonged periods, in non- toxic doses there have been complaints of ill health which ᵐ a fairly distinct picture, Amongst these are sensory loss, especially of touch and ᵇration sense, muscle weakness, loss of muscle mass, excessive fatiguability on ᵉrcise and painful spasms of muscles. These symptoms have been reported after ᵖosure to OP pesticides, especially after chronic exposure associated with sheep dips ᵈ after prolonged use of the anticholinesterase, pyridostigmine, in servicemen during ᵉ Gulf War (the Gulf War Syndrome). The combined working party set up by the ᵖllege of Physicians and the College of Psychiatrists to investigate the association with ᵉep dip (1998) concluded that the frequency and consistency of these reports ᵍgested a common underlying cause. Epidemiological studies found that those most ᵉly to be affected were workers who mixed the dip and who were therefore exposed to ᵉ highest concentrations of the drug, albeit for relatively short periods. They ᵐcluded that it was not possible from these investigations to suggest the likely ᵉchanism by which the pathological changes were produced.

A study by the Rand Corporation in California published in 1999 of 1000 servicemen, given pyridostigmine for prophylaxis against a nerve gas attack during the Gulf War, concluded that this cholinesterase was the probable cause of many of the symptoms of GWS. No mechanism by which these effects are produced has been identified although there is presumptive evidence of pre-synaptic effects on nerves and of axonal degeneration. The symptoms in this group differ from all the other known effects of OPs in that they are not reversible and are usually progressive. If, as seems likely there is a common underlying causal mechanism, it is linked to prolonged inactivation of cholinesterases. In view of their widespread use it is imperative that further studies be conducted to elucidate the aetiology. One problem that arises in planning such a study is that the symptoms described are not dissimilar from those complained of by patients suffering from myasthenic encephalitis (ME) which is a spontaneously occurring syndrome not associated with known exposure to anticholinesterases. Neuromuscular disorders figure prominently in the various syndromes produced by OP poisons. That they should do so is not surprising as neuromuscular transmission involves a highly sophisticated cholinergic mechanism which may be disturbed at any of several levels, the formation of ACh, its packaging into vesicles, its storage, its release from its tied form into the free, available form, its release into the synaptic cleft and its ability to produce a sufficient ion shift on the post synaptic membrane to trigger off an action potential and contraction of muscle. By preventing the hydrolysis of ACh by acetylcholinesterase, OPs prolong its presence at the myoneural junction resulting in a gross disturbance of this delicate balance. The evidence that prolonged and excessive exposure to ACh, following OP poisoning, produces progressive muscle necrosis offers some clues as to why some symptoms, associated with the use of these chemicals, do not become apparent until days or weeks after the exposure.

Appendix 1, The Receptor

Cholinergic receptors are large structures that are 10nm long and that perforate the cell membranes bulging into the extracellular fluid and also extending marginally into the intracellular space. From the surface they appear like a doughnut with a central pore. Around this central channel are the 5 subunits characteristic of this type of receptor.

The central channel is narrowed at the level of the junction between the extracellular and intracellular parts. When the receptor is stimulated it produces conformational changes in the subunits which result in dilatation of the isthmus. There are two ACh recognition sites, one on each of the 2 alpha subunits in the region of amino acids 191–193. The site is a lacuna guarded by two cysteine amino acids presenting sulfydral terminals, the so called disulfide loop. Both of these recognition sites have to be simultaneously activated in order to evoke a response in the receptor.

The composition of the 5 subunits vary. Those in the central nervous system, ganglia and probably the presynaptic site at the neuromuscular junction are composed solely of 2 alpha and 3 beta units. The genes for expressing delta, gamma and epsilon subunits are not present in the CNS. There are at least 7 variations of each of these subunits depending upon the particular alpha subunit (alpha 2–3, 4 or 7– or beta 2 or 4). It is this variability that gives the different characteristics to the various groups of receptors. The post synaptic muscle receptors are composed of 2 alpha, one delta and one gamma or epsilon subunit depending upon the species studied and the maturity of the subject. In the neonate the epsilon unit is replaced by a gamma. As the child matures fewer gamma units are found and epsilon ones come to predominate. Following denervation and die back neuropathies, the gamma units reappear in the receptor in increasing numbers. A receptor containing gamma rather than epsilon units has a longer open time following stimulation by ACh. As a result there is an increased ion flux during activity. One effect of the difference in the composition of the receptor is that muscle fasciculation and repetitive nerve firing are greatly reduced following exposure to ACh or agonist drugs. This possibly could be the basis for the observation that muscle fasciculations are infrequent following OP intoxication in very young children (Sofer et al 1989, Zwiener and Ginsburg 1988).

In order to open the central channel and increase the membrane permeability to sodium, the focal recognition sites, one on each of the 2 alpha subunits, must be simultaneously activated by ACh.

Prolonged exposure to ACh or anticholinesterases causes refractoriness of both t
pre and post synaptic receptors. This has been termed desensitisation. The process h
been most studied in post synaptic receptors as specific ligands for these receptors a
available which makes it possible to isolate them and to express them in oocytes. The
characteristics can be studied in vitro in patch clamp experiments.   Unfortunate
desensitisation develops most readily in the presynaptic receptors, which are difficult
study and where it may be a physiological protective mechanism. The manner by whi
it occurs remains obscure.

It may involve local ionic changes which 'short circuit' the membrane or a structur
alteration in the receptor. Another possibility is that it is a manifestation of open chann
or channel block. This occurs when an ion to which the membrane is not complete
permeable sticks in the central pore at the isthmus preventing the passage of other ion
This type of block occurs most readily in hyperpolarised membranes in which there
prolonged opening of the ion channel.

Appendix Two, Formation of ACh

ACh is synthesised from choline in the mitochondria of the nerve terminals. Cholir
enters the axoplasm from the extracellular fluid by means of a highly specific, sodiu
pump dependent, transport system.   About 50% of the choline comes from th
hydrolysis of ACh in the synaptic cleft which is carried into the nerve by activ
transport. This process can be impeded by hemicholinium which acts as a false substra
for the carrier mechanism. The remainder is formed in the neuronal body and carried
the nerve terminal by axonal transport. Choline is acetylated by the enzyme choline-C
acetyltransferase in the cytoplasm of the nerve terminal. Once formed it is loaded in
the vesicles against the concentration gradient by an ATPase calmodulin activate
process.

This process can be blocked by the piperidinol compound vesamicol and t
tetraphenylboron (Marshall et al 1976).

It is likely that during the course of OP intoxication, the availability of cholir
(which is dependent on hydrolysis of ACh by acetylcholinesterase) would be decrease
It is uncertain as to what effect prolonged lack of choline from the synaptic cleft wou
have on the synthesis of ACh.

pendix Three, Control of the Release of ACh

out 20% of the ACh vesicles present in the nerve terminals take part in the constant
:ase and refilling process of quiet normal activity. The remaining 80%, although
rphologically indistinguishable from the releasable vesicles, do not take part unless
re is a sudden rapid neural discharge, such as that associated with a voluntary muscle
traction.

It is the size of the immediately available pool of vesicles that determines how much
'h is released each time the motor nerve in stimulated. This is a random process and
I follow the law of mass action. The amount released will therefore be related to the
of the ACh concentration of vesicles. When the potential reaches the nerve terminal
pens voltage dependent calcium channels. These are not homogeneous. Some are
trolled by membrane potassium channels which, when activated, hyper-polarise the
mbrane reducing its conductance for calcium. These potassium channels are
mselves activated by a rise in cytoplasmic calcium. This is one part of the complex
tem of negative and positive feed back that controls the release of ACh.

Another even more important system involves the presynaptic cholinoceptors. These
blocked by drugs like hexamethonium but unlike the post synaptic receptors are
iffected by alpha bungarotoxin. The presynaptic receptors respond to stimulation by
:h by opening calcium channels. The resulting influx of calcium activates a calcium
iendent proteinase that acts on the terminal serine in the fine protein filament,
apsin 1 that appears to tether the stored vesicles of ACh to microtubular structures in
axoplasm. The releases of these vesicles massively increases the number of them
ilable to respond to repeated rapid tetanic rates of nerve stimulation. Without this
nsfer from the store of vesicles into the readily available pool the amount of ACh
illable to meet a train of rapid nerve stimuli would tail off causing tetanic fade. A
:ond action of the calcium ions is to react with the synaptotagamin in the vesicular
ll causing it to rotate and dock with the docking protein at the active zone of the
synaptic membrane, Thus, the net result of this presynaptic positive feed back
chanism, activated by rapid neural activity, is to increase both the amount of ACh
ilable for release and the rate at which release takes place.

References

Ariens, A.T., Cohen, E.M., Meeter, E., *et al.* Reversible necrosis of the end-plate regi in striated muscle of the rat poisoned with cholinesterase inhibitors *Experimen* 1969;**9**:2557–9

Baker, D.J., Sedgwick, E.M. Single fibre electromyographic changes in man af organophosphate exposure. *Human and Experimental Toxicology* 1996;**15**:369–75

Bennett, H.M.K., Calakas, N., Scheller, R.H. Syntaxin, a synaptin protein implicated closing of synaptic vesicles on presynaptic active zones. *Science* 1992;**257**:255–9

Besser, R., Vogt, T., Gutmann, L., *et al.* High pancuronium sensitivity of axo nicotinic acetylcholine receptors in humans during organophosphate poisonir *Muscle Nerve* 1991;**14**:1197–1201

Birks, P.I. The role of sodium ions in metabolism of acetylcholine. *Canadian Journal Biochemistry and Physiology* 1963;**39**:787–827

Bowman, W.C. Block by depolarization. Editorial. *Acta Anaesthesiolog Scandanavica* 1994;**38**.529–30

Bowman, W.C. In: Pharmacology of Neuromuscular Function. John Wright 1990:116-

Bowman, W.C. Physiology and pharmacology of neuromuscular transmission. *Jourr of Intensive Care Medicine* 1993;**19**:S45–53

Bowman, W.C. Prejunctional and postjunctional cholinoreceptors at the neuromuscu junction. *Anaesthesia and Analgesia.* 1980;**59**:935–43

Bowman, W.C., Marshal, I.G., Gibb, A.J. Is there a feedback control of transmitt release at neuromuscular junction? *Seminars in Anaesthesia* 1984;**3**:275–283

Bowman, W.C., Webb, S.N. Tetanic fade during partial transmission failure produced depolarizing neuromuscular blocking drugs in the cat. *Clinical and Experimen Pharmacology and Physiology* 1976;**3**:545–555

Bowman, W.C. Prior, C., Marshall, I.G. Presynaptic receptors in neuromuscul transmission. *Annals of the New York Academy of. Sciences* 1990;**604**–669

Braga, H.F.M., Rawn, E.G., Harvey, A.L., *et al.* Prejunctional action of neostigmine neuromuscular preparations. *British Journal of Anaesthesia* 1993;**70**:405–10

Brodsky, J.B., Ehrcnworth, J. Post operative muscle pains and suxamethonium. *Briti Journal of Anaesthesia.* 1980;**52**.215–7

Burns, B.D., Paton, W.D.M. Depolarization of the motor end plate by decamethonium. *Journal of Physiology* 1951;**115**:41–73

Csillik, B., Savay, G. Release of calcium at the myoneural junction. *Nature* 1963;**184**:399–400

Clinical aspects of long term lower dose exposure. Organophosphate Sheep Dip. Report of Joint Working Party of Royal College Physicians and Royal College Psychiatrists 1998.

Churchill Davidson, H.C., Richardson, A.T. The action of decamethonium iodide (C I 0) in myasthenia gravis. *Journal of Neurology, Neurosurgery and Psychiatry* 1952;**15**:129–36

Clementi, F., Meldolesi, J. eds. Neurotransmitter release in the neuromuscular junction. London: Academic Press; 1990

Colquhoun, D., Ogden, D.C. Activation of ion channels in the frog endplate by high concentration of acetylcholine. *Journal of Physiology* 1988;**395**:131–5

Colquhoun , D. On the principles of post synaptic action of neuromuscular blocking agents. In Handbook of Experimental Pharmacology, New Blocking Drugs. Karkevich D. A. ed. Springer Verlag 1986 Berlin p59-113

De Bleecker, J.L. The intermediate syndrome in organophosphate poisoning; *Neurotoxiology* 1995;**33**:683–6

del Castillo, J., Katz, B. Quantal components of end plate potential *Journal of Physiology* 1954;**124**:560–73

Dettbarn, W.D. Pesticide induced muscle necrosis; mechanisms and prevention. *Fundamental and Applied Toxicology* 1984;**4**; S 18-S36

Drachman, D.A., Murphy, S.R., Nigam, M.P., *et al.*" Myopathic changes" in chronically denervated muscle. *Archives of Neurology* 1969;**21**:170–7

Feldman, S. Neuromuscular Block, 1996.:Butterworth–Heinemann; U.K.

Feldman, S. Neuromuscular Transmission, 8.2–8.8. In: Atlas of Anaesthesia vol 1. Churchill Livingstone, 1997 Phil. U.S.A.

Feldman, S., Hood, J. Depolarizing neuromuscular block—a presynaptic mechanism. *Acta Anaesthesiologica. Scandinavica.* 1994;**38**:535–41

He F, Xu, H, Qin, F et al. Intermediate myasthenic syndrome following acute organophosphate poisoning—an analysis of 21 cases. *Human and Experimental Toxicology* 1998;**17**:40–5

Fenichel, G.M., Dettbarn, W.D., Newman, T.M. An experimental myopathy seconda to excessive acetylcholine release. *Neurology* 1974;2:441-5

Fenichel, G.M., Kibler, V., Olsen, W.H. *et al.* Inhibition of cholinesterase as a cause neuropathy. *Neurology* 1972;**22**:1026–37

Galindo, A. Depolarising neuromuscular block. *Journal of Pharmacology a Experimental Therapeutics* 1971;**178**:39–46

Gibb, A.J., Marshall, I.G., Bowman, W.C. Effect of Ionophoretically appli acetylcholine on tubocurarine induced end plate current run down, evidence for nicotinic feedback mechanism at the rat neuromuscular junction. *Proceedings of t Australasian Physiology and Pharmacology Society* 1984. p. 15–88

Ginsborg, B., Jenkinson, D.H. Transmission of impulse from nerve to muscle. I *Neuromuscular Junction. Handbook of Experimental Pharmacology.* Zaimis, E. e Berlin: Springer–Verlag; 1976. p. 229–364.

Goldstein, B.D., Fincher, D.R., Seorley, J.R. Electrophysiological changes in senso neurons following sub chronic soman and sarin: alterations in receptor functio *Toxicology and Applied Pharmacology* 1987;**91**:55–64

Haddad, L.M. Organophosphates and other insecticides. In: *Clinical Management Poisoning and Drug Overdose.* Haddad, L.M., Winchester, J.W.B. eds. Saunde Co; 1990. p. 1076–87

Hubbard, J.I., Wilson, D.P., Miyamoto, M. Reduction of transmitter release by tubocurarine. *Nature* 1969;228.531

Jenerick, H.P., Gerrard, R.W. Membrane potential and threshold of a single musc fibre. *Journal of Cellular and Comparative Physiology* 1953;**42**:79–83

Johnson, M.K., Lauwerys, P. Protection by some carbamates against neurotoxic delaye effects of diisopropyl phosphofluoride. *Nature* 1969;**222**:1066–7

Karalliedde, L. Organophosphate poisoning and anaesthesia. *Anaesthes* 1999;**54**:1089–94

Katamura, S., .Yoshiyo, 1., Tashiro, C. *et al.*. Succinylcholine causes fasciculation by prejunctional mechanism. *Anesthesiology* 1981;**55**:A221

Katz, B., Thesleff, S. A study of 'desensitization' produced by acetylcholine on th motor nerve end plate. *Journal of Physiology* 1975;**138**:63–9

Kimura, I., Katsuya, U., Tsureki, H. Post synaptic nicotinic receptor desensitized b non-contractile Ca metabolism via proteinkinase-C activation at the mous neuromuscular junction. *British Journal of Pharmacology* 1995;**114**:461–7

onard, J.P., Saltpeter, G. Agonist induced myopathy at the neuromuscular junction is mediated by calcium. *Journal of Cell Biology* 1972;**82**:811–9

arshall, I.G., Parsons, R.L., Paul, V.K. Depletion of synaptic vesicles in frog neuromuscular junction by tetraphenylboron. *Experientia* 1976;**32**:1423–5

artyn, J.A.J. The neuromuscular junction basic receptor pharmacology. In: *Muscle Relaxants*. Fukshemaka, A.K., Ochial, P. eds Springer–Verlag; 1995. p. 31–7

artyn, J.A.J., White, P.A., Gronert, G.A. *et al.* Up and down regulation of skeletal muscle acetylcholine receptors. *Anesthesiology* 1992;**76**:822–43

cIntosh, F.C. Formation, storage and release of acetylcholine at nerve endings. *Canadian Journal of Biochemistry and Physiology* 1963;**37**:343–56

oretto, A., Lotti, M. Poisoning by organophosphorus insecticides and sensory neuropathy. *Journal of Neurology Neurosurgery and Psychiatry* 1998;**64**:463–8

tsaka M., Bndo, M., Nonamura, Y. Presynaptic nature of neuromuscular depression. *Japanese Journal of Pharmacology* 1962;**12**:573–84

aton, W.D.M., Zaimis, E.J. The methonium compounds. *Pharmacological Reviews* 1952;**4**:219–53

aton, W.D.M., Zaimis, E.J. The pharmacological actions of polymethylene bistrimethyl ammonium salts. *British Journal of Pharmacology* 1994;**4**:381–400

eter, J.V., Cherian, A.M. Organic pesticides. *Anaesthesia and Intensive Care* 2000;**28**:11–21

iker, W.F. Actions of acetylcholine on mammalian nerve terminal. *Journal of Pharmacology and Experimental Therapeutics* 1966;**152**:397–416

iker, W.F. Prejunctional effects of neuromuscular blockers and facilitating drugs. In: *Muscle Relaxants.* Katz, R.L. ed.North Holland;1975. p. 59–102

oberts, R.B., Wilson, A. *Myasthenia Gravis*. London: Heinemann Medical Books; 1968,

enanayake, N., Karalliedde, L. Neurotoxic effects of organophosphorus insecticides; intermediate syndrome. *New England Journal of Medicine* 1987;**316**:761–3

ofer, S., Tal,A., Shahak, E. Carbamate and organophosphate poisoning in early childhood. *Pediatric Emergency Care* 1989;**5**:222-5

tandaert, F.G. Basic physiology and pharmacology of the neuromuscular junction. In *Anesthesia* 2nd Edition. New York:Churchill Livingstone; 1986. p. 835–70

tandaert, F.G. The mechanism of post tetanic potention in cat soleus and gastrocnemius muscles. *Journal of. General. Physiology* 1964;**47**:987–1001

Standeart, F.G., Adams J.F. The actions of succinylcholine on mammalian nerve terminals. *Journal of Pharmacology and Experimental Therapeutics* 1965;**149**:113–23

Wadia, R.S., Sadagoppan, C., Amin, R.B., *et al.* Neurological manifestations oforganophosphate insecticide poisoning. *Journal of Neurology, Neurosurgery and Psychiatry* 1974;**37**:841–7

Wessler, 1. Acetylcholine at motor nerves : storage, release and presynaptic modulation by autoreceptors and adrenoceptors. *International Reviews of Neurobiology* 1992:34:283-4.

Zaimis, B.J. The neuromuscular junction. Areas of uncertainty. In: *Neuromuscular Junction. Handbook of Experimental Pharmacology* Zaimis, E.J. ed. Springer–Verlag; 1976 Berlin: p. 1–21

Zaimis, E.J. Motor endplate differences as a determining factor in the mode of action of neuromuscular blocking substances. *British Journal of Pharmacology and Chemotherapy* 1953;**5**:486–98

Zaimis, E.J., Head, S.L. Depolarizing neuromuscular blocking drugs. In: *Neuromuscular Junction. Handbook of Experimental Pharmacology* Zaimis, E.J. ed. Springer–Verlag; 1976. Berlin:p. 365–419

Zwiener,R.J.,Ginsburg,M. Organophosphate and carbamate poisoning in infants and children. *Pediatrics* 1988:**81**:121-6

CHAPTER 10

Organophosphates and the Cardiovascular System

A.M. Saadeh

10.1. Introduction

Two groups of people suffer most from the acute harmful effects of organophosphorous (OP) pesticides (Saadeh *et al.* 1996; Litovitz, 1991; Tsao *et al.*, 1990; Kiss and Fazekas, 1979; Bardin, *et al.*, 1987). These are children who are accidentally poisoned by ingestion of these substances and young adults who ingest them for suicidal intent. These substances are highly toxic to humans, affecting almost all body systems. Cardiac complications often accompany poisoning with these compounds, which may be serious and often fatal. These complications are potentially preventable if they are recognised early and treated adequately.

The extent, frequency and pathogenesis of the cardiac toxicity from these compounds has not been clearly defined. Until very recently the current body of knowledge consisted of limited studies and case reports (Kiss and Fazekas, 1979; Lerman *et al.*, 1984; Lyzhnikov *et al.*, 1975; Ludomirsky *et al.*, 1982). This lack of knowledge may be explained by two facts, first, there is no compulsory official notification scheme for adverse effects of acute toxicity from OP pesticides and secondly, many physicians and general practitioners are not fully aware of the cardiac toxicity associated with this poisoning. Apart from neurological and neuropsychiatric complications, chronic sequelae from organophosphate poisoning may also occur.

Cardiac toxicity, like other systemic complications, are acute exposure effects. In the majority, acute poisoning results either in death or full recovery after a relatively short period. Apart from a single case of congestive (dilated) cardiomyopathy occurring after long-term OP exposure (Kiss and Fazekas, 1983), there are no reports of chronic cardiac sequelae in the literature.

10.2. Diagnosis of OP Poisoning

Confirmation of the diagnosis is usually made by measurement of serum cholinesterase levels.

Erythrocyte cholinesterase levels are more reliable, but they are difficult to estimate and usually require more specialised laboratory facilities. See Chapter 15.

10.3. Toxicity of OPs

Organophosphates inhibit acetylcholinesterase (AChE) activity in blood, brain and most other tissues leading to accumulation of acetylcholine (ACh) at ganglionic and postganglionic synapses of the autonomic nervous system and at the end-plates of the skeletal muscles. Muscarinic effects are produced by accumulation of ACh at parasympathetic cholinergic nerve endings and nicotinic effects by accumulation of ACh at the motor end-plates of skeletal muscle and at autonomic ganglia (Taylor, 1980).

Depending upon the predominant muscarinic or nicotinic effects, OPs cause bradycardia, tachycardia, hypotension, hypertension, pulmonary oedema, heart block and other cardiac rhythm disturbances.

10.4. Cardiovascular Manifestations of OP Poisoning

10.4.1. Manifestations of Acute Toxicity

These include clinical and electrocardiographic changes. The clinical manifestations are:

- Muscarinic (pulmonary oedema and cyanosis due to excessive bronchial secretions and bronchoconstriction, bradycardia, hypotension and heart block).
- Nicotinic (tachycardia, hypertension, respiratory muscle paralysis and respiratory failure).
- CNS (nicotinic). Hypotension, respiratory depression and cyanosis.

Electrocardiographic abnormalities of acute toxicity include: prolongation of the QTc interval, ST-T changes, brady and tachyarrhythmias, ventricular fibrillation and asystole and various degrees of AV conduction defects. Electrocardiographic and other cardiac manifestations of acute OP toxicity seen in 46 adult patients reported by the author (Saadeh et al., 1997) are presented in Table 10.1.

Table 10.1. Cardiac manifestations of acute organophosphate and carbamate poisoning seen in 46 adults (From Saadeh *et al.*, 1997), with permission)

	Female	Male	Total (%)
Electrocardiographic manifestations			
Prolonged QTc-interval	18	13	31 (67)
Elevated ST segment	3	8	11 (24)
Inverted T waves	3	5	8 (17)
Prolonged P-R interval	2	2	4 (9)
Atrial fibrillation	-	4	4 (9)
Ventricular tachycardia	1	3	4 (9)
Extrasystoles	2	1	3 (6)
Ventricular fibrillation	-	2	2 (4)
Other Cardiac Manifestations			
Pulmonary oedema (non-cardiogenic)	11	9	20 (43)
Sinus tachycardia	6	10	16 (35)
Sinus bradycardia	6	7	13 (28)
Hypertension	3	7	10 (22)
Hypotension	4	4	8 (17)

This table refers only to the manifestations recorded before the administration of atropine.

Other rare electrocardiographic abnormalities such as transient right ventricular overload due to transient pulmonary hypertension induced by malathion poisoning were reported by Chharba *et al.* (1970). It is important to mention that all electrocardiographic changes were reversible within a few days, the longest remained for 5-days (Saadeh *et al.*, 1997). However, some investigators (Chharba *et al.*, 1970) reported ST-T changes persisting for two months after the acute poisoning.

10.4.2. Manifestations of Long-Term Exposure

Apart from an isolated case report of congestive (dilated) cardiomyopathy (Kiss and Fazekas, 1983), occurring after long-term exposure to organophosphates, there are no other reports of chronic cardiac sequelae in the literature.

10.4.3. Congenital Cardiac Defects

Congenital cardiac defects were reported in children who were exposed in utero, after exposure of their mothers to insect repellents containing OP pesticides (chlorpyrifos and oxydemeton-methyl) (Sherman, 1996; Romero *et al.,* 1989; Hall, *et al.,* 1975). These include atrial septal defects and pulmonary stenosis (Sherman, 1996), right aortic arch (Romero *et al.,* 1989) and coarctation of the aorta (Hall *et al.,* 1975).

A summary of the frequency of the electrocardiographic and other cardiac abnormalities seen after organophosphate poisoning as reported in world literature over the past three decades is given in Tables 5.2. and 5.3.

10.5. Pathogenesis of Arrhythmias and other Cardiac Toxicity seen in Organophosphate Poisoning

The mechanism by which organophosphates induce cardiotoxicity is still uncertain. It seems that it occurs by more than one mechanism. Possible mechanisms include sympathetic and parasympathetic overactivity, hypoxaemia, acidosis, electrolyte derangements, prolongation of the QTc interval and a direct toxic effect on the myocardium.

10.5.1. Animal Studies

As early as 1948, Dayrit *et al.,* reported elevation of blood pressure and increase in heart rate with ST-T changes in the surface electrocardiograms in dogs following exposure to hexaethyltetraphosphate and diethylpropanediol OPs. Robineau and Guitten (1987) reported prolongation of the QT interval associated with torsade de pointes ventricular tachycardia in dogs after subcutaneous injections of the nerve agent VX. This type of arrhythmia was seen only with high doses (6.0 μg/kg). Sinus bradycardia and first-degree heart block were also seen with high doses.

Hassler *et al.* (1988) studied the effect of an intravenous OP compound (soman) on the electrical properties of foxhound hearts. Although significant ventricular ectopic activity, idioventricular rhythm and recurrent bouts of ventricular tachycardia occurred, torsade de pointes ventricular tachycardia was not observed. Singer *et al.* (1987) described histopathologic changes in the myocardium of rats given soman and sarin subcutaneously.

Table 10.2. Electrocardiographic abnormalities, after OP poisoning as reported in various world literature

Author	Journal	Year	No of Patients	ST-T changes	First-degree Hrt Blk	VPCS	T de p VT	QTc prolongation	VF
Chharba et al.	Ind J Med Sci	1967	35	13/35= 37%					
Luzhnikov et al.	Kardiologia	1975	183	3/183= 2%	10/183= 5%				29/183 = 16%
Hayes et al.	S Afr Med J	1978	105	5/105= 4%					
Kiss and Fazekas	Acta Cardiol	1979	168	134/163 = 80%	2/168= 1%		7/168 = 4%	134/168= 80%	6/168= 4%
Ludomirsky	Am J Cardiol	1982	15				6/15= 40%	14/15= 93%	
Agarwal	Envir Reaearch	1993	190	6%					
Saadeh et al.	Heart	1997	46	19/46= 41%	4/46=9 %	3/36= 6%		31/46= 67%	2/46= 4%

Organophosphates and Health

Table 10.3. Other (Other than ECG) cardiac abnormalities seen after OP poisoning as reported in world literature over the past three decades

Author	Journal	Year	No. of Patients	Sinus Tachy-cardia	Sinus Brady-cardia	Hypert-ension	Hypo-tension	Pul Oedema	Resp Failure
Namba	WHO	1971	77			24/77= 31%		22/77= 29%	
Hayes et al.	S Afr Med J	1978	105	22/105= 21%	11/105= 21%	19/105= 18%	7/105= 6%	17/105= 16%	23/105= 22%
Kiss and Fazekas	Acta Cardiol	1979	168		3/168= 2%				
Ludomirsky	Am J Cardiol	1982	15	3/15= 20%	2/15= 13%				
Zweiner et al.	Pediatrics	1988	37	18/37= 49%	7/37= 19%	3/37= 8%			14/37= 38%
Tsao-Chang-yao	Chest	1990	107						43/107= 40%
Agarwal	Environ Research	1993	190	48/190= 25%	12/190= 6%	21/190= 11%	6/190= 3%	38/190= 20%	
Lifhitz et al.	Pediatrics	1994	26						3/26= 12%
Saadeh et al.	Heart	1997	46	16/46= 35%	13/46= 28%	10/46= 22%	8/46= 17%	20/46= 43%	8/46= 17%

These rats were examined periodically from day 2 through day 35 after injection. Necropsy findings revealed a high rate of occurrence of myocardial damage (50%) which started as early as day 2 and began to resolve, rarely persisting beyond day 14.

Diffuse myocardial damage was also induced by parathion (Jaaskelainen and Alha, 1969) and intrathion (Biernat and Giermaziak, 1975) in experimental animals. Worek *et al.* (1995) induced marked sinus bradycardia, second and third-degree heart block in guinea pigs after intravenous injection of tabun, sarin, soman and VX. Atropine alone and atropine plus oxime administration immediately after poisoning restored sinus rhythm in animals with mild respiratory depression (depression of <50% of the base line), but caused deleterious ventricular tachycardia in the guinea-pigs with severe respiratory depression (>50% of the base line). McDonough *et al.* (1989) demonstrated histopathologic manifestations of myocardial fibrosis but they found resolution in the myocardium of rats treated with a combination of atropine and diazepam shortly after exposure to soman subcutaneously. These results demonstrated the ability of these drugs to protect against the myocardial damaging effect of OPs.

10.5.2. Human Studies

Both sympathetic and parasympathetic overactivity have been shown to cause myocardial damage (Weidler, 1974; Hall *et al.*, 1936; Manning *et al.*, 1937). As early as 1974, Yasue *et al.* postulated that parasympathetic overactivity plays a major role in coronary artery spasm. Horio *et al.* (1986) induced coronary artery spasm in adult humans with healthy coronary arteries after intracoronary injection of ACh. Ginsburg *et al.* (1980) and Toda (1983) respectively have demonstrated the ability of ACh to cause spasm in isolated human coronary arteries.

In a series of 168 poisonings reported by Kiss and Fazekas (1979), five had a picture of transient myocardial infarction. Similarly in a series of 46 adult cases of OP and carbamate poisoning reported by the author (Saadeh *et al.*, 1997), elevation of the ST segment (≥2mm above the isoelectric line) was seen in 11 cases (24%). This was most striking (≥3 mm) in the anterior precordial leads (V2-V4). The ST segment remained elevated for two days in seven cases, three days in three cases and five days in one case. Of these 11 cases, five were associated with raised cardiac enzymes (mean value, 516 and 782 IU/L for CK and LDH respectively).

Chharba *et al.* (1970) reported diffuse myocardial damage demonstrated at necropsy in five cases after malathion poisoning in a series of 37 patients.

Subendocardial infarction with prolonged QT interval and raised cardiac enzymes after malathion was also reported by Povoa *et al.* (1997). Foci of myocardial necrosis were found in these cases on histopathological examination at postmortem. Kiss and Fazekas (1983) reported focal myocardial damage with capillary haemorrhage, micronecrosis and patchy fibrosis after OP poisoning.

Ludomirsky *et al.* (1982) described three phases of cardiac toxicity after organophosphate poisoning: phase 1, a brief period of intense increase in sympathetic tone manifested by sinus tachycardia, phase 2, a prolonged period of parasympathetic activity manifested by ST-T segment changes and associated with hypoxaemia and phase 3, in which QT-interval prolongation, polymorphic (torsade de pointes) ventricular tachycardia and then ventricular fibrillation and sudden death occur.

10.6. Discussion

Some investigators (Lyzhnikov *et al.*, 1975; Ludomirsky *et al.*, 1982) have described a polymorphic ventricular tachycardia of the torsade de pointes type attributed to a prolongation of the QT-interval associated with organophosphate poisoning. In spite of the presence of a prolonged QTc-interval in the majority of the patients (67%) reported by the author (Saadeh *et al.*, 1997), none of them had this type of arrhythmia. QTc prolongation which occurs in OP poisoning is not related to hypokalemia as serum potassium was normal in most of the patients reported by Kiss and Fazekas (1979) and in all patients of Ludomirsky *et al.* (1982). Ventricular arrhythmias occurring after poisoning sometimes appears shortly after intoxication, during the hypoxic phase (Saadeh *et al.*, 1997), or may appear late, usually after several days (from day 3 to day 15) after the poisoning (Kiss and Fazekas, 1979).

It is difficult to pinpoint one mechanism as the cause of the late appearance of these arrhythmias. Some investigators attribute them to release of some lipid-soluble OPs (i.e. dichlorfenthion and fenthion) from subcutaneous fat with subsequent redistribution to the blood causing severe relapses after several days after apparent recovery (Merrill and Mihm, 1982; Davies *et al.*, 1975), while others attribute them to a prolongation of the QT-interval (Kiss and Fazekas, 1979; Lyzhnikov *et al.*, 1975; Ludomirsky *et al.*, 1982). Other investigators (Kiss and Fazekas, 1983; Chharba *et al.*, 1970; Jaaskelainen and Alha, 1969; Biernat and Giermaziak, 1975) believe that these arrhythmias are the result of a direct toxic effect of OPs on the heart.

Administration of atropine in high doses during the hypoxic phase has been implicated in the development of ventricular arrhythmias (Worek *et al.* 1995, Durham and Hayes, 1962; Wills *et al.*, 1950). No correlation between high doses of atropine and ventricular arrhythmias was found in larger series reported by others (Lyzhnikov *et al.*, 1975; Ludomirsky *et al.*, 1982; Saadeh *et al.*, 1997). It is doubtful whether hypoxia, pulmonary oedema, acidosis, and electrolyte derangements during the first few hours of the poisoning are the major predisposing factors for the development of these arrhythmias, particularly those appearing early in the cholinergic phase of the poisoning.

10.7. Pathogenesis of Sinus Bradycardia and Bradyarrhythmias

Excess of ACh at parasympathetic nerve fibres causes decreased heart rate and slowing of conduction with a consequent fall in cardiac output and hypotension (Taylor, 1980). Bradyarrhythmias result from stimulation of ACh receptors located trans-synaptically and from parasympathetic fibres to the sino-atrial and atrio-ventricular nodes in the heart (James, 1967; James and Spence, 1966). Higher concentrations of ACh have been shown to abolish phase 4 (resting membrane potential) of the action potential of the cardiac muscle (Hoffmann, 1967). The resultant effect on the heart would be sinus bradycardia, sino-atrial nodal disease and atrio-ventricular heart block (Hoffmann, 1967).

An OP compound isolated from the marine dinoflagellate *Ptychodiscus brevis* caused irreversible hypotension and bradycardia in laboratory rats at elevated doses (Mazumder *et al.* 1997). The toxin showed a dose-dependent cardiovascular depressor effect. Similar findings of dose-dependent depressor response were reported by Futagawa *et al.* (1997) after intravenous injection of physostigmine to laboratory animals (rabbits). Small doses of physostigmine caused a pressor response, while high doses elicited a depressor response (hypotension and bradycardia). The pressor response was significantly inhibited by pretreatment with atropine (Futagawa *et al.*, 1997). While the pressor response of ACh inhibitors is attributed to cholinergic mechanisms, the depressor response is thought to result from non-cholinergic mechanisms (inhibition of excitation-contraction coupling in cardiac muscle and vascular smooth muscle) (Futagawa *et al.*, 1997).

10.8. Pathogenesis of Hypertension and Sinus Tachycardia

Hypertension and sinus tachycardia occur as nicotinic effects, while hypotension and sinus bradycardia are muscarinic manifestations (Lovejoy and Linden, 1991). Although bradycardia was thought to dominate in the early cholinergic phase of the poisoning, sinus tachycardia is a more frequent finding (Bardin *et al.*, 1987; Saadeh *et al.*, 1997; Hayes *et al.*, 1978). Some investigators consider the presence of hypertension and sinus tachycardia to be manifestations of severe poisoning (Namba *et al.*, 1971). Hypertension and sinus tachycardia are thought to result from preganglionic nicotinic receptor stimulation followed by release of adrenaline and noradrenaline from the adrenal gland, leading to a predominance of adrenergic effects on the heart (Lovejoy and Linden, 1991; Namba, 1971). Pulmonary oedema and hypoxia, when present, are also contributory factors to the sinus tachycardia.

10.9. Management of Organophosphate Poisoning

10.9.1. General Supportive Measures

Emergency treatment of OP poisoning should be primarily directed to decontamination and resuscitation. Details of management are discussed in Chapter 12.

General supportive measures should be directed towards cardiovascular and respiratory systems, with particular attention to blood pressure, hypoxia, respiratory irregularities, and cardiac arrhythmias. Oxygen delivery and the establishment of an airway and adequate ventilation in the early cholinergic phase of the poisoning will prevent hypoxia. Patients should preferably be admitted to an area with good monitoring and resuscitative facilitates (i.e. ICU or CCU) where continuous electrocardiographic monitoring, constant observation of the level of consciousness, monitoring of electrolytes and acid-base balance, urine output, pulse rate, respiratory rate and blood pressure is carried out.

Physicians are hesitant to use atropine or tend to use inadequate doses in patients with tachycardia or hypertension, because of fear of arrhythmias and/or increases blood pressure. In fact, the converse is true and virtually all patients studied who had high blood pressure or sinus tachycardia had a decrease in the level of blood pressure and heart rate with time, in spite of continued atropine therapy (Saadeh *et al.*, 1997). The pressor response induced in laboratory animals by injection of physostigmine was significantly inhibited by pretreatment with atropine (McDonough *et al.* 1989).

10.9.2. Management of Ventricular Arrhythmias

Treatment of ventricular tachycardia associated with prolonged QTc interval which was not responsive to lidocaine (lignocaine) infusions or were recurrent after direct electrical cardioversion have been shown to respond to intravenous isoproterenol or magnesium sulfate infusions. In some cases the ventricular tachycardia has only been responsive to overdrive pacing (Ludomirsky *et al.*, 1982; Brill *et al.*, 1984; Dive *et al.*, 1994). Electrical overdrive pacing was able to shorten the QTc interval and terminate the arrhythmias in 4 out of 6 and 2 out of 7 cases with torsade de pointes ventricular tachycardias reported by Ludomirsky *et al.* (1982) and Kiss and Fazekas (1983). Isoproterenol infusion was also able to terminate this arrhythmia in 1 out of 6 and 3 out of 7 cases reported by the same authors (Ludomirsky *et al.*, 1982; Kiss and. Fazekas, 1983). Cardiac pacing attempted in 5 patients with ventricular arrhythmias in the series of OP poisoning reported by Lyzhnikov *et al.* (1975) did not induce any improvement, while complete blood replacement in four of these cases, induced normalization of the QTc interval and disappearance of the arrhythmia. Isoproterenol infusion or cardiac pacing increase the heart rate, produce overdrive suppression and shorten the QTc interval. Intravenous magnesium sulfate has been reported to be effective in relieving the ventricular arrhythmias of the torsade de pointes type by several authors (Kiss and Fazekas, 1983; Wang *et al.*, 1998). It is postulated that magnesium sulfate may counteract the direct toxic inhibitory effect of organophosphates on Na^+-K^+ ATPase or it may reactivate the membrane Na^+-K^+ ATPase (Shine, 1979).

10.10. Prognosis

Death from severe OP poisoning usually occurs within the first few hours in untreated cases. The usual causes of death in fatal poisoning are respiratory failure and/or ventricular arrhythmias. Respiratory failure occurs mostly within the first 24 hours during the early cholinergic crises (Tsao et al., 1990; Saadeh et al., 1997).

Ventricular arrhythmias progressing to ventricular fibrillation and/or ventricular asystole are common causes of death either due to hypoxia in the early stages of poisoning (Kiss and Fazekas, 1979; Lyzhnikov et al., 1975; Ludomirsky et al., 1982; Saadeh et al., 1997; Namba et al., 1971) or to direct toxic myocarditis (Kiss and Fazekas, 1983; Chharba et al., 1970; Jaaskelainen and Alha, 1969; Biernat and Giermaziak, 1975) or prolongation of the QTc interval in the later stages (Kiss and Fazekas, 1979; Lyzhnikov et al., 1975; Ludomirsky et al., 1982).

Some investigators (Durham and Hayes, 1962; Wills et al., 1950) have suggested that the high atropine dose administered to severely hypoxic patients is the possible mechanism of ventricular arrhythmias, while others (Massumi et al., 1972) have reported ventricular arrhythmias, including ventricular tachycardia and fibrillation, occurring as a result of atropine therapy in the absence of hypoxia. Table 10.4. shows the mortality rates after organophosphate poisoning as reported in the world literature over the past three decades.

Table 10.4. Mortality rates as reported in the world literature

Author (Ref.)	Journal	Year	No. of Patients	Mortality Rate
Lyzhnikov, Savina, Shepelev, (1975)	Kardiologia	1975	183	29/183 = 16%
Hayes, Van Der Westhuizen, Gelfand, (1978)	S Afr Med J	1978	105	16/105 = 15%
Kiss and Fazekas, (1979)	Acta Cardiologica	1979	168	50/168 = 30%
Ludomirsky et al. (1982)	Am J Cardiol	1982	15	3/15 = 20%
Saadeh, Farsakh, Al-Ali (1997)	Heart	1997	46	2/46 = 4%

The possible reasons for the lower mortality rates in the recent literature are the production of newer OPs with less toxic properties, and probably the better MICU facilities available today than in the 1970s during which most of the high mortality rates were reported. The type of OP, the severity of the poisoning, the stage at which treatment is started, and the presence or absence of MICU facilities are the main determinant factors for the hospital mortality.

10.11. Conclusion

Cardiac complications associated with organophosphate poisoning are not fully appreciated by many physicians. Most occur during the first few hours after exposure. Hypoxaemia, acidosis, and electrolyte derangements are major factors for the development of these complications.

Once the condition is recognised, the patient should immediately be transferred to an intensive or coronary care unit where appropriate monitoring and resuscitative facilities are available. Intensive supportive treatment, meticulous respiratory care, and administration of atropine in adequate doses very early in the course of the illness are the keys to successful management in these cases.

References

Bardin, P.G., Van Eden, S.F., Joubert, J.R. Intensive care management of acute organophosphate poisoning: A 7-year experience in the Western Cape. *South African Medical Journal* 1987;**72**:593–7.

Biernat, S., Giermaziak, H. Myocardial and endocardial lesions in rabbit after acute poisoning with Intrathion and after treatment with some detoxifying agents. *Polish Medical Sciences and History. Bulletin* 1975;**15**:249–53.

Brill, D., Maisel, A., Prabhu, R. Polymorphic ventricular tachycardia and other complex arrhythmias in organophosphate insecticide poisoning. *Journal of Electrocardiology* 1984;**17**:97–102.

Chharba, M.L., Sepaha, G.C., Jain, S.R., *et al.* ECG and necropsy changes in organophosphorus compound, (malathion) poisoning. *Indian Journal of Medical Sciences* 1970;**24**:424–9.

Davies, J.E., Barquet, A., Freed, V.H., *et al.* Human pesticide poisoning by fat-soluble organophosphate insecticide. *Archives of Environmental Health* 1975;**30**:608–13.

Dayrit, C., Manry, C.H., Seevers, M. On the pharmacology of hexaethyltetraphosphate. *Journal of Pharmacology and Experimental Therapeutics* 1948;**92**:173–86.

Dive, A., Mahieu, P., Van Binst, R., *et al.* Unusual manifestations after malathion poisoning. *Human and Experimental Toxicology* 1994;**13**:271–4.

Du Toit, P.W., Muller, F.O., Van Tonder, W.M., *et al.* Experience with the intensive care management of organophosphate insecticide poisoning. *South African Medical Journal* 1981;**60**:227–9.

Durham, W.F., Hayes, W.J. Organic phosphorus poisoning and its therapy. *Archives of Environmental Health* 1962;**5**:21.

Futagawa, H., Kakinuma, Y., Takahashi, H. Cardiovascular collapse through non-cholinergic mechanism after intravenous injection of N-methylcarbamate insecticide in rabbits. *Toxicology* 1997;**117**:163–70.

Ginsburg, R., Bristow, MR., Harrison, D.C., *et al.* Studies with isolated human coronary arteries. Some general observations, potential mediators of spasm, role of calcium antagonists. *Chest* 1980;**78**:180–6.

Hall, G.E., Ettinger, G.H., Banting, F.G. An experimental production of coronary thrombosis and myocardial failure. *Canadian Medical Association Journal*, 1936;**34**:9–15.

Hall, J.G., McLaughlin, J.F., Stamm, S. Coarctation of the aorta in male cousins with similar maternal environmental exposure to insect repellent and insecticides. *Pediatrics* 1975;**55**:425–7.

Hase N.K., Shrinivasan, J., Divekar, M.V. Atropine induced ventricular fibrillation in a case of diazinon poisoning. *Journal of the Association of Physicians India* 1984;**32**:536.

Hassler, G.R., Moutvic, R.R., Stacey, D.B., *et al.* Studies of the action of chemical agents on the heart: *final report, USAMRDC, NTIS: AD-A* 1988;209–19.

Hayes, M.M., Van der Westhuizen, N.G., Gelfand, M. Organophosphate poisoning in Rhodesia: A study of the clinical features and management of 105 patients. *South African Medical Journal* 1978;**54**:230–4.

Hoffmann, B.F. Autonomic control of the heart. *Bulletin of the New York Academy of Medicine* 1967;**43**:1087–96.

Horio, Y., Yasue, H., Rokutanda, M. *et al.* Effects of intracoronary injection of acetylcholine on coronary arterial diameter. *American Journal of Cardiology*, 1986;**57**:984–9.

Jaaskelainen, A.J., Alha, A. Histochemically observable alterations in enzyme pattern of rat myocardium caused by parathion (E605). *Acta Pharmacologica et Toxicologica* 1969;**27**:112–9.

James, T.N., Spence, C.A. Distribution within the sinus node and AV node of the human heart. *Anatomical Records*, 1966;**155**:151–62.

James, T.N. Cardiac Innervation: anatomic and pharmacologic relations. *Bulletin of the New York Academy of Medicine* 1967;**43**:1041–86.

Kiss, Z., Fazekas, T. Arrhythmias in organophosphate poisonings. *Acta Cardiologica* 1979;**34**:323–30.

Kiss, Z., Fazekas, T. Organophosphates and torsade de pointes ventricular tachycardia. *Journal of the Royal Society of Medicine*, 1983;**76**:984–5.

Lerman, Y., Hirshberg, A., Shteger, Z. Organophosphate and carbamate pesticide poisoning: the usefulness of a computerized clinical information system. *American Journal of Industrial Medicine* 1984;**6**:17–26.

Litovitz, T. 1990 AAPCC Annual Report. *American Journal of Emergency Medicine* 1991;**9**:463–92.

Lovejoy, F.H., Linden, C.H. Acute poison and drug over dosage. In: *Harrison's Principles of Internal Medicine*. Petersdorf, R., Adams, R.D., Braunwald, E. eds. McGraw-Hill; New York. 1991. p. 2178.

Ludomirsky, A., Klein, H., Sarelli, P. *et al.* Q-T prolongation and polymorphous (torsade de pointes) ventricular arrhythmias associated with organophosphorus insecticide poisoning. *American Journal of Cardiology* 1982;**49**:1654–8.

Lyzhnikov, E.A., Savina, A.S., Shepelev, V.M. Pathogenesis of disorders of cardiac rhythm and conductivity in acute organophosphate insecticide poisoning. *Kardiologia* 1975;**15**:126–9.

Manning, G.W., Hall, G.E., Banting, F.G. Vagus stimulation and the production of myocardial damage. *Canadian Medical Association Journal* 1937;**37**:314–8.

Massumi, R.A., Mason, D.T., Amsterdam, E.A. *et al.* Ventricular fibrillation and tachycardia after intravenous atropine for treatment of bradycardia. *New England Journal of Medicine* 1972;**287**:336–8.

Mazumder, P.K., Gupta, A.K., Kaushik, M.P., *et al.* Cardiovascular effects of an organophosphate toxin isolated from *Ptychodiscus brevis*. *Biomedical and Environmental Sciences* 1997;**10**:85–92.

McDonough, L.H., Jaax, N.K., Crowley Mays, M.Z., *et al.* Atropine and/or diazepam therapy protects against soman-induced neural and cardiac pathology. *Fundamental and Applied Toxicology* 1989;**13**:256–76.

Merrill, D.G., Mihm, F.G. Prolonged toxicity of organophosphate poisoning. *Critical Care Medicine* 1982;**10**:550–1.

Namba, T., Nolte, C.T., Jackrel, J., *et al.* Poisoning due to organophosphate insecticides: Acute and chronic manifestations. *American Journal of Medicine* 1971;**50**:475–92.

Povoa, R., Cardoso, S.H., Luna Filho, B., *et al.* Organophosphate poisoning and myocardial necrosis. *Arquivos Brasileiros de Cardiologia* 1997;**68**:377–80.

Robineau, P., Guitten, P. Effects of an organophosphorous compound on cardiac rhythm and hemodynamics in anaesthetized and conscious beagle dogs. *Toxicology Letters* 1987;**37**:95–102.

Romero, P., Barnett, P.G., Midtling, J.E. Congenital anomalies associated with maternal exposure to oxydemeton-methyl. *Environmental Research* 1989;**50**:256–61.

Saadeh, A.M., Al-Ali, M.K., Farsakh, N.A. et al. Clinical and sociodemographic features of acute carbamate and organophosphate poisoning: A study of 70 adult patients in north Jordan. *Journal of Toxicology Clinical Toxicology* 1996;**34**:45–51.

Saadeh, A.M., Farsakh, N.A., Al-Ali, M.K. Cardiac manifestations of acute carbamate and organophosphate poisoning. *Heart* 1997;**77**:461–4.

Sherman, J.D. Chlorpyrifos (Dursban)-associated birth defects: Report of four cases. *Archives of Environmental Health* 1996;**51**:5–8.

Shine, K.I. Myocardial effects of Magnesium. *American Journal of Physiology* 1979;**237**:413–23.

Singer, A.W., Jaax, N.K., Graham, J.S., *et al.* Cardiomyopathy in soman and sarin intoxicated rats. *Toxicology Letters*, 1987;**36**:243–9.

Taylor, P. Anticholinesterase agents. In: *The Pharmacological Basis of Therapeutics.* Gilman, A.S., Goodman, L.S., Gilman, A. eds. MacMillan Publishing Co. Inc; New York:1980. p. 91–119

Toda, N. Isolated human coronary arteries in response to vasoconstrictor substances. *American Journal of Physiology* 1983;**245**:937–41.

Tsao, T.C., Juang, Y., Lan, R., *et al.* Respiratory failure of acute organophosphate and carbamate poisoning. *Chest* 1990;**98**:631–6.

Wang, M.H., Tseng, C.D., Bair, S.Y. QT-interval prolongation and polymorphic ventricular tachyarrhythmia (torsade de pointes) in organophosphate poisoning: report of a case. *Human and Experimental Toxicology* 1998;**17**:587–90.

Weidler, D.J. Myocardial damage and cardiac arrhythmias after intracranial hemorrhage: a critical review. *Stroke* 1974;**5**:759–64.

Wills, J.H., McNamara, B.P., Fine, E.A. Ventricular fibrillation in delayed treatment of TEPP poisoning. *Federation Proceedings* 1950;**9**:136.

Worek, F., Kleine, A., Falke, K., *et al.* Arrhythmias in organophosphate poisoning: effect of atropine and bispyridinium oximes. *Archives Internationales de Pharmacodynamie et de Therapie* 1995;**329**:418–35.

Yasue, H., Touyama, M., Shimamoto, M., *et al.* Role of autonomic nervous system in the pathogenesis of Prinzmetal's variant form of angina. *Circulation* 1974;**50**:534–9.

CHAPTER 11

Gulf War Syndrome, Idiopathic Environmental Intolerance and Organophosphate Compounds: Diseases in Search of Causal Hypotheses

Jeffrey Brent and Laura Klein

11.1. Introduction

Organophosphate (OP) pesticides are known to be capable of producing a prodigious variety of acute and chronic health effects, which are described in their respective chapters. In addition to the well-characterised and generally accepted effects of OPs, these compounds have been implicated, by some, as causing a variety of other vague and poorly characterised health effects. These include so-called idiopathic environmental intolerance (IEI, Multiple Chemical Sensitivity [MCS]) and the Gulf War Syndrome (GWS). The organic solvents, which are in some formulation of OP insecticides, have also been implicated as causing a solvent-induced encephalopathy. This is unlikely because the toxicity profile of OP pesticides is such that any reasonable exposure to an organic solvent-based preparation of OPs would be unlikely to cause a chronic encephalopathy. This chapter will review the relevant features of IEI and GWS and critically assess the evidence that OPs play a causative role in the genesis of these conditions.

Because organophosphates are commonplace and may cause profound clinical effects, it is no surprise that these agents have been associated with syndromes beyond the scope of that which the scientific evidence supports as being causally related to their exposure. Organophosphates are frequently solubilised in organic solvents, have odours, are irritants, and cause significant morbidity following major exposure. It is not surprising therefore that they have been natural targets for several vague, ill-defined, human syndromes.

11.2. Gulf War Syndrome

The Iraqi invasion of Kuwait in August of 1990 lead to the deployment of in excess of 700,000 troops over the several months. Most of these troops came from the United States, United Kingdom, and Canada. In February of 1991, in an operation referred to as Desert Storm, this aggregation of troops mounted an effort to evict Iraq from Kuwait. Because of the threat of chemical or biological retaliation a large number of casualties were anticipated to result from such an invasion. Although less than 200 battle-related casualties actually occurred, the expectation of larger numbers of fatalities due to chemical agent attacks may have led to fear of sequelae from exposure. Those fears would be expected to have had the greatest impact on those who were characterised as "suggestible". Shortly after the return of these troops to their native countries, many veterans of the Persian Gulf complained of a large array of different symptoms. The variety of symptoms reported among these troops is given in Table 11.1.

Table 11.1 Symptoms Commonly Articulated by Gulf War Veterans

Fatigue
Joint and muscle aches
Cognitive disturbances
Headaches
Various respiratory complaints
Various gastrointestinal complaints
Sleep disturbances
Rashes and other dermatologic problems

The large number veterans of the Persian Gulf complaining of ill-health resulted in the development of case registries, databases, and high level commissions charged with determining the cause of these symptoms. As reviewed below, many epidemiological studies were spurred to test the hypotheses that there might be a connection between some factor in serving in the Persian Gulf and the symptoms in Gulf War veterans.

In addition, these studies attempted to determine whether there was a unique medical condition related to service in the Persian Gulf. The possible novel medical condition hypothesised to exist was referred to as the Gulf War Syndrome.

Epidemiologic studies have consistently found that veterans that served in the Persian Gulf have a higher rate of symptoms than either the general population (Kang *et al.*, 2000; Hodgson and Kipen, 1999; NIH, 1994) or veterans who were deployed at the same time but did not serve in that location (Kang *et al.*, 2000; Unwin *et al.*, 1999; Proctor *et al.*, 1998; The Iowa Persian Gulf Study Group, 1997; Klaustermeyer *et al.*, 1998). However, the symptoms reported by the Gulf War veterans are diverse and do not tend to fall into a specific pattern (Table 11.1).

In addition, these symptoms are remarkably similar to those frequently seen in primary care medical practices among the general population (Dunn *et al.,* 1993; Hammond, 1964; Lees-Haley and Brown, 1993; Fox *et al.,* 1995). Other than the symptoms, no epidemiologic study has provided any objective evidence of an increased frequency of any particular generally accepted medical diagnosis in Gulf War veterans.

The diverse and subjective nature of the complaints of Gulf War veterans argues against a unique condition as a result of service in the Persian Gulf. However, those findings by themselves certainly do not rule out an increase in either some known illness or illnesses, a novel illness, or both, associated with the Gulf War. A fundamental component of any epidemiological investigation is the assessment of a dose-response relationship. The veracity of epidemiologic results related to the assessment of toxic exposures is dependent upon a demonstration that there is a relationship between the dose to which individuals were exposed and the likelihood of disease. Several epidemiologic studies have attempted to assess whether such a dose-response relationship exists between exposures and symptoms in Gulf War veterans. These studies have all demonstrated that service in the Gulf region was associated with symptoms, but none could be correlated with any particular chemical exposure in a dose response relationship.

Since there has been no demonstration of a unique syndrome that could properly be called GWS, the term has come to imply the increased number of non-specific symptoms in Gulf War veterans.

Those studies that have attempted to make exposure assessments (Kang *et al.*, 2000; Wolfe *et al.*, 1998; Haley *et al.*, 1997a; Haley and Kurt, 1997) have never correlated an objective measure of exposure with any sign or symptom.

Rather, they have demonstrated that individuals with GWS who have symptoms are more likely to subjectively believe that they were in a higher exposure situation.

The experience of serving in the Gulf was highly stressful. Prominent in the sources of stress associated with serving in the Persian Gulf was the fear of exposure to nerve agents. Surveys before the actual Persian Gulf War indicated that the most common fear before deployment was the threat of attack by chemical or biological weapons (Wright *et al.*, 1995). This fear was substantially heightened by the monitoring protocols used in the Gulf, which utilized both ionization and colorimetric detectors (Noble, 1994). The ionization alarm, known as the M8A1, was used as a screening device because it possessed the important properties of a high sensitivity for nerve agents (0.1–0.2 mg/m^3) and a time to alarm of less than 2 minutes. Ionization detectors were located at the perimeter of each military base. Because the M8A1 detectors had a low specificity for nerve agents, the alarms would sound frequently alerting troops to don full protective gear in anticipation of possible nerve agent exposure. In contrast to the ionization detectors, the colorimetric detector, known as the M256A1, was used to confirm the actual presence of nerve agent. This device, which determined the presence of nerve agents by a colorimetric cholinesterase-based reaction, was considerably more specific than the M8A1 ionization detector but required approximately 15 minutes to respond. Thus troops were forced to rely on the non-specific ionization detector for warnings. Although the confirmatory colorimetric detector never went off during the Persian Gulf War, military personnel were repeatedly stressed by the presumed threat of imminent chemical weapons attack from the time the ionization detectors sounded an alert until the absence was confirmed by the colorimetric detection some 13 minutes later. A variety of non-specific influences, such as exhaust from trucks, and the burning of latrine waste, apparently caused the ionization detectors to go off. Thus, although there was constant and considerable stress concerning the possibility of a nerve agent attack, there was no evidence that most troops were ever exposed to nerve agents.

The stresses described above undoubtedly contributed to the variety of psychiatric diagnoses that resulted in Gulf War veterans, including anxiety, depression, and post-traumatic stress disorders (Proctor *et al.* 1998; The Iowa Persian Gulf Study Group, 1997; Engle *et al.*, 1999; Fukuda *et al.*, 1998; Labbate *et al.*, 1998; Gray *et al.*, 1996; Department of Defense, Washington, D.C., 1995). Most of these diagnoses are commonly associated with somatic complaints. The Epidemiologic Catchment Area Study demonstrated that for the general population, having a large number of somatic symptoms is strongly associated with expression of psychological distress or psychiatric symptoms (Reiger *et al.*, 1984).

The etiology of the increased symptoms in Persian Gulf Veterans must be explained. A large part of the explanation for this may come from a study of the experience with prior wars. Major military campaigns since the Crimean War (DaCosta, 1871) have shown that there is a correlation between a large number of physical symptoms and serving in a warfare environment. At the time of the United States Civil War a syndrome occurred in veterans, called "Irritable Heart Syndrome" (DaCosta, 1871), involving a large number of symptoms without any consistency or objective signs of disease in many patients. Similar syndromes have been described related to World War I (Hyams *et al.*, 1996), World War II (Elder *et al.*, 1997), the Korean War (Hyams *et al.*, 1996) and the Vietnam War (Hyams *et al.*, 1996; Haley *et al.*, 1997). The results of these studies have shown that it is expected that there would be some increase in typical infectious syndromes related to the conditions of warfare. However, for soldiers that do not have identifiable infectious disease, the multitude of symptoms following warfare is remarkably predictable and similar from conflict to conflict. Thus, it appears that the very act of sending soldiers into war is sufficient to cause a large number of physical symptoms to occur.

In 1997 a series of publications by Haley *et al.*, using factor analysis, attempted to correlate self-reported symptoms in Persian Gulf veterans with potential chemical exposures during the Gulf War (Haley *et al.*, 1997a, 1997b; Haley and Kurt, 1997). This study solicited volunteers from a naval reserve battalion that had been activated to serve in the Gulf War. This particular battalion consisted of 606 veterans and was selected because of the high prevalence of symptoms in its members.

From this group, 249 participants were recruited, most of whom (70%) felt that they had serious health problems attributable to service in the Gulf War. This was a unique group known for its frequent medical evaluations, media contacts, and extensive internal dialogue about health problems they perceived to be war related. (Gray *et al.*, 1998) Using factor analysis, Haley *et al.* determined a series of clusters of symptoms, which they hypothesised were due to 6 individual syndromes, 3 of which were major clusters (Haley *et al.*, 1997a, 1997b; Haley and Kurt, 1997). Psychological assessment using the Personality Assessment Inventory showed that unlike the veterans who perceived themselves as healthy, those with symptoms which they attributed to the Gulf War tended to have higher scores on a number of scales, including striking elevations in conversion and somatisation scales. They also tended to have elevated scales related to a variety of psychological disorders and problems (Haley *et al.*, 1997a). This suggests that those symptomatic Persian Gulf Veterans, without an explanatory medical diagnosis, may have a personality structure predisposing them to somatic manifestations of emotional stresses.

The factor analyses technique used by Haley *et al.* attempts to group symptoms into clusters that tend to occur in the same individuals. A given cluster is, therefore, hypothesised to represent a syndrome. Using a similar technique Ismail *et al.* (1999) failed to confirm the existence of novel symptom clusters. Methodological factors may be responsible for this discrepancy. The Haley study was an uncontrolled observational analysis on a 606-person single unit known for its high prevalence of symptoms (Presidential Advisory Committee on Gulf War Veterans' Illnesses, 1996b). The response rate on this small group was only 41% (Haley *et al.*, 1997a). A striking 70% of Haley's subjects complained of being symptomatic after the war. By contrast, Ismail's study was a controlled epidemiologic evaluation with a sample size in excess of 3,000, and had a 70% response rate (Ismail *et al.*, 1999). However, since the Ismail study did not precisely replicate that of Haley *et al.* (1997a, 1997b; 1997c), the latter may still be considered hypotheses-generating.

Haley *et al.* physically evaluated 23 symptomatic veterans and compared them to 20 healthy controls. Despite the prevalence of neurological symptoms in this group, they only did nerve action potential studies on five patients. An independent panel of neurologists could not diagnose any neurologic disease in the symptomatic veterans.

Any study attempting to demonstrate the existence of a causal nexus between a chemical exposure and a biological effect should demonstrate a dose-response relationship. Although Haley attempted to do so, it was based on an after-the-fact self-report, a technique that is well known for its high error rate and susceptibility to recall bias. Haley *et al.* report no attempt to verify the reported exposures.

11.2.1. Were Persian Gulf veterans exposed to cholinesterase inhibiting nerve agents?

Based on the U.S. Department of Defense Incidence Analyses there was an opportunity for exposure to nerve agents in the Persian Gulf. This occurred after the warfare ended, when an Iraqi arsenal was identified at Khamisiyeh. In March of 1991 allied troops exploded the bunker at Khamisiyeh, causing the release of a plume of sarin, to which troops were exposed over an approximately 3-day period. No exposed soldier became symptomatic. The estimated amount of sarin in this plume (Central Intelligence Agency, Washington, D.C., 1997) was sufficiently low that no health consequences would have been expected to occur. An epidemiologic study of the exposed troops has failed to reveal any evidence that they suffered any adverse effect from this exposure (Gray *et al.*, 1999). That these veterans did not appear to suffer any adverse effects of the exposure to nerve agents at Khamisiyeh is not surprising since sarin tends not to cause long-term sequelae, particularly in the absence of acute symptoms at the time of exposure.

Various surrogate markers have been used in an attempt to define those circumstances that put soldiers at theoretical risk of nerve agent exposure. A major one is service in the Gulf at the time of Desert Storm, as opposed to before or after the war. It would be reasonable to assume that any unidentified nerve agent exposure would have happened at the time of the war. A relevant study to this point is the Danish Gulf War (DGW) Study, (Ishoy *et al.*, 1999) which evaluated neuropsychological symptoms in Danish Persian Gulf veterans. This study found a high prevalence of neuropsychological symptoms, fatigue, and headaches in these soldiers. Despite the similarity in symptoms between the U.S. and Danish troops, the risk of exposure to nerve agents was markedly different. 95% of the Danish troops' involvement in the Persian Gulf was related to peace-keeping and humanitarian activities after the conclusion of Desert Storm.

The major factor found to correlate with developing these symptoms in the Danish Cohort was having had stressful experiences in the Gulf (Suadicani *et al.*, 1999) Similarly, in another epidemiologic study, there was no demonstrable difference in reported symptoms among veterans present during Desert Shield, Desert Storm, or the post war period (Staudenmayer *et al.*, 1993).

A fundamental principle in toxicologic analyses of causation is that defined chemical exposures have a specifically definable, and limited, set of consequences. If Persian Gulf veterans were suffering from nerve agent exposure, it would be predicted that they would suffer from long-term consequences typical of OP poisoning. An epidemiologic study from the U.S. Veterans Administration on 15,000 randomly selected veterans with GWS and an equivalent number of non-deployed controls found that Persian Gulf veterans reported an increased rate of every one of the 48 symptoms queried (Kang *et al.*, 2000). A similar study on British Persian Gulf veterans came had similar findings (Coker *et al.*, 1999). This lack of specificity is better understood as an endorsement of symptoms, which commonly accompany the diagnosis of PTSD depression, and somatoform disorder (Reiger *et al.*, 1984).

11.2.2. Psychiatric diagnoses in symptomatic Persian Gulf veterans

Many studies have indicated that psychological factors may play a major role in many of the symptoms expressed by Persian Gulf veterans. A British study (Unwin *et al.*, 1999 of veterans deployed either to Bosnia or to the Persian Gulf demonstrated that duty in either unfamiliar environment caused similar symptoms. However, the frequency of reporting these symptoms was significantly higher in those soldiers serving in the more hostile environment of the Persian Gulf. This pattern is similar to that observed after World War II (Straus, 1999). A high rate of psychiatric morbidity was also noted in the U.S. Department of Defense Comprehensive Clinical Evaluation Program (CCEP) of over 13,000 Persian Gulf veterans (Engle *et al.*, 1999; Labbate *et al.*, 1998; Department of Defense, Washington, D.C., 1995). The most common primary diagnosis in the CCEP was psychiatric.

A similar pattern was noted in the DGW Study, which concluded that having a
essful experience in the war was a major determinant of reporting neuropsychiatric
mptoms up to as long as six years later (Suadicani *et al.*, 1999). A study by the U.S.
nters for Disease Control, comprehensively looking for any infectious element in the
tiology of the symptoms reported, found that having a high rate of symptoms after
rving in the Persian Gulf was not predictive of an established medical diagnosis.
owever, symptoms did predict an increased likelihood of having a diagnosis of
pression, somatoform disorders, or PTSD (Fukuda *et al.*, 1998).

Support for psychiatric diagnoses as an explanation for the high prevalence of
mptoms in Persian Gulf veterans can also be found in the Iowa Persian Gulf Study,
hich was a population-based epidemiologic study of Gulf War veterans demonstrating
 increased prevalence of depression, PTSD, and anxiety in symptomatic veterans (The
wa Persian Gulf Study Group, 1997).

.2.3. Is there a unifying diagnosis explaining the Gulf War Syndrome?

here are many factors that may explain the symptoms reported by some Gulf War
eterans. Kang *et al.* (2000) summarised the various self-reported factors that may
ontribute to the symptoms reported. Although there may be a small group of veterans
at have specific symptoms related to these factors, the epidemiologic studies make it
ear that the act of sending otherwise well men and women into the hostile combat
nvironment is sufficient to provoke large numbers of non-specific symptoms. This is as
ue of all the wars studied as it is of Persian Gulf veterans.

1.3. Idiopathic Environmental Intolerance

he initial articulation of the concept of MCS derives from the theories of an allergist,
heron G. Randolph, MD (1906–1995) who espoused that multiple problems such as
atigue, emotional disorders, and neuro-psychological syndromes derived from allergies
 environmental chemicals (Randolph, 1945, 1947).

Randolph's theories led him ultimately to become disenfranchised from the established medical community, causing him to lose his medical school appointment and hospital privileges (Moss, 1982).

Although frequently referred to as "multiple chemical sensitivity", the most generally accepted current terminology of IEI is based on recommendations of the World Health Organization. This is a syndrome that has been given many names. An abbreviated list of the most popular designations are:

- chemical AIDS
- chemical allergy
- environmental illness
- 20th century disease
- universal reactivity
- cerebral allergy

None of these names truly describe this syndrome, which has been universally attributed to all chemical agents including OPs. The name that is used most commonly is MCS, a designation that was promulgated by Mark Cullen, MD, at Yale University. Many studies have shown that the major factor that individuals with these diagnoses respond to is a demonstrated ability to detect the presence of a chemical substance by either olfactory or irritant properties.

The established medical community does not generally accept IEI as a bona fide medical diagnosis. The lists of professional organizations that have taken a formal position indicating that there is not data to support IEI as a unique medical diagnosis are listed in Table 11.2.

A unifying common complaint of individuals labelled as having IEI is an intolerance to environmental factors at levels that are below that which causes any symptoms in the general population. A requisite requirement for accepting this diagnosis therefore would be whether it is possible for these patients to discriminate, the presence or absence of a chemical to which they believe they respond, by way of symptoms, especially when that chemical is provided to them at low levels in a massed fashion. The latter can be achieved by utilising masking odours or nose clips. Selner and Staudenmayer, who have pioneered the use of these double-blind provocation challenges have published their results on 20 cases labelled as having IEI, encompassing a total of 145 different challenges (Staudenmayer et al., 1993).

ble 11.2. Professional societies and organisations which have taken the position that IEI should not be
nsidered an established medical diagnosis.

merican Academy of Allergy, Asthma and Immunology
merican Academy of Clinical Toxicology
merican College of Occupational and Environmental Medicine
merican College of Physicians
merican Council on Science and Health
merican Medical Association
alifornia Medical Association
anadian Psychiatric Association
ternational Society of Regulatory Toxicology and Pharmacology
ational Academy of Sciences
oyal College of Pathologists
oyal College of Physicians
orld Health Organization

No patient in their series was able to discriminate between implicated chemicals and
acebo.

Several factors have lead to the conclusion that it is unlikely that IEI is a unique
edical diagnosis. Virtually any chemical can be implicated as provoking symptoms.
here has never been a patient published in the peer-reviewed literature who has been
le to discriminate between implicated chemicals in a valid double-blind provocation
allenge. IEI has no objective findings. Unlike most accepted toxicologic conditions,
I defies dose-response relationships. Therefore, a psychogenic theory of IEI has been
veloped suggesting that pre-morbid personality disorders predispose individuals to
nbrace this diagnosis (Staudenmayer, 1999). The symptoms expressed by patients
belled as having IEI are often encouraged by the clinical ecology community, support
oups, and multiple evolving Internet sites. Unconscious psychological factors appear
 be significantly more common than are either conscious attempts at articulating these
mptoms for secondary gain or malingering. There are a number of psychiatric
agnoses that have overlapping features with many of the complaints of patients with
I. These include: somatoform, anxiety, and mood disorders.

Associated with complaints labelled as IEI is a high likelihood of having a series other diagnoses including:

- fibromyalgia
- chronic fatigue syndrome
- irritable bowel syndrome
- vocal chord dysfunction
- sick building syndrome
- Gulf War syndrome.

A WHO/IPCS workshop in 1996 recommended dropping the term MCS in that "makes an unsupportable judgment on causation" for which there is no scientific ba (IPCS/WHO, 1996). In its most recent Position Statement the American Academy Allergy, Asthma and Immunology (AAAAI) declined to reach a formal definition of I stating that its "varied and subjective nature" precluded valid diagnostic criteria bei specified. The AAAAI further recommended that medical approaches to treatme practiced by clinical ecologists, such as multi-dose vitamins, intravenous gamm globulin, "desensitisation" treatment, "detoxification" treatment with saunas, etc. abandoned because they are of no proven benefit and may be harmful. Rather, th recommended a psychotherapeutic approach for these patients (AAAI Board Directors, 1986).

The American College of Occupational and Environmental Medicine, in its mo updated Position Statement on IEI reiterated that, in their opinion, there appears to be case definition that can embrace the various features of MCS as promulgated by proponents (ACOEM, 1999). However, we believe that such a definition is possible if encompasses the criteria of discrimination in a properly conducted double-bli exposure chamber challenge. To date no such patient has been described in the pee reviewed medical literature that has ever been able to discriminate between provokir chemicals and placebo in such a challenge test.

Organophosphate pesticides have odours and can provoke acute symptoms wi exposure. Both of these qualities make them a prime target for allegations of triggerir IEI.

However, to date there has never been a scientific study published which supports the provocation of a pathologically definable condition leading to IEI by organophosphates. For a further discussion regarding IEI the reader is referred to the excellent treatise by Staudenmayer (1999).

References

AAAI Board of Directors. Physician reference materials: position statement 35 Idiopathic environmental intolerances. 1986.

ACOEM. ACOEM updates position on multiple chemical sensitivities. *American College of Occupational and Environmental Medicine* 1999;June:1–3.

Central Intelligence Agency, Washington, D.C. Modelling the chemical agent release at the Khamisiyah Pit. 1997.

Coker, W.J., Bhatt ,B.M., Blatchley, N.F. *et al.* Clinical findings for the first 1000 Gulf war veterans in the Ministry of Defence's medical assessment programme. *British Medical Journal* 1999;**18**:290–4.

DaCosta, J.M. On irritable heart: a clinical study of a form of functional cardiac disorder and its consequences. *American Journal of Medical Science* 1871;**61**:17–52.

Department of Defense, Washington, D.C. Comprehensive clinical evaluation program for Gulf War veterans: report on 10,020 participants. 1995.

Dunn, J.T., *et al.* Neurotoxic and neuropsychologic symptom base rates: a comparison of three groups. Poster presented at the 13th Annual Conference of the National Academy of Neuropsychology, Phoenix, Arizona, October 28–30, 1993.

Elder, G.H., Shanahan, M.J., Clapp, E.C. *et al.* Linking combat and physical health: the legacy of World War II in men's lives. *American Journal of Psychiatry* 1997;**154**:330–6.

Engle, C.C., Ursano, R, Magruder, C. *et al.* Psychological conditions diagnosed among veterans seeking Department of Defense care for Gulf War-related health concerns. *Journal of Occupational and Environmental Medicine* 1999;**41**:384–92.

Fox, D.D., *et al.* Base rates of postconcussive symptoms in health maintenance organization patients and controls. *Neuropsychology* 1995;**9**:606–11.

Fukuda, K., Nisenbaum, R., Stewart, G. *et al.* Chronic Multisymptom illness affecting Air Force veterans of the Gulf War. *Journal of the American Medical Association* 1998;**280**:981–8.

Gray, G.C., Knoke, J.D., Berg, S.W. *et al.* Counterpoint: responding to suppositions and misunderstandings. *American Journal of Epidemiology* 1998;**148**:328–33.

Gray, G.C., Smith, T.C., Knoke, J.D. *et al.* The postwar hospitalization experience of Gulf War veterans possibly exposed to chemical munitions destruction at Khamisiyah, Iraq. *American Journal of Epidemiology 1999*;**150**:532–40.

Gray, G.C., Coate, B.D., Anderson, C.M. *et al.* The postwar hospitalization experience of U.S. veterans of the Persian Gulf War. *The New England Journal of Medicine* 1996;**335**:1505–14.

Haley, R.W., Kurt, J.L., Hom, J. *et al.* Is there a Gulf War syndrome? Searching for syndromes by factor analysis of symptoms. *Journal of the American Medical Association* 1997a;**277**:215–22.

Haley, R.W., Hom, J., Roland, P.S. *et al.* Evaluation of neurologic function in Gulf War veterans. *Journal of the American Medical Association,* 1997b;**277**:223–30.

Haley, R.W., Kurt, T.L. Self-reported exposure to neurotoxic chemical combinations in the Gulf War. *Journal of the American Medical Association* 1997c;**277**:231–7.

Hammond, E.C. Some preliminary findings on physical complaints from a prospective study of 1,064,004 men and women. *American Journal of Public Health,* 1964;**54**:11–23.

Hodgson, M.J., Kipen, H.M. Gulf war illnesses: causation and treatment. *Journal of Occupational and Environmental Medicine* 1999;**41**:443–52.

Hyams, K.C., Wignall, F.S., Roswell, R. *et al.* War syndromes and their evaluation: from the U.S. Civil War to the Persian Gulf War. *Annals of Internal Medicine* 1996;**125**:398–405.

IPCS/WHO (International Programme on Chemical Safety/World Health Organization) Conclusions and recommendations of a workshop on multiple chemical sensitivities (MCS). Regulatory Toxicology and Pharmacology 1996;**24**:S188–9.

Ishoy, T., Suadicani ,P., Guldager, B. *et al.* State of health after deployment in the Persian Gulf. *Danish Medical Bulletin,* 1999;**46**:416–9.

Ismail, K., Everitt, B., Blatchley, N. *et al.* Is there a Gulf War syndrome? *Lancet* 1999;**353**:179–82.

Kang, H.K., *et al.* Illnesses among United States Veterans of the Gulf War: A population-based survey of 30,000 veterans. *Journal of Occupational and Environmental Medicine* 2000;**42**:491–501.

Klaustermeyer, W.B., Kraske, G.K, Lee, K.G. *et al.* Allergic and immunologic profile of symptomatic Persian Gulf war veterans. *Annals of Allergy, Asthma, and Immunology* 1998;**80**:269–73.

Labbate, L.A., Cardena , E., Dimitreva, J. *et al.* Psychiatric syndromes in Persian Gulf War veterans: an association of handling dead bodies with somatoform disorders. *Psychotherapy and Psychosomatics* 1998;**67**:275–9.

Lees-Haley, P.R., Brown, R.S. Neuropsychological complaint base rates of 170 personal injury claimants. *Archives of Clinical Neuropsychology* 1993;**8**:203–9.

Moss, R.W. An alternative approach to allergies. Forword to Randolph, T.G. *et al.* Bantam Books, New York. 1982

NIH Technology Assessment Workshop Panel. The Persian Gulf experience and health. *Journal of the American Medical Association* 1994;**272**:391–5.

Noble, D. Back into the story reanalyzing health effects of the Gulf War. *Analytical Chemistry* 1994;**66**:805A–8A.

Presidential Advisory Committee on Gulf War Veterans' Illnesses. Final Report. U.S.Govt. Printing Office, Washington, DC. 1996b

Proctor, S.P., Heeven, T., White, R.F. *et al.* Health status of Persian Gulf War veterans: self-reported symptoms, environmental exposures and the effect of stress. *International Journal of Epidemiology* 1998;**27**:1000–10.

Randolph, T.G. Allergy as a causative factor in fatigue, irritability and behavior problems in children. *Journal of Pediatrics* 1947;**31**:560–72.

Randolph, T.G. Fatigue and weakness of allergic origin (allergic toxemia) to be differentiated from "nervous fatigue" or neurasthenia. *Annals of Allergy* 1945;**3**:418–30.

Reiger, D.A., Myers, J.K., Kramer, M. *et al.* The NIMH Epidemiologic Catchment Area (ECA) program: historical context, major objectives and study population characteristics. *Archives of General Psychiatry* 1984;**41**:934–41.

Spencer, P.S., McCauley, L.A., Joos, S.K. *et al.* U.S. Gulf War veterans: service periods in theater, differential exposures, and persistent unexplained illness. *Toxicology Letters* 1998;**102-103**:515–21.

Staudenmayer, H. *Environmental illness: myth and reality*. Boca Raton, Florida: Lewis Publishers; 1999

Staudenmayer, H., Selner, J.C., Buhr, M.P. *et al*. Double-blind provocation chamber challenges in 20 patients presenting with "MCS". *Regulatory Toxicology and Pharmacology* 1993;**18**:44–53.

Straus, S.E. Bridging the gulf in war syndromes. *Lancet* 1999;**353**:162–3.

Suadicani, P., Ishoy, T., Guldager,B. *et al*. Determinants of long-term neuropsychological symptoms. *Danish Medical Bulletin* 1999;**46**:423–7.

The Iowa Persian Gulf Study Group. Self-reported illness and health status among Gulf War Veterans. *Journal of the American Medical Association* 1997;**277**:238–45.

Unwin, C., Blatchley ,N., Coker, W. *et al*. Health of UK servicemen who served in Persian Gulf War. *Lancet* 1999;**353**:169-178.

Wolfe, J., *et al*. Health symptoms reported by Persian Gulf War veterans two years after return. *American Journal of Industrial Medicine* 1998;**33**:104–13.

Wright, K., *et al*. *Operation Desert Shield/Desert Storm*. Washington, D.C.: Walter Reed Institute of Research; 1995

CHAPTER 12

Management of Organophosphorus Compound Poisoning

Lakshman Karalliedde and Ladislaus Szinicz

The management of organophosphorus (OP) compound poisoning depends very much on its severity. In mild cases removing the patient from area of exposure and a low dose of atropine may suffice. However, in severe cases artificial respiration, oxygen, high doses of antidotes and resuscitation become necessary

12.1. Treatment of Organophosphorus Compound Poisoning

12.1.1. General Measures

a. Removal of the patient from contaminated environment.
b. Decontamination
    removal of contaminated clothing
    skin: decontamination with water and soap
    eye: irrigation with water
c. Establishment of airway. Removal of food, vomit or secretion from mouth and airway.
d. Restoration and maintenance of respiration to give a $PO_2 > 10kPa$, $SaO_2 > 94\%$. This may require supplementary oxygen, positive pressure ventilation and PEEP.
e. Restoration of adequate circulation to maintain a heart rate >50 beats per minute and a mean blood pressure >50 mm Hg.
    Establishment of venous access for infusion of fluids and drugs
    Give catecholamines to support blood pressure (dobutamine 2.5–10 µg/kg/min, dopamine 2.5 µg/kg/min)
    Correct any acidosis and maintain electrolyte and fluid balance
    Correct serious arrhythmias. If QT interval exceeds half the R-R interval, consider use of pace maker (Finkelstein *et al.*, 1989).

f. CNS function

Monitor level of consciousness

Control convulsions using diazepam 5–10 mg IV slowly over 3 min. If necessary repeat every 10–15 min (maximum 30 mg); children 0.2–0.3 mg/kg IV every 10–15 min (maximum 5 mg for 1 month to 5 years old and 10 mg for 5 years and older)

12.1.2. Antidote Treatment

Give- **atropine** after correcting any hypoxia

Bolus injections: IV 2 mg (0.05 mg/kg) every 5–10 min in adults. Children: 0.02 mg/kg body weight

Or

Infusions of atropine: 0.02–0.08 mg/kg/hr

Aim is to achieve adequate atropinisation i.e. dry mouth (tongue) and skin, no bronchial rales. Pulse rate over 80 beats per minute, dilatation of pupils. (Avoid heart rates of over 120 beats per minute after atropine)

Give- **Pralidoxime**: slowly IV – 30mg/kg body weight, children 20–40 mg/kg. Repeat 4–6 hourly (Therapeutic concentration 50-100 µmol/l)

Or

Give a 30 mg/kg body weight bolus followed by an **infusion** of 8–10 mg/kg/hour (in some countries obidoxime is used - 250 mg bolus IV, children 3–6 mg/kg, followed by a 0.5mg/kg/h infusion –therapeutic concentration 10-20 µmol/l))

12.1.3. Protective measures for those involved in treatment

Solvent resistant gloves (neoprene nitril), if necessary doubled and changed frequently

No mouth to mouth respiration should be used

If possible, use activated charcoal filter equipped protective mask or self sustained (re-circulating low flow) respirator to prevent contamination of surroundings with highly toxic compounds such as nerve agents. In severe cases a protective suit may be indicated.

Decontamination by washing oneself thoroughly and discarding contaminated clothing to prevent secondary contamination of personnel and equipment. Patients and helpers must not enter medical facilities prior to decontamination in order to prevent secondary decontamination.

12.2. General Measures

OP compounds can cause toxicity following absorption from the skin, via the lungs or following ingestion. Some OP insecticides, such as parathion exhibit high toxicity, similar to nerve agents and pose a threat to both the patient and the helper. Contamination of the surroundings by such compounds, as in the case of the sarin attack in Tokyo, necessitates adequate protection of the helpers and thorough decontamination of the victims as early as possible.

12.3. Decontamination

Exposure of the skin may be managed by removing and discarding contaminated clothing (particularly leather which absorbs pesticides) in to sealed bags. The exposed skin should be repeatedly washed with soap and plenty of warm water. Special attention should be given to washing skin creases, around the ears, around the external auditory canals, the umbilicus, genitalia and under the nails. (AAP, 1983). OP agents can be deactivated with a dilute hypochlorite (bleach) solution. Some OP agents are likely to be less stable in alkaline solution and the addition of baking soda to the fluid helps breakdown of the OP (Garcia-Repetto et al., 1994).

Contamination of the eyes should be managed by continuous irrigation of the affected eye for 10–15 min with clean water or saline. Contact lenses must be removed and washed before re-use.

Gordon et al. (1999) described the decontamination of sensitive skin and medical equipment using immobilized enzymes. These are made of sponges which can be moulded to any form, where ChE is immobilized to a polyurethane matrix. They stated that in addition to treatment of OP-contaminated soldiers, the sponge could protect medical personnel from secondary contamination while attending medical casualties.

12.4.   Minimising Further Absorption of OP Agent

12.4.1. Gastric Decontamination

Ingested OPs should be removed as quickly as possible. Various gastric decontamination procedures such as gastric aspiration and lavage, induced emesis, administration of activated charcoal and cathartics have all been widely used.

Induced emesis has now become obsolete (Bateman, 1999) as it carries an unacceptable risk of pulmonary aspiration. There is no acceptable role for cathartics alone in the management of the poisoned patient, nor is there evidence that they are useful in combination with activated charcoal (Anonymous, 1997a).

12.4.2. Gastric Aspiration followed by Lavage

Gastric aspiration followed by lavage should only be carried out after protecting the airway. Most OPs are dissolved in aromatic hydrocarbons which can cause serious harm if aspirated in to the lungs. Lavage and the administration of activated charcoal are contraindicated without protection of the airways, especially in patients with depressed consciousness. Although gastric lavage is most effective within 30 minutes of ingestion it might still be useful up to 4 h.

OP pesticide may persist in the gut for long periods (Willems, 1981), especially in patients with an impaired circulation. Gastric lavage should therefore be performed in all severe cases, on admission to hospital, after the airways have been protected to prevent aspiration.

12.4.3. Oral Activated Charcoal

Administration of oral activated charcoal in conventional doses should also be considered for reducing further absorption of OP pesticides (Haddad, 1987; IPCS WHO, 1986). However, the capacity of charcoal to adsorb most OP compounds has not been established. Activated charcoal should not be administered if there has been an injury involving the gastro-intestinal tract. Continuous lavage with activated charcoal for several days has been advocated, but its usefulness has not been proven.

In acute fenthion poisoning, evacuation of the gastro-intestinal tract followed by activated charcoal administration, repeated until the absence of anticholinesterase activity in the gastro-intestinal fluid could be demonstrated, was advocated by clinicians in Belgium (Mahieu *et al.*, 1982). These clinicians found that in vitro, 1g of charcoal powder can adsorb 55mg of fenthion at 25°C. However, a rectal ulcer with massive haemorrhage caused by activated charcoal treatment in oral OP poisoning was reported from Japan (Mizutani *et al.*, 1991).

12.4.4.   Intestinal Lavage and Whole Bowel Irrigation (WBI).

Intestinal lavage is carried out in cases of severe intoxication in some Russian centers (Ostapenko, 1999) when patients present with CNS depression and a marked lowering of cholinesterase activity. A stomach tube is introduced endoscopically in to the duodenum and 30 litres of normal saline with added magnesium and potassium is used for the lavage, which is carried out over 2 hours, until the effluent is clear and free from smell of OP agent.

A similar procedure, Whole Bowel Irrigation (WBI) using a polyethylene glycol-electrolyte solution (PEG–ES) is routinely carried out in some centers in Europe and North America.

There is no evidence that there is improved clinical outcome using either of these methods though the use of WBI in cases of poisoning with compounds not adsorbed by activated charcoal has been recommended. WBI is contraindicated in the presence of ileus, bowel obstruction, bowel perforation, clinically significant haemorrhage, haemodynamic instability, intractable vomiting, and an unprotected or compromised airway (Anonymous, 1997b).

12.4.5.   Haemodialysis, haemoperfusion, forced diuresis

These procedures are not considered to be effective in OP poisoning. Haemodialysis with or without charcoal in OP poisoning is controversial in view of the large volume of distribution of OPs and their high affinity for binding to body tissues. In a study of 10 patients who underwent 1–3 haemoperfusions, the procedure failed to remove >0.1% of the total absorbed poison (Martinez-Chuecos *et al.*, 1992).

In these patients, the fat tissue concentrations were 20–50 times higher than the concentration in the plasma. However, clinicians from Japan □reported halving of blood concentration of fenitrothion using charcoal haemoperfusion (Kamijo *et al.*, 1999).

12.5.   Diagnosis

The clinical diagnosis depends upon observing the smell of OPs, constricted pupils, salivation, lachrymation, increased tracheo-bronchial secretions, muscle fasciculations, decreased levels of ChE's in the blood and the finding of metabolites of OPs in the urine (there is a relatively small number of the alkyl phosphate/phosphorothioate metabolites compared to the potential number of different OPs). A measure of six of these 'alkyl phosphates' will cover about 85% of likely encountered OPs in the UK and can be quantified in a single gas chromatographic (GC) analysis after extraction with pentafluorobenzylbromide, using a flame photometric detector (Health and Safety Executive Guidance Notes MS 17, 2000). See Chapter 5.

12.6.   Monitoring

12.6.1.   Basic Monitoring of Physiological Parameters

This should include continuous measurement of oxygen saturation (pulse oximetry), blood pressure, ECG (12 lead ECG twice a day and continuous ECG monitoring), level of consciousness (it is preferable to use a standard scale such as the Glasgow coma scale or Edinburgh scale), respiratory rate and minute volume, fluid balance (measure or estimate urine output, vomitus, diarrhoea, sweating, intravenous fluids). Continuous wave form monitoring of end-tidal carbon dioxide (capnography) may be useful in detecting return of bronchospam and the need for atropine therapy. Polish clinicians (Kolarzyk *et al.*, 1997) monitored respiratory regulation by synchronic measurements of respiratory patterns and of occlusion pressures and recommended the measurement of respiratory tract resistance to detect any increase in airway resistance.

Arterial blood: for assessment of PaO_2, $PaCO_2$ and pH.

Venous blood: A sample of the patient's blood should be collected in EDTA bottles as soon as possible and separated plasma and erythrocytes stored at 4°C until the cholinesterase activities can be measured ((Health and Safety Executive Guidance notes MS 17,2000) in red blood cells and plasma. (RBC AChE and BuChE levels). To prevent erroneous results because of ongoing inhibition of the ChEs by remaining poison in the sample or reactivation by the oxime used, it was recommended (Worek *et al.*, 1997) that the blood sample be diluted immediately (1:100) with ice cold phosphate buffer and the sample be frozen until measurement. RBC AChE activity measurement is useful for confirmation of diagnosis and for monitoring the therapeutic effect of oximes. Recovery of BuChE activity may be used as evidence of the clearance of OP agents from the blood. Taken together with an improving clinical status, this would help in deciding when to stop artificial respiration.

Venous blood to measure levels of OP compound and biochemical profiles: (electrolytes, glucose, amylase, lipase, creatinine, creatine phosphokinase) and **haematology** including white cell count (as leucocytosis is common). Renal and hepatic function tests should be performed at least three times a week. Profuse diarrhoea necessitates maintenance of fluid and electrolyte (particularly potassium) balance (Karalliedde and Senanayake, 1989).

Estimation of cholinesterase in gastric aspirate to decide whether gastric aspiration should be stopped (Mahieu *et al.*, 1982).

Chest X-Rays: Initially daily chest X-rays as aspiration pneumonia is a frequent complication of severe OP poisoning.

Monitoring of body temperature: Both hypothermia (rectal temperatures as low as 27.5°C) and hyperthermia (temperatures of 40°C) have been reported following OP poisoning (Hantson *et al.*, 1996).

Urine analysis for estimation of metabolic/excretory products of OP agents e.g. urinary p-nitrophenol (excretory products of parathion). Urinary levels of p-nitrophenol have been used to estimate parathion exposure. The concentration of p-nitrophenol falls rapidly after cessation of exposure and a brief delay in collecting the sample may result in a value that would not be representative of maximal absorption and excretion (el-Refai *et al.*, 1971) (See chapter 5).

Electromyography (EMG) and train of four responses (TOF), Single fibre E.M.G: See chapters 6 and 9. Singh *et al.* (1998) reported the administration of 0.1 mg of edrophonium to reveal EMG changes when not demonstrable initially in mild intoxications. Electrical studies and especially the response to 10–50 Hz stimuli gives evidence of the degree of neuromuscular involvement. They also provide an objective method of assessment of the response of the neuromuscular junction to cholinesterase reactivators- the oximes (See annexe and Chapter 5). Single fibre E.M.G. may show abnormalities for up to two years after intoxication (Baker and Sedgwick, 1996).

CAT Scan, PET, EEG. In patients with cortical visual loss following OP poisoning along with respiratory failure, conventional neuro-imaging techniques may fail to visualize damage that can be detected by Positron Emission Tomography (PET) (Wang *et al.*, 1999)

Others: Ultra-sound scan of the abdomen for pancreatic involvement. Indirect laryngoscopy may be required to confirm vocal cord paralysis,

12.7. Antidote Treatment

Antidote treatment should be started concurrently with establishment of adequate oxygenation.

12.7.1. Counteracting the Muscarinic Effects of Excess Acetylcholine

12.7.1.1. Atropine

Atropine antagonises the muscarinic actions of excessive AChE. It has little if any beneficial effect at the nicotinic effector sites such as the neuromuscular junction (Heath and Meredith, 1992; Karalliedde and Senanayake, 1989). Although atropine is not very lipophilic, it crosses the blood brain barrier (BBB) to a sufficient degree at recommended dosage to counteract the effects of excess ACh in the central nervous system.

Mild to moderate poisoning: Adults: Initial dose of 2 mg intravenously should be repeated at five to ten minute intervals until signs of atropinisation occur- dry tongue, dry skin (arm pits), no nasal secretions, pulse rate over 80 beats/min (bpm). Adequate oxygenation and correction of acidosis are essential to limit the risk of arrhythmias.

Children: doses of 0.015–0.05 mg/kg should be given every 10–30 min (Sofer *et al.,* 1989; Mortensen, 1986)). After atropinisation is achieved, it should be maintained until there is complete clinical recovery. The usual maintenance dose is 0.5 mg/hour.

If respiratory arrest occurs artificial ventilation with high inspired oxygen concentrations followed by rapid atropinisation is desirable; 5 or 10 mg may be administered initially. In massive exposures- hundreds of milligrams of atropine may be needed over few hours. Significant reductions in mortality using infusions of atropine (0.02–0.08 mg/kg/h) rather than intermittent bolus doses has been reported (Tafuri and Roberts, 1987) and is emerging as the method of choice for atropine therapy. If only isolated pulmonary manifestations are observed, nebulised atropine or ipratropium may relieve these signs and symptoms. In a study from China, the use of a lower than traditional doses of atropine over a shorter duration was associated with a lower complication and fatality rate (Fang *et al.,* 1997). However, comparison of regimens of atropine therapy requires considerations of OP agents involved, severity of intoxication, physical status of patient prior to poisoning, the range of physiological and biochemical parameters measured etc before comparisons could be made.

It has been suggested that very high doses of atropine may enhance neuromuscular transmission and/or transmitter release, possibly by acting on muscarinic presynaptic inhibitory receptors (Wali *et al.,* 1987; Bradshaw *et al.,* 1986).

This observation raises the possibility of high doses of atropine increasing the concentration of ACh at the neuromuscular junction. In animal experiments, following poisoning with tabun or soman, use of atropine and oxime (Hl-6 or Hlö 7) therapy resulted in the conversion of sinus rhythm to dangerous ventricular tachycardia within one minute of treatment (Worek *et al.*, 1995). Atropine-containing antidote combinations may induce lethal arrhythmias in nerve agent poisoning and thus close monitoring is necessary.

The role of atropine in OP induced seizures with nerve agents was evaluated in animals. The results showed a probable beneficial effect with sarin and VX poisoning (Shih and McDonough, 1999). A case of OP poisoning refractory to atropine and in which glycopyrrolate was successfully used to manage the intermediate syndrome was reported recently (Choi *et al.*, 1998). In certain centres in South Africa atropine is combined with glycopyrrolate to limit the central stimulation produced by atropine (Beverly Hoffman, 1999).

Atropine and 2-PAM given together are synergistic and oximes are considered to possess an atropine sparing effect (Eyer *et al.*, 1999).

12.7.1.2. Glycopyrrolate

Glycopyrrolate (more selective for peripheral cholinergic sites than atropine) has been useful for controlling secretions with fewer side-effects such as flushing, tachycardia and depression of the level of consciousness which may be experienced with atropine (Bardin and Van Eeden, 1990; Tracey and Gallagher, 1990).

However, it is less effective in countering bradycardia and is less effective as an antidote to the central neurologic effects of OPs. A combination of glycopyrrolate and atropine adequately controlled bronchorrhoea and bradycardia without causing tachycardia (Tracey and Gallagher, 1990). A double-blind randomised trial comparing glycopyrrolate and atropine showed no differences in clinical outcomes and complications (Bardin and Van Eeden, 1990).

Other antimuscarinic compounds (e.g. lipophilic compounds like scopolamine and benactyzine, G3063 and less lipophilic agents which act mainly in the periphery like methyl-atropine) have been used in animal experiments and in human OP poisoning. Most OP compounds are lipophilic, especially the nerve gases. As a result they penetrate the blood brain barrier causing central effects such as respiratory depression.

In such instances an anti-muscarinic compound that reaches the brain will be needed. Kassa and Bajgar (1994) found benactyzine and G 3063 more advantageous due to their central effect in the treatment of GV poisoning than atropine. However, atropine sulphate which acts both peripherally and centrally and is relatively cheap, remains the antimuscarinic of choice amongst the majority of clinicians for the treatment of OP compound poisoning (Grob, 1963; Karalliedde and Senanayake, 1989; Heath and Meredith, 1992).

Cyanotic patients should be oxygenated, if necessary following endotracheal intubation, at the same time that atropine is administered. This minimises the risk of ventricular arrhythmias.

In young children, Sofer et al. (1989) observed that atropine had an obvious beneficial effect on the presenting signs which were related to the CNS. The central cholinergic synapses were considered to be more sensitive to atropine in the very young. Further, atropine may pass through the blood brain barrier more easily in children.

12.7.2. Counteracting the Nicotinic Effects of Inhibition of Cholinesterase

12.7.2.1. Oximes (see also appendix 2)

Pralidoxime available as different salts (PAM chloride, iodide, mesylate) is a monopyridinium compound whilst obidoxime, trimedoxime and HI-6 are bispyridinium compounds (Marrs, 1993). Oximes reactivate inhibited AChE by cleavage of phosphorylated or phopshonylated active sites of the enzyme (Howland and Aaron, 1998; Bismuth et al., 1992, Thiermann et al., 1997,1999). Reactivation by oximes is most marked at the neuromuscular junction. They do not reverse the muscarinic manifestations of OP poisoning and they have a short half-life (1.2 h) when administered intravenously. Other effects, attributed to oximes (in very high doses) are:

1. anticholinergic effect similar to that of atropine,
2. sympathomimetic effect potentiating the pressor effect of epinephrine.
3. depolarising effect at the neuromuscular junction
4. weak ability to inhibit cholinesterase.
5. direct influence on synaptic transmission by mechanisms which are not known precisely at present. (Bismuth et al., 1992).
6. direct reaction with sarin, soman and tabun (Becker et al., 1997).

Oximes, being ionized compounds, do not easily cross the blood brain barrier. The approximately 10% reactivation of brain acetylcholinesterase claimed, following oxime therapy is considered to be an overestimation (Hobbiger and Vojrodic, 1967: Rump *et al.*, 1978). However, some workers believe that even the limited passage of the oxime to the brain may have a significant, albeit small effect. Prompt improvement has been reported in the level of consciousness (Lotti and Becker, 1982) and in the EEG in an intoxicated child following an iv. infusion of pralidoxime chloride. They are ineffective, by themselves, in counteracting the central effects of OPs. The therapeutic effect of atropine together with an oxime, where the latter is effective (see later) is more than merely additive (Grob, 1963; Howland and Aaron, 1998). In English speaking countries, the oxime, pralidoxime is preferred. In Central Europe, obidoxime is the oxime of choice.

The main circumstance limiting oxime efficacy is the so called 'ageing' phenomenon (see chapter 1). The time during which a functionally significant portion of the enzyme can be reactivated (i.e. is not aged) is 4 times its half life. In the case of poisoning with dimethyl compounds, oximes will become ineffective 16 hours after poisoning, and with diethyl compounds after 124 hours (or about 5 days). This means that patients with dimethyl OP poisoning arriving at the hospital on the second day are unlikely to benefit from oxime treatment. These assumptions have been shown to apply in clinical cases (Thiermann *et al.*, 1997). However, in a case of parathion poisoning, treated with obidoxime, an increase in the ageing half life time from 31 to 66 hours was observed (Thiermann *et al.*, 1997). This was explained by suggesting that reactivation reduced the portion of the enzyme available for ageing.

Studies have shown that significant reactivation occurs only after the OP concentration in the body falls below a critical value: only where the reactivation rate exceeds the inhibition rate, does significant reactivation occur (Thiermann *et al.*, 1997). In the above case of parathion poisoning complete recovery of the non-aged portion of the enzyme was observed by the fifth day, by which time AChE inhibitory activity in the plasma was undetectable. This probably indicates that even when there is no immediate clinical evidence for oxime efficacy, where reactivation is possible, i.e. the inhibited enzyme is not completely aged, oxime therapy should be continued until clinical recovery occurs.

The effective concentration of oxime would depend on the oxime used and the OP agent causing intoxication (Willems *et al.*, 1993; Worek *et al.*, 1997).

In animal experiments, a plasma concentration of 4mg/l pralidoxime was reported to be the minimum concentration required to counteract neuromuscular block in cats poisoned by a quaternary sarin-analogue (Sundwall, 1961). This value was uncritically promulgated by other authors without considering the type of oxime and the type of OP. The experimental work by Worek *et al.* (1997) demonstrated unequivocally that oximes are not equi-effective and rank order of effectiveness changes with the OP compound involved. These workers found obidoxime to be the most potent and efficacious oxime in reactivating AChE inhibited by OP insecticides but was inferior to HI-6 against the nerve agents with the exception of tabun. One possible reason for this specificity is the inevitable formation of phosphonyloximes during reactivation. These metabolites are highly potent anticholinesterases by themselves and are possibly more reactive than the parent OP compounds. The 2-pyridinium aldoximes such as PAM and HI-6 form very unstable phosphonyloximes which lose their ChE enzyme-inhibiting activity much faster than the more stable phosphonyloximes formed with 4–pyridinium salts like obidoxime. Recent theoretical calculations have shown (Worek *et al.*, 1997) that a much higher concentration of pralidoxime is necessary for effective treatment of poisoning in man i.e. 20–40mg/l. Thompson *et al.* (1987) had demonstrated that intermittent doses in adults of 1 g of 2-PAM, 8 hourly, would maintain the desired target concentration for less than 5 hours in a 24-hour period. After an i.v infusion dose of 1g of 2-PAM, the plasma level was less than 4mg/l after 1.5 h. A continuous infusion of 500mg/h of 2-PAM leads to a level greater than 4mg/l after 15 minutes, which is maintained throughout the infusion (Thompson, 1987b). Intravenous administration of 2-PAM in 15–30 mg/kg doses initially, intravenously, together with a continuous infusion, using a dose of 550mg/h, would provide levels >4mg/l and has been advocated for severe poisoning. Two intravenous bolus doses of 30mg/kg, 4 h apart, has also been recommended prior to the infusion (Medicis *et al.*, 1996). Continuous infusions were shown to be effective following exposure to large quantities of OP compound (Tush and Anstead, 1997). Continuous infusion protocols have now been used safely and effectively in children and adults (Aaron and Howland, 1998; Howland and Aaron, 1998).

12.8. Anticonvulsants

There are reports on the use of barbiturates and hydantoins in OP poisoning (Sellström, 1992).

However, the most important anticonvulsant in present use is the benzodiazepine, diazepam (Sellström, 1992; Aaron and Howland, 1998; Lallement et al., 1998). Benzodiazepines are useful adjuncts to atropine (and oximes) in the treatment of OP poisoning (Karalliedde and Senanayake, 1989). They increased survival and decreased the incidence of associated neuropathies (McDonough et al., 1995; Shih and McDonough, 1999). Lipp (1973) found that diazepam produced an immediate decrease in cerebral electrical activity and terminated the convulsions produced in rhesus monkeys by soman. The combination of atropine and diazepam was more effective than atropine alone in reducing mortality due to soman (McDonough et al., 1989). Intravenous administration of either clonazepam or nitrazepam also effectively suppressed soman-induced seizure activity and terminated convulsions in monkeys. The latter benzodiazepines were effective when given prophylactically (Lipp, 1973; 1974).

Johnson and Lowndes (1974) found that diazepam abolished the convulsive syndrome and appeared to reduce or abolish miosis and salivation in animals indicating possible anticholinergic actions.

Diazepam decreased the cardiac and brain damage resulting from OP seizures (Johnson and Wilcox, 1975). Diazepam is also useful in sedating patients during ventilatory care, together with morphine analogues. Experiments with the nerve agent soman, in guinea-pigs, indicate that midazolam was the most potent and fastest acting anticonvulsant, when compared with many other benzodiazepines, but its effects are short-lived.

A total of eight anticholinergic drugs (aprophen, atropine, azaprophen, benactyzine, biperiden, procyclidine, scopolamine, trihexyphenidyl) were tested in parallel with diazepam for the ability to terminate seizures induced by soman. With the exception of atropine, all anticholinergic drugs were effective at a lower doses than diazepam in terminating seizures when given 5 min after seizure onset. Benactyzine, procyclidine and aprophen terminated seizures most rapidly. When given 40 min after seizure onset, diazepam was most effective (McDonough et al., 2000).

12.9. Magnesium and Pancuronium

Kiss and Fazekas (1983) reported that i.v. magnesium sulphate eliminated ventricular premature contractions.

Magnesium infusions were also used with good result in the management of hypertension associated with acute OP poisoning (Petroianu *et al.*, 1992).

12.10. Sodium Bicarbonate Infusions

Correction of acidosis is an essential therapeutic measure in severe OP poisoning. Alkalinisation of the blood to pH 7.5 with sodium bicarbonate may be useful as hydrolysis of the esteratic portion of some OP molecules increase as the pH increases. One animal study suggested that sodium bicarbonate therapy favourably affected mortality rates (Cordoba *et al.*, 1983). Clinicians in Brazil (Wong, 1999) and Iran (Balali-Mood, 1999) report successful management of OP intoxicated patients using infusions of sodium bicarbonate. Sodium bicarbonate 3–5 MEq/kg is administered intravenously as an infusion over 30 minutes and a similar amount in 500–1000ml of 5% dextrose every 24 h until recovery. The average duration of such a regimen of treatment was 5–7 days. In a study on the influence of pH on the degradation kinetics of some OP pesticides in aqueous solution, Garcia-Repetto *et al.* (1994) showed that dimethoate, parathion-methyl, malathion and trichlorfon were more stable in acidic than basic solution, and that diazinon was less stable in an acidic solution. The pH changes had greater effects on the stability of trichlorfon than on the rest of pesticides studied by them.

Balali-Mood and Shariat (1998) reported from Iran that respiratory complications were more common in the group of patients treated with obidoxime when compared to those treated with alkalinisation regimens. They also found that high doses of 2-PAM (12g over 3 days) were associated with a higher mortality, increased ventilatory requirements and a greater incidence of the intermediate syndrome.

Szinicz and Eyer (2000) consider that though most OPs will hydrolyse more rapidly at an alkaline pH, the range of pH change possible in the living organism is very limited. The calculation of the maximal change in the rate of hydrolysis relative to pH change which is possible showed a negligible increase in elimination velocity. Thus this regimen may be of limited benefit.

12.11. Phenothiazines

The use of phenothiazines in the management of OP poisoning is controversial (Hayes Jr, 1982).

The potentiation of OP insecticides by phenothiazines has been suggested (Arterberry et al., 1962). Phenothiazines have anticholinergic properties and some may inhibit AChE (Szinicz, 2000). Montoya-Cabrera et al. (1999) reported the successful use of diphenhydramine intravenously in the management of extrapyramidal symptoms which followed acute parathion methyl poisoning. However, a specific therapeutic role for phenothiazines in the management of acute OP poisoning cannot be identified at present.

12.12. Respiratory Stimulants

Lerman and Gutman (1988) concluded that respiratory stimulants should not be used in the treatment of acute OP poisoning in humans. They will not reverse the bronchospasm, neuromuscular block and may induce convulsions.

12.13. Extracorporeal Cardiopulmonary Support (ECPS)

Kamijo et al. (1999) considered ECPS useful in the treatment of severe OP poisoning particularly in the presence of hypothermia resistant to usual forms of treatment.

12.14. Management of Poisoning during Pregnancy

Only six case reports of OP poisoning during pregnancy had been published until 1997 (Bailey, 1997) and only three women received oximes. One of them, in the third month of pregnancy, received obidoxime but opted for a therapeutic abortion (Gadoth and Fisher, 1978). Karalliedde et al. (1988) treated two patients (16th week of gestation and the other during the 36th week of gestation) with atropine, pralidoxime and ventilatory support. They recovered and progressed to have normal deliveries. However, the subsequent status, mental and physical, of the babies is not known. The experience with pralidoxime or other oximes during pregnancy is limited. It would appear that no reason exists to withhold an oxime, a drug which may decrease morbidity and prevent mortality. It has been stated that the basic management of OP poisoning in a pregnant woman should not differ from that in the non-pregnant patient (Tenebein, 1994).

12.15. Psychiatric Counselling

The need for psychiatric intervention generally occurs at two points (Parker and Brown, 1989). Firstly, when symptoms of the central nervous system of confusion and agitation may confound the medical management. Secondly, in instances of self-harm where such counseling would be of benefit to the patient. In the South East Asian countries (Karalliedde, 2000), there is a tendency for the patients to resent psychiatric help after recovery from poisoning as many patients yearn for anonymity after such an event.

12.16 Prevention of Further Exposure

Following symptomatic occupational exposure, patients should not work with OP pesticides until BuChE or AChE levels have returned to at least 75% of normal.

Of increasing concern particularly to the residents in developed countries is the exposure to OP residues in food and exposure during recreational activities such as gardening. Chlorpyrifos residue estimations in tomatoes and tomato products (Aysal *et al.*, 1999), and that of parathion-methyl in field-sprayed apples (Pappas *et al.*, 1999), following indoor spraying (Davis and Ahmed, 1998) and during manual operations on pesticide treated ornamental plants (Aprea *et al.*, 1999) have been the subject of recent publications. Further, a study has shown that semi-volatile pesticides would accumulate on toys and other sorbent surfaces in a home following application (Gurunathan *et al.*, 1998). These studies are important and need to be standardized to provide appropriate information to the public and health care personnel in order for the general population to adhere to safety precautions.

12.17. Monitoring and Prevention of Occupational Exposure

Constant monitoring of the health status of those involved in manufacture, formulation and application of OP insecticides is mandatory. Monitoring should include periodic measurements of ChEs (Fenske *et al.*, 1999; Lu and Fenske, 1999). These would ensure the use of adequate protective measures such as clothing, ventilation and health education which are an important aspect of management.

It is recommended that anyone who mixes, loads, applies or expects to handle or come in contact with OP insecticides and anyone who is in contact with these chemicals for more than 30 hours at a time in one 30 day period should be tested for ChE. **For methods see chapter 15.** There is no set formula for deciding the frequency of ChE testing. It may be carried out monthly or weekly during the active season Baseline samples should be taken when a worker has not been exposed for at least 30 days.

Appendix 1

Additional Data on Clinically and Experimentally Used Antidotes

1. NMDA receptor channel blockers, adenosine receptor agonists
There is interest in the role of glutamate in sustained OP-induced seizure activity and therefore the possible therapeutic role of non-selective glutamate receptor antagonists, such as felbamate and of selective N-methyl-D-aspartate (NMDA) receptor-channel blockers, such as dizocilpine in the management of OP poisoning (Meredith, 1999). Another agent of interest is the tertiary amine antimuscarinic procyclidine (Meredith 1999). Initially, the convulsions following OP poisoning are considered to be due to excess ACh in the brain. A few minutes after the onset of seizures several transmitter systems such as those for excitatory amino acids (e.g. glutamate, aspartate) and catecholamines are progressively disrupted (van Helden and Bueters, 1999). It has been suggested that glutamate plays a role in the maintenance of OP-induced seizures. Glutamate when present in sufficiently high concentrations mediates cell death via the NMDA receptor. Gacyclidine was useful in the management of nerve agent poisoning and produced rapid normalization of EEG activity, clinical recovery and neurprotection (Lallement et al., 1999)

Adenosine has a specific neuroprotective function under circumstances of enhanced neuronal activity which is thought to be a result of post-synaptic modulatory effect on K^+ and Cl^- channel activity via the post-synaptic A1 receptor. Adenosine also inhibits adenylate cyclase and phospholipase C - effects that might contribute to its neuroprotective properties (van Helden and Bueters, 1999).

Activation of the presynaptic A1 receptor results in a reduction in neurotransmitter release in several systems including ACh and excitatory amino acids. Preliminary experiments using adenosine A1 receptor agonists 5'-N-ethylcarboxamido-adenosine (NECA) and N6-cyclopentyl adenosine (CPA) administered by intramuscular injection 1 min following subcutaneous soman poisoning (1.5–2 LD50) in rats resulted in postponement of chewing, salivation, convulsive activity and respiratory distress (symptoms produced by excess ACh) and the mortality rate was reduced (van Helden *et al.*, 1998).

2. Clonidine and Medetomidine

Clonidine inhibits the release of ACh from central and peripheral cholinergic neurons in addition to being a centrally active alpha-2-adrenergic agonist. In rodents, clonidine pre-treatment (0.3mg/kg) delayed the onset of tremor from 5 to 20 min, delayed death from 12 to 24 min and increased the percentage of survivors to 50% following poisoning with physostigmine. It was suggested that central cholinergic neurones involved in the regulation of respiration and fine motor control (not peripheral motor neurons) are inhibited by clonidine acting on alpha-receptors (Buccafusco and Aronstam, 1986). Mice pre-treated with clonidine (0.1–1 mg/kg), were protected from several of the toxic manifestations of soman (Buccafusco, 1982). The protection resulted in increased survival rates and a reduction in centrally mediated symptoms of soman intoxication. Pre-treatment with atropine (25mg/kg) also protected against soman toxicity. When atropine was combined with clonidine, the degree of protection afforded by the combination was greater than that predicted for a simple additive effect. The protective effects of clonidine are likely to involve multiple sites of action, including blockade of ACh release and on muscarinic receptors (Yang *et al.*, 1993). Yakoub and Mohammad (1997) studied the effects of alpha 2 agonist medetomidine in diazinon-induced poisoning in mice. Subcutaneous injection of medetomidine at 0.05, 0.1 and 0.3 mg/kg, 15 minutes before administration of diazinon (75 mg/kg orally) significantly and dose dependently decreased the incidence of toxic manifestations, delayed the onset of tremors and death and increased 24 hour survival rates to 70, 80 and 100% respectively. Similarly, medetomidine pretreatments (0.1 and 0.3 mg/kg, sc) significantly protected mice from the toxicity of a high dose (100mg/kg orally) of diazinon and increased the 24 hour survival rates.

The authors observed that the alpha 2 antagonist atipamezole significantly abolished the protective effect of medetomidine. When atropine sulphate (6mg/kg, s.c.) was combined with medetomidine (0.3 mg/kg s.c) the degree of protection against diazinon toxicosis was more than that produced by either drug alone. Thus the role of alpha 2 agonists in the treatment of OP poisoning merits further study.

3. Fluoride

Pretreatment of mice with atropine (17mg/kg) and sodium fluoride (NAF) (5 or 15mg/kg) had a significantly better effect than atropine alone against the toxic effects of soman and sarin. Atropine + NAF (15 mg/kg) was effective against tabun, whereas a lower dose of NAF was not. It was hypothesized that the effect of NAF was due to a reduction of the desensitising action at nicotinic receptors in the neuromuscular junction and/or sympathetic ganglia in addition to the proposed increased hydrolysis of sarin and direct detoxification of tabun (Clement and Filbert, 1983).

AChE and NTE which had been inhibited with either mipafox or with a di-n-butylphosphorodiamidate has been shown to be reactivated by prolonged treatment with aqueous potassium fluoride (Milastovic and Johnson, 1993). It is interesting to note that increased cholinesterase levels were observed in workers in a plastic factory handling fluorine compounds (Xu et al., 1992). On the other hand fluoride has reactivating potency and, in the case of fluorinated compounds like most of the nerve agents, the original poison can be reconstituted and inhibition of the esterases may occur again.

4. Lidocaine

Lidocaine (lignocaine) was found to be ineffective in the treatment of arrhythmias following OP intoxication by Kiss and Fazekas (1979) and Ludomirsky et al. (1982) (see chapter 10). Rump with Kaliszan (1969) and earlier with Edelwein (1966) studied the effect of lidocaine as an anticonvulsant. Later Lowndes and Johnson (1971) studied the effect of lidocaine on twitch potentiation and repetitive neural activity produced by soman and neostigmine.

Lidocaine was found to abolish the repetitive nerve impulses in motor nerves following OP intoxication. Further, lidocaine abolished the post OP potentiation of twitch tension. Rump and Edelwein (1966) observed that lidocaine blocked the epileptiform patterns due to DFP in the rabbit brain. These observations in animals have not been studied in man.

5. Annealed Red Cells

Ihler *et al.* (1973) reported that enzymes and drugs could be encapsulated within erythrocytes. Cannon *et al.* (1994) first reported that murine carrier erythrocytes containing rhodanase (rhodanese) and thiosulfate protected mice against the lethal effects of cyanide.

The primary advantage of this cell carrier system is that it would enhance the persistence and stability of the enzyme.

By placing phosphotriesterase within the resealed annealed erythrocytes in the circulation by a single injection, this enzyme can theoretically persist for the life of an erythrocyte (120 days), and can constantly remove OP which is being slowly released in to the blood stream from fatty tissues, thereby minimizing the incidence of the delayed polyneuropathy.

Intravenous administration of the free enzyme has been reported to protect mice from soman poisoning (Raveh *et al.*, 1992).

Presently the annealed erythrocytes are a convenient carrier system which has the potential utility as a prophylactic agent by autologous transfusion to individuals who are at risk to OP agents e.g. aerial crop dusters, agricultural workers, soldiers exposed to nerve gases. This would not be suitable therapy for acute poisoning as a delay is incurred in which blood typing would be required before encapsulation of the enzyme within the erythrocyte is initiated. However, by using an alternative carrier system e.g. stable liposome, such an approach may be practical for the actual treatment of poisoning. With the use of a protein-containing carrier system, there exists a potential for immunological reactions. However, the long-term use of this system to treat inborn errors of metabolism in humans and other clinical uses suggest that this has not been a major problem (Pei *et al.*, 1995).

Resealed cells containing a recombinant phosphotriesterase provided protection against the lethal effect of paraoxon. Phosphotriesterase hydrolyses paraoxon to the much less toxic 4-nitrophenol and diethylphosphate.

Carrier red cells increased the protection against paraoxon by over 1000-fold. When these carrier cells were administered in combination with 2-PAM and/or atropine a marked synergism was observed.

6. Glucoside Extracted from Root of *Astragalus membranaceus*

Li *et al.* (1998) observed that the survival time of guinea pigs intoxicated with dimethoate (600mg/kg) was increased, from an average of 70 minutes to an average of 235 minutes, when the animals were treated with the glucoside extracted from the root of *Astragalus membranaceus*. They also observed that arrhythmias were either delayed or minimized along with muscle fasciculations, seizures and secretions within the respiratory tract.

Appendix 2

Oximes

Pralidoxime

Pralidoxime chloride (2-PAM) and methyl sulfate and the methanesulphate or mesylate (P2S) are usually used as the iodide increases the risk of adverse cardiac events and of iodism. Although 2-PAM is effective when administered orally or intramuscularly, intravenous administration is the preferred route. Traditional dosing for pralidoxime in OP poisoning was 1–2g (20–40 mg/kg) of 2-PAM dissolved in 0.9% saline administered over 30 minutes, every 12 hours intravenously in adults. The dose for children was 25–50mg/kg (Johnson and Vale, 1992; Mortensen, 1986).

The pharmacokinetics of pralidoxime is characterised by a two compartment model with a steady-state volume of distribution of about 0.8 l/kg (Medicis *et al.*, 1996). Pralidoxime is renally excreted. Within 12 h, 80% of the dose can be recovered, unchanged in the urine. In poisoned patients, the pharmacokinetics of 2-PAM appears to be altered.

A volume of distribution of 2.77 l/kg and an elimination half-life of 3.44 h has been reported. The pharmacokinetics of pralidoxime in poisoned children following continuous infusion vary widely and differ from those reported both in healthy and poisoned adults (Schexnayder *et al.*, 1998).

The volume of distribution (Vd) and the plasma clearance of pralidoxime was found to be greater in children. A loading dose of 20mg/kg in children, should achieve plasma pralidoxime concentrations of approximately 7 mg/l. Larger loading doses will be required in patients with seizures, coma, bradycardia or respiratory depression. A loading dose of 50mg/kg in a severely ill patient with a Vd of 8–9 l/kg should result in a pralidoxime serum concentration of approximately 5–6mg/l. As clearance does not appear to vary with the severity of poisoning, a continuous infusion rate of 10–20mg/kg/h would be expected to maintain a plasma pralidoxime concentration of 11 to 22 mg/l in most children, and in excess of 4mg/l in children with increased clearance. Such dose regimens would result in pralidoxime concentrations of 30–60mg/l in subjects with low clearance. However, concentrations up to 30 mg/l in 3 of their patients was not associated with any clinical toxicity. Thus, the recommended regimen in children was a loading dose of 20–50 mg/kg based on symptom severity followed by a continuous infusion of 10–20mg/kg/h (Schexnayder et al., 1998). Earlier, Farrar et al. (1990) stated that continuous infusions of 2-PAM should be initiated with 25mg/kg intravenous dose given for 15–30 minutes, followed by a continuous infusion of 10–20 mg/kg/h in children and be continued for at least 18 hours or longer, depending on the patients clinical status.

Other regimens advocated are a loading dose of 4.42 mg/kg administered over 30 minutes followed by 2.14 mg/kg/h for pralidoxime methylsulphate or an initial dose of 4 mg/kg over 15 minutes followed by 3.2 mg/kg/h (Willems, 1992).

Different regimens of pralidoxime were also studied by Cherian et al. (1997) and Johnson et al. (1996) in India.

Besser et al. (1995) observed dramatic improvement in neuro-electrophysiological function when obidoxime was administered within the first 12 h of intoxication. When administered 24 h after intoxication, obidoxime produced little or no improvement or even worsening (Maselli and Soliven, 1991).

Adverse effects of therapeutic doses of 2-PAM in humans have been minimal, occurring only when the plasma level was greater than 400mg/l. Calesnick et al. (1967) found that intravenous 2-PAM doses of 15–30 mg/kg in adults produced transient, dose-dependent, increases in blood pressure but no adverse symptoms. However, at doses of 45 mg/kg marked hypertension (diastolic blood pressure >110 mm Hg) and electrocardiographic changes (increased T wave amplitude and PR interval duration) were observed. Additionally, pupillary light reflexes were sluggish and subjects complained of supraorbital headache, alterations in visual accommodation and epigastric discomfort.

Jager and Stagg (1958) did not observe significant variations in blood pressure, electrocardiographic changes or respiratory patterns after administering 15–30 mg/kg of 2-PAM intravenously for 2–4 minutes. Dizziness (100%), blurred vision (72%) and diplopia (50%) were commonly reported in this study along with headaches, impaired accommodation and nausea. Namba *et al.* (1959) reported no side effects with doses of 2-PAM as high as 26g for 54 hours in adults. Transient dizziness, blurred vision and elevation of diastolic pressure may be related to rapid administration, which has also caused sudden cardiac and respiratory arrest. Pralidoxime in large doses (producing concentrations of $2x\ 10^{-3}$ M in humans) can produce neuromuscular block and even inhibition of AChE (Hayes Jr, 1982).

Thiamine administered intravenously at 100 mg/h for 2.5 h prolonged the half-life, increased the volume of distribution and peak plasma concentrations and decreased renal clearances, when pralidoxime 5 mg/kg was given intravenously and concomitantly (Josselson and Sidell, 1978). The purported benefit of thiamine in poisoned patients is that it prolongs the plasma half-life of pralidoxime although this has never been tested. To improve the central effects of pralidoxime, the dihydropyridine derivative was synthesized. This derivative known as pro-2PAM acts as a 'pro drug' which is able to pass through membranes, such as the blood brain barrier and once across the membranes, in vivo oxidation converts the pro-2-PAM to PAM to give a 13 fold higher level of 2-PAM in the brain. The use of sugar oximes (the molecular combination of glucose with 2-PAM derivatives) to promote CNS penetration has also been considered (Bodor *et al.*, 1975).

There exists some controversy regarding the use of pralidoxime in OP poisoning (De Silva *et al.*, 1992; Singh *et al.*, 1995; Du Toit *et al.*, 1981; Gnanendran *et al.*, 1974) and the specific temporal sequence for administration of atropine and pralidoxime (Du Toit *et al.*, 1981). In vitro studies with human sera by Gnanendran *et al.* (1974) showed that PAM made no significant improvement in the overall outcome following OP insecticide poisoning and that there was a risk of producing harmful and more potent phosphorylated oximes. In one study using pralidoxime methylsulphate, it was found that following parathion-methyl and parathion poisoning, enzyme reactivation occurred in some subjects at oxime concentrations as low as 2.88mg/l. In others, however, oxime concentrations as high as 14.6 mg/l were present without effect. These workers concluded that the therapeutic effect of oximes seemed to depend on the plasma concentration of the OP agent with minimal benefit when the levels of OP in the blood were high (Willems *et al.*, 1993).

After reporting repeated asystole following PAM in OP self-poisoning, Scott (1986) concluded that the "time honoured eminence of PAM as an antidote in OP poisoning is undeserved". It should be noted that until now no controlled clinical study has been carried out to assess the clinical efficacy of the oximes.

Obidoxime

The effective therapeutic plasma concentration of obidoxime was anticipated to be 4mg/L i.e. about 10 μmol/l, corresponding to an administration of a IV bolus of 250 mg followed by 750 mg/day or after the bolus, a continuous infusion of 0.4mg/kg/h (Eyer, 1996; Worek et al., 1997; Thiermann et al., 1997).

In a multi-hospital study, a high incidence of cardiac arrhythmias was observed in patients who received high cumulative doses of atropine and obidoxime. The impairment of liver function was also significantly higher in these patients, (Finlkelstein et al., 1989) compared to those receiving pralidoxime. Thiermann et al. (1997) reported that even the low dose regimen (which produced plasma concentrations of 10–20 μmol/l) impaired liver function transiently in patients with multi-organ failure.

In 1999, scientists from Munich (Thiermann et al., 1999) developed a monitoring system to assess RBC AChE, reactivability of RBC AChE, ex-vivo plasma cholinesterase activity, the plasma concentrations of AChE inhibiting compounds and their potential precursors, plasma obidoxime and atropine levels. Obidoxime was given as an IV bolus of 250mg followed by a continuous infusion of 750mg/24h producing a steady-state plasma concentration of 10–20 μmol/l. Obidoxime was administered until plasma ChE activity increased and AChE inhibiting material was no longer detectable. The following conclusions were based on the preliminary results:

1. Obidoxime was highly effective in life-threatening parathion poisoning when the dose absorbed was relatively low
2. In poisoning with excessive doses of parathion, significant net reactivation was not achieved until several days after ingestion when the concentration of parathion had declined below 0.2 μmol/l
3. Reactivation of diethyl-phosphoryl RBC AChE in vivo lasted up to 5 days
4. With dimethoxy-phosphoryl-RBC AChE, obidoxime was effective when administered within 12 h of ingestion of oxydemeton-methyl

5. The effectiveness of obidoxime was indicated by a drastic reduction of atropine demand. Usually 1 mg of atropine sulfate/h or less (resulting in plasma concentrations of approximately 20nM), was sufficient to limit muscarinic signs and this could be discontinued when RBC AChE was reactivated by >30% of normal.
6. Signs of transiently impaired liver and kidney functions were observed in severely poisoned patients with transient multi-organ failure.

More recently, Worek *et al.* (1999) found that efficacy of obidoxime in reactivating dimethylphosphoryl-AChE (phosphorylation produced by OP agents containing two methoxy groups such as malathion, paraoxon-methyl, dimethoate and oxydemeton-methyl) was 40, 9 and 3 times higher than that of HI-6, pralidoxime and HLö respectively. In addition, OP concentrations up to 10^{-6} M (paraoxon-methyl) and 10^{-4} M (oxydemeton-methyl) could be counteracted at clinically relevant oxime concentrations of 10microM. Further, the potency of oximes to reactivate dimethylphosphoryl-BuChE was much lower than that of the corresponding AChE. Thus these workers concluded that BuChE estimations would not provide reliable information on AChE status either at diagnosis or during therapeutic monitoring.

A recent review (Johnson *et al* 2000), recommended that plasma concentrations of 85-170 μmol/l of pralidoxime or 10-20 μmol/l of obidoxime should be achieved during any regimen of oxime therapy.

Other oximes used in man and in experimental animals include methoxime, the H-oximes (Hl-6 and HLö-7) and BI-6 (1-(2-hydroxyiminomethylpyridinium)-4-(-carbamoylpyridinium)-2-butene dibromide). In a comparison of the efficacy of oximes against GF, it was found that in vitro, methoxime seemed to be the most efficacious reactivator, whilst pralidoxime and obidoxime appeared to be very poor reactivators. *In vivo*, H-oximes were the most efficacious antidotes (Kassa and Cabal, 1999).

Oximes are contraindicated in patients with myasthenia gravis who are being treated with anticholinesterases, as the oximes may precipitate a myasthenic crisis (Bismuth *et al.*, 1992).

References

AAP 1983

Aaron, C.A., Howland, M.A. Insecticides: Organophosphates and carbamates. In:. *Goldfrank's Toxicological Emergencies.* Goldfrank, L.R., Flomenbaum, N.E., Lewin, N.A., *et al.* eds. Appleton and Lange; Stamford, Connecticut:1998 p. 1429–44.

Anonymous. Position statement: Cathartics. *Journal of Toxicology Clinical Toxicology* 1997a;**35**:743–52.

Anonymous. Position Statement: Whole Bowel Irrigation. *Journal of Toxicology Clinical Toxicology* 1997b;**35**:753–62.

Aprea, C., Sciarra, G., Sartorelli, P., *et al.* Multi-route exposure assessment and excretion of urinary metabolites of fenitrothion during manual operations on treated ornamental plants in greenhouses. *Archives of Environmental Contamination and Toxicology* 1999;**36**:490–7.

Atterberry, J.D., Bonifaci, R.W., Nash, E.W., *et al.* Potentiation of phosphorus insecticides by phenothiazine derivatives. *Journal of the American Medical Association* 1962;**182**:848–50.

Aysal, P., Goxek, K., Artik, N., *et al.* 14C-chlorpyrifos residues in tomatoes and tomato products. *Bulletin of Environmental Contamination and Toxicology* 1999;**62**:377–82.

Bailey, B. Organophosphate poisoning in pregnancy. *Annals of Emergency Medicine* 1997;**29**:299.

Baker, D.J., Sedgwick, E.M. Single fibre electromyographic changes in man after organophosphate exposure. *Human and Experimental Toxicology* 1996;**15**:369–75.

Balali-Mood, M. Personal communication 1999.

Balali-Mood, M., Shariat, M. Treatment of organophosphate poisoning. Experience of nerve agents and acute pesticide poisoning on the effects of oximes. Abstract *Journal Physiology (Paris)* 1998;**92**:375–8.

Bardin P.G., Van Eeden, S.F. Organophosphate poisoning: grading the severity and comparing treatment between atropine and glycopyrrolate. *Critical Care Medicine* 1990:**18**:956-60.

Bateman, D.N. Gastric decontamination—a view for the millennium. *Journal of Accident and Emergency Medicine* 1999; **16**:84–6.

Becker, G., Kawan, A., Szinicz, L. Direct reaction of oximes with sarin, soman, or tabun *in vitro. Archives of Toxicology* 1997; **71**:714–8.

Besser, R., Weilemann, L.S., Gutman, L. Efficacy of obidoxime in human organophosphate poisoning: determination by neuromuscular studies. *Muscle Nerve* 1995; **18**:15–22.

Bismuth, C., Inns, R.H., Marrs, T.C. Efficacy, toxicity and clinical use of oximes in anticholinesterase poisoning. In: *Clinical and Experimental Toxicology of Organophosphates and Carbamates.* Ballantyne, B., Marrs, T.C. eds: Butterworth–Heinemann, .Oxford 1992. 555–77.

Bodor, N., Shek, B., Higuchi, T. Delivery of a quaternary pyridinium salt across the blood-brain barrier by its dihydropyridine derivative. *Science* 1975;**90**:155–6.

Bradshaw, B.C., Dark, C.H., Suer, A.H. *et al.* Atropine sulphate enhances neuromuscular transmission in anaesthetized patients. *Proceedings of the British Pharmaceutical Society* 1986;**23**:636.

Buccafusco, J.J. Mechanism of the clonidine induced protection against acetylcholinesterase inhibitor toxicity. *Journal of Pharmacology and Experimental Therapeutics* 1982;**222**:595–9.

Buccafusco, J.J., Aronstam, R.S. Clonidine protection from the toxicity of soman, an organophosphate acetylcholinesterase inhibitor, in the mouse. *Journal of Pharmacology and Experimental Therapeutics* 1986;**239**:43–7.

Calesnick, B., Christensen, J.A., Richter, M. Human toxicity of various oximes.2 pyridine aldoxime methyl chloride, its methane sulphonate salt and 1,1' trimethylenbis –(4 formylpyridinium chloride). *Archives of Environmental Health* 1967; **15**:599–608.

Cannon, E.P., Leung, P., Hawkins, A. *et al.* Antagonism of cyanide intoxication with murine carrier erythrocytes containing rhodanase and sodium thiosulfate. *Journal of Toxicology and Environmental Health* 1994; **41**:267–74.

Cherian, A.M., Peter, J.V., Samuel, J., *et al.* Effectiveness of P2AM in the treatment of organophosphorus poisoning. A randomised double blind placebo controlled clinical trial. *Journal of the Association of Physicians India* 1997;**45**:22–4.

Choi, P.T.L., Quinonez, L.G., Cook, D.J. *et al.* The use of glycopyrrolate in a case of intermediate syndrome following acute organophosphate poisoning. *Canadian Journal of Anaesthesia* 1998; **45**:337–40.

Clement, J.G., Filbert, M. Antidote effect of sodium fluoride against organophosphate poisoning in mice. *Life Sciences* 1983;**32**:1803–10.

Cordoba, D., Cadavid, S., Angulao, D., *et al.* Organophosphate poisoning: modifications in acid-base equilibrium and use of sodium bicarbonate as an aid in the treatment of toxicity in dogs. *Veterinary and Experimental Toxicology* 1983:**25**:1–3.

Coye, M.J., Barnett, P.G., Midtling, J.E., *et al.* Clinical confirmation of organophosphate poisoning by serial cholinesterase analysis. *Archives of Internal Medicine* 1987; **147**:438–42.

Davis, D.L., Ahmed, A.K. Exposures from indoor spraying of chlorpyrifos pose greater health risks to children than currently estimated. *Environmental Health Perspectives* 1998; **106**:299–301.

De Silva, H.J., Wijewickrema, R., Senanayake, N. Does pralidoxime affect outcome of management in acute organophosphorus poisoning? *Lancet* 1992;**339**:1136–8.

Du Toit, P.W., Muller, F.O., Van Tonder, W.M., *et al.* Experience with the intensive care management of organophosphate insecticide poisoning. *South African Medical Journal* 1981;**60**:227–9.

el-Refai, A.R., el-Essawi, M., el-Esnair, N. *et al.* Hazards from aerial spraying in cotton culture area of the Nile river. *Archives of Environmental Health* 1971;**22**:328–33.

Eyer, P. Optimal oxime dosage regimen, a pharmacokinetic approach. In: *Role of oximes in the treatment of anticholinesterase agent poisoning.* Szinicz, L., Eyer, P., Klimmek, R. eds.: Spektrum Akademischer Verlag; Heidelberg 1996. p. 33–51.

Eyer, P., Worek, F., Thiermann, H., *et al.* The role of atropine and oximes in the treatment of organophosphate poisoning. Abstract, *European Congress of Toxicology* 1999. p. 369.

Fang, Y., Pei, Z.I., Li, Z. Study on observation indexes of rational dosage of atropine in treatment of acute OP insecticide poisoning (Chinese). *Chung-Hua Hu Li Tsa Chih. Chinese Journal of Nursing* 1997;**32**:311–5.

Farrar, H.C., Wells, T.G., Kearns, G.L., Use of continuous infusion of pralidoxime for treatment of organophosphate poisoning in children. *Journal of Pediatrics* 1990;**116**:658–61.

Fenske, R.A., Simcox, N.J., Camp, J.E. *et al.* Comparison of three methods for assessment of hand exposure to azinphos-methyl (Guthion) during apple thinning. *Applied Occupational and Environmental Hygiene* 1999;**14**:618–23.

Finlkelstein, V., Kushnir, A., Raikhlin-Eisenkraft, B., *et al.* Antidotal therapy of severe acute organophosphate poisoning: a multihospital study. *Neurotoxicology and Teratology* 1989;**11**:593–6.

Gadoth, N., Fisher, A. Late onset of neuromuscular block in organophosphorus poisoning. *Annals of Internal Medicine* 1978;**88**:654–5.

Gallagher, H., Tracey, J.A. Organophosphorus insecticide poisoning. (Letter). *British Journal of Anaesthesia* 1990;**65**:293–4.

Garcia-Repetto, R., Martinez, D., Repetto, M. The influence of pH on the degradation kinetics of some organophosphorus pesticides in aqueous solutions. *Veterinary and Human Toxicology* 1994;**36**:202–4.

Gnanendran, A., Balabaskaran, Chea, U.J. The role of pyridine-2-aldoxime methiodide in the management of organophosphate insecticide poisoning. *Proceedings 4th Asian-Australasian Congress of Anaesthesiologists* 1974.

Gordon, R.K., Feaster, S.R., Russell, A.J., *et al.* Organophosphate skin decontamination using immobilized enzymes. *Chemico Biological Interactions* 1999;**119–120**:463–70.

Grob, D. Anticholinesterase intoxication in man and its treatment. In: *Cholinesterases and Anticholinesterase agents*, Koelle, G.B. ed Springer Verlag, Berlin. 1963.

Gurunathan, S., Robson, M., Freeman, N. *et al.* Accumulation of chlorpyrifos on residential surfaces and toys accessible to children. *Environmental Health Perspectives* 1998;**106**:9–16.

Haddad, L.M., The emergency management of poisoning. *Pediatric Annals* 1987;**16**:900–12.

Hagerstrom-Portnoy, G., Jones, R., Adams, A.J. *et al.* Effects of atropine and 2-PAM chloride on vision and performance in humans. *Aviation Space and Environmental Medicine* 1987;**10**:47–53.

Hantson, P., Hainaut, P., Vander Stappen, M., *et al.* Regulation of body temperature after acute organophosphate poisoning. *Canadian Journal of Anaesthesia* 1996;**43**:755.

Hayes, W.J. Jr. *Pesticides studied in man.* Baltimore: Williams and Wilkins 1982.

Health and Safety Executive Guidance notes MS 17. Medical Aspects of work-related exposures to organophosphates. May 2000.

Heath, J.W., Meredith, T. Atropine in the management of anticholinesterase poisoning. In: *Clinical and Experimental Toxicology of Organophosphates and Carbamates.* Ballantyne, B., Marrs, T.C. eds. Butterworth–Heinemann; Oxford: 1992. p. 543–554

Hobbiger, P., Vojvodic, V. The reactivation by pyridine aldoximes of phosphorylated acetylcholinesterase in the central nervous system. *Biochemical Pharmacology* 1967;**16**:455–62.

Hoffman, B. Personal communication 1999.

Howland, W.A., Aaron, C. Antidotes in depth: Pralidoxime In: *Goldfrank's Toxicologic Emergencies*. Goldfrank, L.R., Flomenbaum, N.E., Lewin, N.A., et al. eds. Appleton and Lange; Stamford, Connecticut: 1998. p. 1429–44

Ihler, G.M., Glew, R.H., Schnure, F.W. Enzyme loading erythrocytes. *Proceedings of National Academy of Sciences of the USA* 1973;**70**:2663–6.

IPCS. Environmental Health Criteria 63. *Organophosphorus Insecticides: A General Introduction.* Geneva: World Health Organization (WHO) 1986; 17–111.

Jager, B.V., Stagg, G.N. Toxicity of diacetyl monoximine and of pyridine-2-aldoxime methiodide in man. *Bulletin of the Johns Hopkins Hospital* 1958;**102**:203–11.

Johnson, D.D., Lowndes, H.E. Reduction by diazepam of repetitive electrical activity and toxicity resulting from soman. *European Journal of Pharmacology* 1974;**28**:245.

Johnson, D.D., Wilcox, C.W. Studies on the mechanism of the protective and antidotal actions of diazepam in organophosphate poisoning. *European Journal of Pharmacology*.1975;**34**:127–32.

Johnson ,M.K., Jacobsen, D., Meredith, T.J. et al. Evaluation of antidotes for poisoning by organophosphorus pesticides. *Emergency Medicine* 2000;**12**:22-37

Johnson, M.K., Vale, J.A. Clinical management of acute organophosphorus insecticide poisoning: an overview. In:. *Clinical and Experimental Toxicology of Organophosphates and Carbamates.* Ballantyne, B., Marrs, T.C. eds Butterworth–Heinemann; Oxford: 1992. p. 555–77.

Johnson, S., Peter, J.V., Thomas, K. *et al.* Evaluation of two treatment regimens of pralidoxime (1 g single bolus dose vs 12g infusion) in the management of organophosphorus poisoning. *Journal of the Association of Physicians India* 1996;**44**:529–31.

Josselson, I., Sidell, F.R. Effect of intravenous thiamine on pralidoxime kinetics. *Clinical Pharmacology and Therapeutics* 1978;**24**:95–100.

Kamijo, Y., Soma, K., Uchimiya, H. *et al.* A case of serious organophosphate poisoning treated by percutaneous cardiopulmonary support. *Veterinary and Human Toxicology* 1999;**41**:326–8.

Karalliedde, L. Personal observation 2000.

Karalliedde, L., Senanayake, N. Organophosphorus insecticide poisoning. *British Journal of Anaesthesia* 1989;**63**:736–50.

Karalliedde, L., Senanayake, N., Ariaratnam, A. Acute organophosphorus insecticide poisoning during pregnancy. *Human Toxicology* 1988;**7**:363–4.

Kassa, J., Bajgar, J. Comparison of the effect of selected anticholinergic agents on cholinergic and noncholinergic effects of GV substances during acute poisoning in rats. *Ceskoslovenska Farmacie* 1994;**43**:222–5.

Kassa, J., Cabal, J. A comparison of the efficacy of acetylcholinesterase reactivators against cyclohexyl methylphosphonofluoridate (GF agent) by in vitro and in vivo methods. *Pharmacology and Toxicology* 1999;**84**:41–5.

Kiss, Z., Fazekas, T. Organophosphates and torsade de pointes ventricular tachycardia. *Journal of the Royal Society of Medicine* 1983;**76**:983–4.

Kolarzyk, E., Szpak, D., Pach, D. The influence of acute poisoning with an organophosphate compound on the regulation of breathing and respiratory system efficiency. *Przeglad Lekarski* 1997;**54**:745–9.

Lallement, G., Baubichon, D., Clarencon, D. *et al.* Review of the value of gacyclidine (GK-11) as adjuvant medication to conventional treatments of organophosphate poisoning: primate experiments mimicking various scenarios of military or terrorist attack by soman. *Neurotoxicology* 1999;**20**:675–84.

Lallement, G., Dorandeu, F., Filliat, P. *et al.* Medical management of organophosphate-induced seizures. *Journal of Physiology (Paris)* 1998;**92**:369–73.

Lerman, Y., Gutman, H. The use of respiratory stimulants in organophosphorus intoxication. *Medical Hypothesis* 1988;**26**:267–9.

Li, Y., Liu, X., Xue, S.Z. Antidotal effect of glucoside extracted from *Astragalus membranaceus* on dimethoate intoxication in guinea pigs. *Medicina del Lavoro* 1998;**89** Suppl 2:S136–41.

Lipp, J.A. Effect of benzodiazepine derivatives on soman-induced seizure activity and convulsions in the monkey. *Archives Internationales de Pharmacodynamie et de Therapie* 1973;**202**:244.

Lipp, J.A. Effect of small doses of clonazepam upon soman-induced seizure activity and convulsions. *Archives Internationales de Pharmacodynamie et de Therapie* 1974;**210**–49.

Ludomirsky, A., Klein, H.O., Sarelli, P. *et al.* QT prolongation and polymorphous ("Torsade de pointes") ventricular arrhythmias associated with organophosphorus insecticide poisoning. *American Journal of Cardiology* 1982;**49**:1654–8.

Lotti, M., Becker, C.E. Treatment of acute organophosphate poisoning, evidence of a direct effect on nervous system by 2-PAM (pyridine-2-aldoxime methyl chloride). *Journal of Toxicology Clinical Toxicology* 1982;**19**:121–7.

Lowndes, H.E., Johnson, D.D. The effect of lidocaine on twitch potentiation and repetitive neural activity produced by soman and neostigmine. *Canadian Journal of Physiology and Pharmacology* 1971;**49**:464.

Lu, C., Fenske, R.A. Dermal transfer of chlorpyrifos residues from residential surfaces: comparison of hand press, hand drag, wipe and polyurethane foam roller measurements after broadcast and aerosol pesticide applications. *Environmental Health Perspectives* 1999;**107**:463–7.

Mahieu, P., Hassoun, A., Van Binst, R., *et al.* Severe and prolonged poisoning by fenthion. Significance of the determination of the anticholinesterase capacity of plasma. *Journal of Toxicology-Clinical Toxicology* 1982;**19**:425–32.

Maselli, R.A., Soliven, B.C. Analysis of the organophosphate-induced electromyographic response to repetitive nerve stimulation: paradoxical response to edrophonium and D tubocurarine. *Muscle Nerve* 1991;**14**:1182–8.

Marrs, T.C. Organophosphate poisoning. *Pharmacology and Therapeutics* 1993;**58**:51–66.

Martinez-Chuecos, J., del Carmen Jurado, M., Paz Gimenez, M., *et al.* Experience with hemoperfusion for organophosphate poisoning. *Critical Care Medicine* 1992; **20**:1538–43.

McDonough, J.H., Jaax, N.K., Crowley, P.A., *et al.* Atropine and/or diazepam therapy protects against soman-induced neural and cardiac pathology. *Fundamental and Applied Toxicology* 1989;**13**:256–76.

McDonough J.H., Dochterman L.W., Smith C.D., *et al.* Protection against nerve-agent induced neuropathy, but not cardiac pathology, is associated with the anticonvulsant action of drug treatment. *Neurotoxicology* 1995;**16**:123–32.

McDonough J.H., Zoeffel, L.D., McMonagle, J., *et al.* Anticonvulsant treatment of nerve agent seizures: anticholinergics versus diazepam in soman-intoxicated guinea pigs. *Epilepsy Research* 2000;**38**:1–14.

Medicis, J.J., Stork, C.M., Howland, M.A., *et al.* Pharmacokinetics following a loading dose plus a continuous infusion of pralidoxime compared with the traditional short infusion regimen in human volunteers. *Journal of Toxicology Clinical Toxicology* 1996;**34**:289–95.

Meredith, T.J. Mechanisms of toxicity of organophosphorus insecticides. *EAPCCT XIX International Congress* 1999 p. 366.

Milastovic, D., Johnson, M.K. Reactivation of phosphorodiamidated acetylcholinesterase and neuropathy target esterase by treatment of inhibited enzyme with potassium fluoride. *Chemico Biological Interactions* 1993;**87**:425–30.

Mizutani, T., Naito, H., Dohashi, N. Rectal ulcer with massive haemorrhage due to activated charcoal treatment in oral organophosphate poisoning. *Human and Experimental Toxicology* 1991;**10**:385–6.

Montoya-Cabrera, M.A., Escalante-Galindo, P., Rivera-Rebolledo, J.C., *et al.* Acute methyl parathion poisoning with extrapyramidal manifestations not previously reported (Spanish). *Gaceta Medica de Mexico* 1999;**135**:79–82.

Mortensen, M.C. Management of acute childhood poisonings caused by selected insecticides and herbicides. *Pediatric Clinics of North America* 1986;**33**:421–445.

Ostapenko Yuri, N. Personal communication: 1999.

Pappas, C.J., Kyriakidis, N.B., Athnasopoulos, P.E. Degradation of parathion-methyl on field sprayed apples and stored apples. *Journal of AOAC International* 1999; **82**:359–63.

Parker, P.E., Brown, F.W. Organophosphate intoxication: Hidden Hazards. *Southern Medical Journal* 1989;**82**:1408–10.

Pei, L., Petrikovics, I, Way, J.L. Antagonism of the lethal effects of paraoxon by carrier erythrocytes containing phosphotriesterase. *Fundamental and Applied Toxicology* 1995;**28**:209–14.

Petroianu, G., Ruefer, R. Beta blockade or magnesium in organophosphorus insecticide poisoning. *Anaesthesia and Intensive Care* 1992; **20**:538–9.

Raveh, L., Segall, Y., Leader, H., *et al.* Protection against tabun toxicity in mice by prophylaxis with an enzyme hydrolysing organophosphate ester. *Biochemical Pharmacology* 1992;**44**:397–400.

Rump, S., Edelwejn, Z. Effects of lignocaine on epileptiform patterns of bioelectrical activity of the rabbit's brain due to diisopropyl phosphorofluoridate (DFP). *International Journal of Neuropharmacology* 1966;**5**:401–3.

Rump, S., Faff, J., Borkowska, G., *et al.* Central therapeutic effects of dihydro-derivative of pralidoxime (pro-2-PAM) in organophosphate intoxication. *Archives Internationales de Pharmacodynamie et de Therapie* 1978;**232**:321–31.

Rump, S., Kaliszan, A. Anticonvulsive effects of intravenous local anaesthetics in organic phosphate intoxication. *Archives Internationales de Pharmacodynamie et de Therapie* 1969;**182**:178.

Schexnayder, S., James, L.P., Kearns, G.L., *et al.* The pharmacokinetics of continuous infusion pralidoxime in children with organophosphate poisoning. *Journal of Toxicology Clinical Toxicology* 1998;**36**:549–55.

Scott, R.J. Repeated asystole following PAM in organophosphate self-poisoning *Anaesthesia and Intensive Care* 1986;**14**:458–60.

Sellström, Å. Anticonvulsants in anticholinesterase poisoning In: *Clinical and Experimental Toxicology of Organophosphates and Carbamates.* Ballantyne, B., Marrs, T.C. eds. Butterworth–Heinemann; Oxford: 1992. p. 578–86.

Shih, T.M., McDonough, J.H. Jr. Organophosphorus nerve agents-induced seizures and efficacy of atropine sulfate as anticonvulsant treatment. *Pharmacology, Biochemistry and Behaviour* 1999;**64**:147–53.

Singh, G., Avasthi, G., Khurana, D., *et al.* Neurophysiological monitoring of pharmacological manipulation in acute organophosphate (OP) poisoning. The effects of pralidoxime, magnesium sulphate and pancuronium. *Electroencephalography and Clinical Neurophysiology* 1998;**107**:140–8.

Singh, S., Batra, Y.K., Singh, S.M., *et al.* Is atropine alone sufficient in acute severe organophosphorus poisoning? Experience of a North West Indian Hospital. *International Journal of Clinical Pharmacology and Therapeutics* 1995;**33**:628–30.

Sofer, S., Tal, A., Shahak, B. Carbamate and organophosphate poisoning in early childhood. *Pediatric Emergency Care* 1989;**5**:222–5.

Sundwall, A. Minimum concentrations of N-methylpyridinium-2-aldoxime methane sulphonate (P2S), which reverse neuromuscular block. *Biochemical Pharmacology* 1961;**8**:413–7.

Szinicz., L.. Personal observation 2000

Szinicz, L., Eyer,P. Personal observations 2000.

Tafuri, J., Roberts, J. Organophosphate poisoning. *Annals of Emergency Medicine* 1987;**16**:193–202.

Tenebein, M. Poisoning in pregnancy, in Koren G ed. *Maternal-Fetal* Toxicity 2nd Ed, New York; Marcel Dekker, 1994. p. 223.

Thiermann, H., Mast, U., Klimmek, R., *et al.* Cholinesterase status, pharmacokinetics and laboratory findings during obidoxime therapy in organophosphate poisoned patients. *Human and Experimental Toxicology* 1997;**16**:473–80.

Thiermann H, Szinicz I, Eyer P., *et al.* Modern strategies in therapy of organophosphate poisoning. *Toxicology Letters* 1999;**107**:233–9.

Thompson, D.F., Thompson, C.D., Greenwood, R.B. *et al.* Therapeutic dosing of pralidoxime chloride. *Drug Intelligence and Clinical Pharmacy* 1987a;**21**:1590–3.

Thompson, D.F. Pralidoxime chloride continuous infusions. *Annals of Emergency Medicine* 1987b;**16**:831–2.

Tracey, J.A., Gallagher, H. Use of glycopyrrolate and atropine in acute organophosphorus poisoning. *Human and Experimental Toxicology* 1990;**9**:99–100.

Tush, G.M., Anstead, M.I. Pralidoxime continuous infusion in the treatment of organophosphate poisoning. *Annals of Pharmacotherapy* 1997;**31**:441–4.

Van Helden, H.P., Bueters, T.J. Protective activity of adenosine receptor agonists in the treatment of organophosphate poisoning. *Trends in Pharmacological Sciences* 1999;**20**:438–41.

Van Helden, H.P.M., Groen, B., Moor, E. *et al.* New generic approach to the treatment of organophosphate poisoning: adenosine receptor mediated inhibition of ACh release. *Drug and Chemical Toxicology* 1998;**21**:171–81.

Wali, F.A., Bradshaw, B.C., Suer, A.J.E. *et al.* Atropine enhances neuromuscular transmission in humans. *Fundamental Clinical Pharmacology* 1987;**1**:59–66.

Wang, A.G., Liu, R.S., Liv, J.H. *et al.* Positron emission tomography scan in cortical visual loss in patients with organophosphate intoxication. *Ophthalmology* 1999;**106**:1287–91.

Willems, J.L. Poisoning by organophosphate insecticides: analysis of 53 human cases with regard to management and drug treatment. *Acta Clinica Belgica* 1981;**134**:7–14.

Willems, J.L., De Bisschop, H.C., Verstraete, A.G. *et al.* Cholinesterase reactivation in organophosphorus poisoned patients depends on the plasma concentrations of the oxime, pralidoxime methylsulphate and of the organophosphate. *Archives of Toxicology* 1993;**67**:79–84.

Willems, J.L., Langenberg, J.P., Verstraete, A.G., *et al.* Plasma concentrations of pralidoxime methylsulphate in organophosphorus poisoned patients. *Archives of Toxicology* 1992;**66**:260–6.

Wong, A. Personal communication 1999.

Worek, F., Backer, M., Thiermann, H. *et al.* Reappraisal of indications and limitations of oxime therapy in organophosphate poisoning. *Human and Experimental Toxicology* 1997;**16**:466–72.

Worek, F., Diepold, C., Eyer, P. Dimethylphosphoryl-inhibited human cholinesterase: inhibition, reactivation and ageing kinetics. *Archives of Toxicology* 1999;**73**:7–14.

Worek, F., Kleine, A., Falke, K., *et al.* Arrhythmias in organophosphate poisoning: effect of atropine and bispyridinium oximes. *Archives Internationales de Pharmacodynamie et de Therapie* 1995;**329**:418–35.

Xiong, S., Rodgers, K. Effects of malathion metabolites on degranulation of and mediator release by human and rat basophilic cells. *Journal of Toxicology and Environmental Health* 1997;**51**:159–75.

Xu, B., Zhang, J., Mao, G., *et al.* Elevated cholinesterase activity and increased urinary excretion of inorganic fluorides in the workers producing fluorine containing plastic (polytetra fluoroethylene). *Bulletin of Environmental Contamination and Toxicology* 1992;**49**:44–50.

Yakoub, L.K., Mohammad, F.K. Medetomidine protection against diazinon-induced toxicosis in mice. *Toxicology Letters* 1997;**93**:1–8.

Yang, X. H., Li, W., Erwin, L., *et al.* Regulation of central muscarinic receptors after cholinesterase inhibition: effect of clonidine. *Brain Research Bulletin* 1993;**32**:681–4.

CHAPTER 13

Carcinogenicity and Mutagenicity of Organophosphates

Michael D. Waters, H. Frank Stack and Marcus A. Jackson

13.1. Introduction

Since the late 1930s, when organophosphorus compounds were first synthesised as potential warfare agents, numerous OPs have been formulated for use in agriculture, industry, and medicine. Currently, more than two hundred OP pesticides have been developed for agricultural and residential use (Ecobichon, 1996). Additionally, OPs have been used as flame retardants, gasoline additives, plasticisers, cleaning agents, water treatment chemicals and chemotherapeutic agents (Woo *et al.*, 1996). Because of their widespread use, particularly as pesticides, and their toxic properties, there is concern that adverse health effects could be associated with human exposures to these compounds. Individuals who are at the greatest risk of exposure are pesticide applicators and workers in industries where OPs are manufactured or are used in textile and other manufacturing processes. However, the general population is also at risk of low-level exposure to OP pesticides due to chemical residues on plants and soil, vaporisation during application, and/or contamination of water from leaching and runoff (Racke, 1992). Many of the OP pesticides, as well as the non-pesticides, have been evaluated over the past 20 years for their carcinogenic and mutagenic effects in various test systems. The results from these studies have provided valuable information for assessing the carcinogenic/mutagenic potential of OPs in humans in the absence of adequate human data from occupational and/or accidental exposures.

There is evidence that gene mutations, gene amplifications, chromosomal rearrangements, and aneuploidy are associated with numerous types of tumours (Barrett, 1992). Results from short-term tests that measure these types of genetic and related effects (mutagenicity), which could potentially damage genes involved in carcinogenesis, can provide valuable insight into the carcinogenic potential of a chemical agent, especially in the absence of adequate carcinogenicity data.

The carcinogenicity and mutagenicity data for a selected group of OPs will be presented in this chapter. The results will be discussed with regard to the evaluation of potential human carcinogenicity as presented by the U.S. Environmental Protection Agency's (EPA), Office of Pesticide Programs and/or by the International Agency for Research on Cancer (IARC).

13.2. Approach

Over fifty OPs, mostly pesticides, were identified for which carcinogenicity data are available from the National Toxicology Program's (NTP) technical reports (see the NTP web page ntp-server.niehs.nih.gov/htdocs/pub.html), the EPA registration data (see the EPA web page www.epa.gov/pesticides/op/status.htm), or the published literature (Woo *et al.,* 1996). Twenty three of these OPs, including 16 pesticides, also have mutagenicity data in the EPA/IARC Genetic Activity Profile (GAP) database (Waters *et al.,* 1991). The organophosphorus chemotherapeutic agents (i.e., cyclophosphamide, thiotepa, and related compounds) were not included here because of their well established carcinogenic and mutagenic properties. The database was developed through a collaborative effort between the EPA and IARC in the evaluation of mutagenicity data used in cancer risk evaluation. Data reported in the open literature for about 700 chemical agents have been compiled in the database from volumes 1–73 of the *IARC Monographs* as well as from several EPA priority projects.

The carcinogenicity and mutagenicity test results for the 23 OPs in the EPA/IARC GAP database are presented in Table 1 and summarised below. Only results from tests for gene and chromosomal mutation are presented and they are arranged according to the phylogeny and endpoint of the test system used. The chemicals in Table 1 are organised by OP subclass and then by the evidence of carcinogenicity and mutagenicity. A chemical was determined positive for rodent carcinogenicity if it clearly induced tumours in either sex of either species. Also in Table 13.1. for each chemical that showed evidence of carcinogenicity, the sites of tumor induction are listed for each rodent sex/species. The underlying mutagenicity data and source bibliographies for each chemical are available in the current version of the GAP database. (A personal computer program, GAP2000, with the database may be downloaded from the Internet at www.epa.gov/gapdb).

13.3. Results

Only 15 of the 58 OPs that have been evaluated in rodent cancer bioassays showed positive evidence of carcinogenicity, while 16 others gave equivocal results. The overview of carcinogenicity test results presented in Table 13.1. include six pesticidal and five non-pesticidal OPs in the GAP database that showed some evidence of carcinogenicity. Details of the carcinogenicity and mutagenicity test results for each chemical in Table 13.1. are summarised below.

13.4. Two Unique OPs

Two non-pesticidal carcinogens that are members of unique subclasses of OPs are included in this group. Hexamethylphosphoramide (HMPA) is a phosphoramide that has been used as a polymer solvent, a jet fuel additive, and a chemical stabilizer. Dimethyl hydrogen phosphite, a dialkyl phosphonate, is a flame retardant, primarily used for nylon products, and it is a degradation product of other pesticides, including malathion and trichlorfon.

13.4.1. Hexamethylphosphoramide

HMPA was classified by the IARC as possibly carcinogenic to humans (IARC, 1999) based on evidence that HMPA induced tumours in rat nasal epithelium. Metabolism studies showed that HMPA is metabolised to formaldehyde, which is also carcinogenic to rat nasal epithelium. Both formaldehyde and HMPA induce DNA-protein cross links in the target tissue which may be an important factor in their carcinogenic mechanisms. However, other factors may be more critical, such as cell proliferation via cytotoxicity or mitogenesis.

Data from one published study showed no evidence of carcinogenicity in rats given HMPA *per os* (po), but there was increased tumour incidence of squamous cell carcinomas in the nasal epithelium in rats exposed to HMPA by inhalation (Lee and Torchimowicz, 1982).

Tumours were induced in both male and female rats, but no carcinogenicity studies in mice were available.

Table 13.1. Summary of the mutagenicity and carcinogenicity test results for OPs in the EPA/IARC GAP database

OP subclass / Compound Name[c]	Mutagenicity[a]										Rodent Carcinogenicity[b]				
	Nonmamm		Mammalian Cells In Vitro					Mamm. in vivo			Eval.	Tumour sites			
	Gene Mut.		Rodent			Human			Rodent			Rat		Mouse	
	Sal	Dros	GM	SCE	CA	SCE	CA	SCE	MN	CA		Male	Female	Male	Female
Unique OPs															
Hexamethylphosphoramide	-	+	+	+	-	(+)	(-)	?	+	?	Pos	nas	nas	-	-
Dimethyl hydrogen phosphite	(-)	(-)	(+)	(+)	(+)						Pos	lun;for	(lun;for)	-	for
Phosphates															
Dichlorvos	+	-	?	+	+	(+)	(-)	(-)	(-)	-	Pos	pan;leu	mam	for	for
Tris (2,3-dibromopropyl) phosphate	+	+	+	+	+	(+)		(+)	+	?	Pos	kid	kid	lun;kid;for	lun;liv;for (har)
Tris (2-chloroethyl) phosphate	?	+	(-)	?	(-)				?	(+)	Pos	kid;(thy;leu)	kid;(thy;leu)	(kid)	ute
Trimethylphosphate	(+)								+	+	Pos	sub	-	-	
Phosphorothioates															
Parathion	-	(-)	(+)	(+)		(+)			?	?	Pos	pan;(adr)	(adr)	lun	(lym)
Parathion-methyl	+	?	+	+		+			+	+	Neg				
Methamidophos	-	(-)	(+)	(+)	(+)	(+)			(+)		Neg				
Chlorpyrifos	-		(-)						+		Neg				
Diazinon	-		-								Neg				
Pirimphos-methyl	+			(+)			(+)			(-)	Neg				
Phosphoramidates															
Acephate	+	-	(+)	(+)	+	(+)	+		?	?	Equiv	(pan)			(liv)
Glyphosate	-		(-)							(-)	Equiv			(kid)	-
Phosphorodithioates															
Dimethoate	+	(+)		+	(+)	+			(+)	?	Equiv	(spl;lym)		(lun;lym)	(liv)
Malathion	-	-	(+)	+	+	+	+		(+)	?	Equiv	(thy;adr)	(thy;adr)	(liv)	(liv)
Disulfoton	-	(-)	(+)	(-)					(-)		Neg				
Phorate	?	(-)	?	?	(+)				?	(+)	Neg				
Fonofos	-	+									Neg				
Terbufos	?										Neg				
Bensulide	(-)										Neg				
Phosphonium salts															
THPC	-		(+)	+	+				(-)	(-)	Neg				
THPS	-		(+)	+					(-)	(+)	Neg				

The carcinogenic classification of HMPA is supported by mutagenicity data in rodent cells *in vitro* and *in vivo*. HMPA was negative for the induction of gene mutation in *Salmonella typhimurium (S. typhimurium)*, but it induced sex-linked recessive lethal mutation, heritable translocation, and somatic mutation in *Drosophila melanogaster (D. melanogaster)*. In mammalian systems *in vitro*, HMPA induced gene mutation in mouse lymphoma and sister chromatid exchange (SCE) in Chinese hamster cells in the presence of metabolic activation only. It also induced micronuclei (MN) and SCEs in human cells *in vitro* without metabolic activation. In single studies *in vivo*, HMPA induced SCEs in mouse bone marrow and chromosomal aberrations (CA) in rat but not mouse bone marrow. It also induced MN in mouse and rat bone marrow. Conflicting results were seen for the induction of dominant lethal mutation in mice.

13.4.2. Dimethyl hydrogen phosphite

The IARC evaluated dimethyl hydrogen phosphite as not classifiable as to carcinogenicity in humans (IARC, 1999). There were no data available from human carcinogenicity studies, and the results from rodent carcinogenicity bioassays were evaluated as showing limited evidence of carcinogenicity in animals (significant evidence of tumour induction was reported for the male rat only). The specific mechanism of action for this dialkyl phosphonate is not certain, but it may involve its potential alkylating properties (Woo *et al.*, 1996). Dimethyl hydrogen phosphite has not been well tested for mutagenicity, but results from two *in vitro* mammalian studies were positive for gene mutation and chromosomal damage.

Dimethyl hydrogen phosphite, administered to B6C3F1 mice via gavage at doses up to the MTD, was not carcinogenic. However, gavage treatment of F344 rats caused a significant increase in lung squamous cell carcinomas, alveolar/bronchiolar carcinomas, and forestomach squamous cell adenomas/carcinomas in the males, and a marginal increase in lung and forestomach tumours in the females (NTP, 1985). The NTP concluded that there is clear evidence of carcinogenicity in the male rat and equivocal evidence of carcinogenicity in the female rat.

In single studies, dimethyl hydrogen phosphite did not induce gene mutation in *S. typhimurium* or sex-linked recessive lethal mutation in *D. melanogaster*. It did cause gene mutation in mouse lymphoma in the presence of metabolic activation. It also induced SCEs and CAs in Chinese hamster ovary (CHO) cells in a single study *in vitro*.

13.5. Phosphates

This subclass contains the dimethyl vinyl phosphate pesticide, dichlorvos, and three phosphoric acid triesters which have been used as flame retardants or gasoline additives. The data reported for each of these agents showed some evidence of carcinogenicity in both rats and mice following *po* exposures. With the exception of dichlorvos, the phosphates also showed some evidence of mutagenicity in most of the mammalian tests in which they were evaluated. Two of the phosphoric acid triesters, trimethylphosphate and tris(2-choroethyl)phosphate, were not as thoroughly tested as tris(2,3-dibromopropyl)phosphate or the OP pesticide, dichlorvos.

13.5.1. Dichlorvos

Both the IARC and the EPA classified dichlorvos as possibly carcinogenic to humans (IARC, 1991; EPA, 1998). There was inadequate evidence from one epidemiological study that dichlorvos is carcinogenic to humans, but there was sufficient evidence that it is carcinogenic in both sexes of rats and mice treated by gavage. Dichlorvos is one of the stronger alkylating agents among the OPs and this appears to be an important factor in its carcinogenic potential (Woo *et al.,* 1996).

One case-control study of leukemia in the U.S. reported a significant excess of leukemia among farmers who used dichlorvos, however, other pesticides, including additional OPs, were also used by the study group (Brown *et al.,* 1990). The contribution of dichlorvos to the excess of leukemia could not be determined. This was the only data available on the potential carcinogenicity of dichlorvos in humans.

Dichlorvos was not carcinogenic to Osborne–Mendel rats or B6C3F1 mice exposed to this OP in the diet (NCI, 1977a). However, there was evidence of carcinogenicity in F344 rats and B6C3F1 mice exposed to dichlorvos via gavage (NTP, 1989). Increased incidences of pancreatic acinar cell adenomas and mononuclear cell leukemia were reported for male rats, while a marginal increase in mammary gland fibromas was seen in females. The incidence of squamous cell papillomas of the forestomach was increased in male and female mice from the high dose group only. Forestomach squamous cell carcinomas were also seen in two high dose female mice.

There was evidence *in vitro* that dichlorvos is mutagenic in mammalian cells, but this was not confirmed *in vivo*. Dichlorvos increased point mutations in *S. typhimurium,* however, the mutagenicity was found only in the presence of metabolic activation. It induced CAs but not sex-linked recessive lethal mutation in *D. melanogaster*. Dichlorvos induced gene mutation in mouse lymphoma cells and SCEs and CAs, but not gene mutation, in Chinese hamster cells *in vitro*. In single studies, dichlorvos did not induce SCEs or CAs in human cells *in vitro*. Results from mammalian *in vivo* tests were confirmed negative for the induction of CAs and dominant lethal mutation and were negative in single studies for the induction of SCEs and MN.

13.5.2. Tris(2,3-dibromopropyl) phosphate

Tris(2,3-dibromopropyl) phosphate (tris-DBP) was produced in low volumes in the 1970s for use in the textile industry as a flame retardant but does not appear to have been produced since then. It has been classified by the IARC as a probable human carcinogen (IARC, 1999). Evidence from one cohort mortality study of workers exposed to tris-DBP was inadequate for assessing carcinogenicity in humans, but there was sufficient evidence of carcinogenicity in both sexes of mice and rats. The positive mutagenicity test results reported for a wide range of mammalian test systems were also taken into consideration in making the overall evaluation of carcinogenicity (IARC, 1999). The potent carcinogenic and mutagenic activity of tris-DBP is apparently related to its potential cross-linking capabilities and/or the electrophilic reactivity of its hydrolysis products (Woo *et al.,* 1996).

Tris-DBP is reported to be a multi-site, multi-species carcinogen (NCI, 1978a). It induced squamous cell adenomas/carcinomas of the forestomach, renal tubule cell adenomas/carcinomas, and hepatocellular and bronchiolar/alveolar neoplasms in both sexes of B6C3F1 mice given tris-DBP in their feed. It also increased the incidence of renal tubule cell adenomas in male and female F344 rats exposed via the feed. Results from one study reported in the open literature for female mice, showed that dermal exposure to tris-DBP induced tumours at multiple sites, including dorsal skin, lung, liver, forestomach, oral cavity, and kidney (Woo *et al., 1985)*.

Tris-DBP was mutagenic in virtually every test in which it was evaluated. It induced gene mutation in *S. typhimurium* in the presence of metabolic activation. In *D. melanogaster,* it was mutagenic in somatic and germ cells and induced cytogenetic damage. Tris-DBP induced gene mutation, sister chromatid exchanges and chromosomal aberrations in Chinese hamster cells *in vitro.* It also induced SCEs but not CAs in human lymphocytes in a single study *in vitro.* It induced gene mutation in mouse kidney and micronuclei in rat liver and in mouse and hamster bone marrow *in vivo.* Tris-DBP induced SCEs but gave conflicting results for the induction of CAs in mouse bone marrow *in vivo.*

13.5.3. Tris(2-chloroethyl) phosphate

The IARC evaluated tris (2-chloroethyl) phosphate (tris-CP) as not classifiable as to its carcinogenicity to humans (IARC, 1999). No data from human studies of carcinogenicity were available for evaluation and data from studies with experimental animals were evaluated as showing limited evidence of carcinogenicity (tumours were induced at a single site in male and female rats). The mutagenicity data were not influential in the evaluation because there were no confirmed positive results. As with tris-DBP, the carcinogenic activity of tris-CP is most likely associated with its cross-linking potential and/or its electrophilic hydrolysis products (Woo *et al.,* 1996).

Results from the NTP two year rodent bioassay showed that there was clear evidence of carcinogenicity in male and female F344 rats and equivocal evidence of carcinogenicity in B6C3F1 mice exposed to tris-CP via gavage. Tris-CP induced renal tubule adenomas and, to a less extent, thyroid follicular cell tumours and mononuclear cell leukemia in both sexes of rats. A marginal increase was reported in renal tubule and harderian gland neoplasms in male and female B6C3F1 mice, respectively (NTP, 1991).

Only one of three studies reported evidence of mutagenicity with tris-CP in *S. typhimurium* with the addition of metabolic activation. Gene mutation was not induced in Chinese hamster V79 cells in a single study. Tris-CP gave equivocal results for induction of SCEs and was negative for the induction of CAs in Chinese hamster cells *in vitro.* In single studies, tris-CP gave equivocal results in the MN test in Chinese hamsters and caused dominant lethal mutations in rats *in vivo.*

13.5.4. Trimethylphosphate

Trimethylphosphate has not been evaluated by the IARC for its carcinogenicity in humans. The evidence of carcinogenicity in rodents is not as strong as that shown for tris-DBP and tris-CP. Tumours were induced in male, but not female, F344 rats and in female, but not male, B6C3F1 mice treated with trimethylphosphate via gavage. The incidence of benign fibrosarcomas of the subcutaneous tissue increased in a dose-related manner in male rats while the incidence of malignant adenocarcinomas of the endometrium increased in a dose-related manner in female mice (NCI, 1978b). The weak alkylating activity reported for trimethylphosphate appears to be responsible for its weaker carcinogenic potential compared to tris-DBP and tris-CP (Woo et al., 1996).

In a single study, trimethylphosphate induced gene mutation in S. typhimurium strain TA100 with and without the addition of a metabolic activation system. It induced MN in mouse bone marrow and CAs in rat bone marrow. It also induced dominant lethal mutations and heritable translocations in mice in vivo.

13.6. Phosphorothioates

Of the six OP pesticides in this subclass, only one, parathion, has been reported to show evidence of carcinogenicity in rodents. In general, the phosphorothioates, with the exception of parathion-methyl and methamidophos, tended to exhibit mixed results in short-term tests for mutagenicity. It should be noted, however, that most of the agents in this group were not as thoroughly tested as parathion-methyl and methamidophos.

13.6.1 Parathion

Parathion was evaluated by the IARC as not classifiable as to its carcinogenicity to humans (IARC, 1987). This evaluation was based on there being no data available from epidemiological studies and limited evidence of carcinogenicity in experimental animals at the time (positive in rats only). The data from mutagenicity tests were also limited. Registration data submitted to EPA since the time of the IARC evaluation showed that parathion is also carcinogenic to mice. EPA has classified parathion as a possible human carcinogen (EPA, 1999).

Like trimethylphosphate, the weaker carcinogenic response to parathion may reflect its weak alkylating potential (Woo *et al.,* 1996).

Parathion given in the diet was not carcinogenic to B6C3F1 mice and only produced a marginal increase in adrenal cortical adenomas in male and female Osborne–Mendel rats (NCI, 1979a). More recent data submitted to EPA showed that although parathion in the diet was not carcinogenic in Sprague–Dawley rats it did induce a small but significant increase in pancreatic islet cell adenomas in male Wistar rats. Results from exposure of B6C3F1 mice to parathion in the feed showed significant increases in lung adenomas in males and malignant lymphomas in females at the low dose only (EPA, 1991a).

Parathion did not induce gene mutation in *S. typhimurium,* nor sex-linked recessive lethals, CAs, or aneuploidy in *D. melanogaster.* It did induce SCEs in human lymphoblastoid and CHO cells *in vitro,* in single studies. Parathion did not cause dominant lethal mutations nor CAs in germ cells of mice. It gave conflicting results for the induction of CAs in mouse bone marrow *in vivo.*

13.6.2. Parathion-methyl

Parathion-methyl was evaluated by the IARC as not classifiable as to its carcinogenicity to humans (IARC, 1987). According to EPA there was no evidence of carcinogenicity in humans and parathion-methyl was characterised as not likely to be carcinogenic in humans via relevant routes of exposure (EPA, 1999). Administration of parathion-methyl in the diet up to the maximum tolerated dose (MTD) was not carcinogenic in Osborne–Mendel, Sprague–Dawley, or Wistar rats nor in B6C3F1 mice (NCI, 1979b; EPA, 1999).

Parathion-methyl induced gene mutation in *S. typhimurium* in the presence and absence of exogenous metabolic activation. It gave conflicting results for the induction of sex-linked recessive lethal and somatic cell mutations in *D. melanogaster.* It induced gene mutation in the mouse lymphoma TK+/- assay in the presence of metabolic activation and SCEs in Chinese hamster cells *in vitro.* Parathion-methyl also induced SCEs in human lymphocytes and lymphoblastoid cells and CAs in human lymphocytes *in vitro.* Positive test results were reported for the induction of MN in rat and mouse bone marrow and for CAs in rat but not mouse bone marrow *in vivo.* One of two studies also reported weak induction of CAs in lymphocytes of patients suffering from acute insecticide intoxication.

13.6.3. Methamidophos

Methamidophos was classified by EPA as not likely to be carcinogenic in humans via relevant routes of exposure. No treatment-related increases in tumor incidence compared to controls were reported in the EPA registration data for F344 rats or CD-1 mice exposed to methamidophos in the diet (EPA, 1999).

Methamidophos induced SCEs and CAs in mouse splenocytes but not Chinese hamster V-79 cells *in vitro*. It also induced SCEs and MN in mouse bone marrow in a single *in vivo* study. Results from registration data submitted to EPA (not included in Table 1) showed that methamidophos was not mutagenic to *S. typhimurium* but did induce gene mutations in cultured mammalian cells in the presence of high levels of metabolic activation. Evidence of clastogenicity *in vitro* was also reported when high concentrations of methamidophos were tested. Methamidophos was negative for the induction of CAs *in vivo* (EPA, 1999).

13.6.4. Chlorpyrifos

Chlorpyrifos was classified as showing evidence of non-carcinogenicity for humans. Results from two carcinogenicity studies in F344 rats and two studies in CD-1 mice were negative in both males and females treated with chlorpyrifos in their feed (EPA, 1993).

Chlorpyrifos did not induce gene mutation in *S. typhimurium*. It did not induce sex-linked recessive lethal mutation in *D. melanogaster*. Chlorpyrifos did not induce SCEs in CHO cells *in vitro* but did induce MN in mouse bone marrow *in vivo*.

13.6.5. Diazinon

The carcinogenicity data reported by the National Cancer Institute (NCI) were negative for male and female F344 rats and CD-1 mice given diazinon in their feed (NCI, 1979c).

Diazinon was not mutagenic in *S. typhimurium*. It did not induce SCEs in CHO cells, but did induce a small, though significant, increase in CAs in human lymphocytes *in vitro*.

13.6.6. Pirimiphos-methyl

EPA could not determine the carcinogenic potential of pirimiphos-methyl in humans because the results from studies with Wistar rats were deemed unacceptable (EPA, 1999). There was no evidence of carcinogenicity in CD-1 mice fed diets containing pirimiphos-methyl.

Pirimiphos-methyl was mutagenic to *S. typhimurium* and it did not induce MN or CAs in mouse bone marrow *in vivo*. EPA registration data (not included in Table 1) showed that pirimiphos-methyl was negative in the mouse lymphoma TK+/- gene mutation assay, negative for the induction of CAs in human lymphocytes and positive for the induction of SCEs in Chinese hamster fibroblasts *in vitro* (EPA, 1999).

13.7. Phosphoramidates

There are two phosphoramidates included in this chapter, acephate and glyphosate. Both chemicals are pesticides and both gave equivocal results for carcinogenicity in feeding studies with rats and mice. Acephate may have some alkylating potential but glyphosate does not since it has no terminal alkyl groups. Results from mutagenicity testing with acephate were positive *in vitro* and equivocal *in vivo*. Glyphosate was negative in the three tests in which it was evaluated.

13.7.1. Acephate

Acephate was classified by the EPA as a possible human carcinogen (EPA, 1999). This classification was based on the statistically significant increase in hepatocellular carcinomas reported for female mice. Results from the EPA registration data showed that acephate given in the feed was not carcinogenic in Charles Rivers CD rats or in male CD-1 mice but it did increase the incidence of hepatocellular carcinomas and adenomas/carcinomas in female CD-1 mice at the lowest and highest dose tested.

Acephate was positive for gene mutation in *S. typhimurium* strain TA 100 at the highest dose tested but was negative in all other strains. It did not induce sex-linked recessive lethal mutation, CAs or aneuploidy in *D. melanogaster*.

It induced gene mutation in mouse lymphoma cells and SCEs in CHO cells *in vitro*. Acephate did not increase the frequency of SCEs in mouse bone marrow but gave conflicting results for the induction of MN, CAs and dominant lethal mutations in mice *in vivo*.

13.7.2. Glyphosate

EPA placed glyphosate between two classification categories, not classifiable as to carcinogenicity in humans and not likely to be carcinogenic in humans via relevant routes of exposure (EPA, 1991b). The data from feeding studies with glyphosate that were submitted to EPA showed equivocal evidence of carcinogenicity in rats and mice. High dose exposures were required in both species to produce any positive response. The lowest dose of glyphosate tested was equal to or greater than the highest acephate dose tested. An increase in the incidence of pancreatic islet cell adenomas was reported for male Sprague–Dawley rats, but the increase was not dose-dependent and the tumor incidence in concurrent controls was low. Similarly, a slight increase in renal tubular adenomas was reported for male B6C3F1 mice exposed to high doses of glyphosate, but the response was not considered biologically significant because of the high doses requirement.

Glyphosate was not mutagenic in *S. typhimurium*. It did not induce gene mutation in CHO cells *in vitro*. In separate studies, glyphosate did not induce CAs in rat bone marrow or dominant lethal mutations in mice.

13.8. Phosphorodithioates

This subclass consists of seven OP pesticides. Two of these pesticides, dimethoate and malathion, showed equivocal evidence of carcinogenicity in rats and mice. The other phosphorothioates showed no evidence of carcinogenicity. Dimethoate, malathion and phorate were clastogenic in mammalian tests *in vitro* and *in vivo*. Disulfoton was positive in a single study for gene mutation at the *tk* locus in the mouse lymphoma assay. Only test results from non-mammalian systems were available in the GAP database for the other three agents.

13.8.1. Dimethoate

Dimethoate was classified by the EPA as a possible human carcinogen based primarily on equivocal evidence of carcinogenicity in male Wistar rats and B6C3F1 mice and the evidence of mutagenicity induced by dimethoate (EPA, 1999). Dimethoate has alkylating capabilities (Woo *et al.*, 1996) which directly parallel its weak carcinogenic activity in rodents.

Results from early rodent carcinogenicity studies published in the literature reported positive results for spleen reticulum cell sarcomas, forestomach papillomas and lung adenomas in Wistar rats given dimethoate PO (Gibel *et al.*, 1973). The data from the NCI feeding studies using Osborne–Mendel rats and B6C3F1 mice, however, were negative (NCI, 1977a). Equivocal results were reported in the EPA registration data from feeding studies using rats and mice. A significant, dose-related, increasing trend in spleen hemangiomas/hemagiosarcomas and a significant increase in lymph angiomas/angiosarcomas were reported in male Wistar rats in the low dose group. In B6C3F1 male mice, dimethoate was associated with a significant dose-related increase in combined lung adenomas and/or adenocarcinomas and with combined incidence of lymphoma, reticular sarcoma and leukemia. In female mice, an increased incidence of liver adenomas and combined adenomas and/or carcinomas was also reported (EPA, 1999).

Dimethoate induced gene mutation in *S. typhimurium*. It did not cause somatic mutation in *D. melanogaster* but did cause weak induction of sex-linked recessive lethal mutations. It induced SCEs and CAs in Chinese hamster cells *in vitro*. Dimethoate induced SCEs in human fibroblasts and lymphoid cells and CAs in human lymphocytes but not fibroblasts *in vitro*. It was positive in the mouse bone marrow MN assay but did not induce dominant lethal mutations nor CAs in mouse germ cells *in vivo*. Conflicting results were reported for CAs in mouse bone marrow.

13.8.2. Malathion

EPA reported that the potential carcinogenicity of malathion to humans was not classifiable. The NCI carcinogenicity data from feeding studies with malathion were negative for both sexes of Osborne–Mendel and F344 rats and for B6C3F1 mice (NCI, 1978c; 1979d). Results from feeding studies submitted to the EPA were equivocal, showing an apparent increase in tumours in the thyroid and adrenal glands of Osborne–Mendel rats and in the liver of B6C3F1 mice (EPA, 1990). Like dimethoate, malathion has been shown to be weak compared to other OP pesticides with alkylating activity (Woo *et al.*, 1996).

Presumably, such activity is associated with its carcinogenic potential. Malathion was not mutagenic in *S. typhimurium*. It did not induce sex-linked recessive lethals nor somatic mutation in *D. melanogaster*. SCEs and CAs were induced in Chinese hamster cell cultures, but MN were not. Malathion also induced SCEs and CAs in human lymphocytes and fibroblasts *in vitro*. It induced MN but not CAs in mouse bone marrow and did not induce CAs in mouse germ cells *in vivo*. A slight, but significant, increase in CAs in peripheral blood lymphocytes of 14 patients suffering from insecticide intoxication was reported in one study.

13.8.3 Disulfoton

The carcinogenic potential of disulfoton to humans was determined as not classifiable by the EPA. The data submitted for review showed that there were no treatment-related increases in tumor incidence in either sex of F344 rats or CD-1 mice given disulfoton in the diet (EPA, 1999). Rats were treated with doses up to the MTD.

Disulfoton was not mutagenic in *S. typhimurium* or in the sex-linked recessive lethal assay in *D. melanogaster*. It induced gene mutations in mouse lymphoma at the *Tk+/-* loci in a single study and it gave conflicting results for the induction of SCEs in CHO cells in the presence of exogenous metabolic activation (one of three studies reported a weak positive response). One study reported that disulfoton did not induce MN in mouse bone marrow *in vivo*.

13.8.4. Phorate

It was determined that phorate is not likely to be carcinogenic in humans via relevant routes of exposure. Registration data submitted to the EPA showed that phorate given in the diet is not carcinogenic in either sex of rats or mice (EPA, 1999).

Phorate was not mutagenic in *S. typhimurium*. It did not induce sex-linked recessive lethals in *D. melanogaster*. It caused a weak induction of CAs in CHO cells but not human lymphocytes *in vitro*. Phorate was positive in the rat but not mouse bone marrow MN assay. It induced CAs in mouse bone marrow but not dominant lethal mutations *in vivo*.

13.8.5. Terbufos, Fonofos and Bensulide

There is no evidence from feeding studies that any of these three phosphorodithioates is carcinogenic in either sex of rats or mice (EPA, 1999). It was concluded that these OP pesticides are not likely to be carcinogenic in humans via relevant routes of exposure.

Only data from non-mammalian tests were available in the GAP database for these chemicals. One of two studies reported that fonofos was positive in *S. typhimurium* strains TA1535 and TA1538 in the presence of metabolic activation, but negative in all other strains tested. Terbufos and bensulide were not mutagenic to *S. typhimurium*. Registration data from mammalian tests submitted to EPA for terbufos were negative for the induction gene mutation (CHO/Hprt) and CAs *in vitro*. Equivocal test results were reported for the rat dominant lethal assay. Data submitted for bensulide was also negative for gene mutation (*Tk* locus, mouse lymphoma) and for the induction of MN in mouse bone marrow (EPA, 1999).

13.9. Phosphonium Salts

Two chemicals are included in this subclass, tetrakis(hydroxymethyl)phosphonium chloride (THPC) and tetrakis(hydroxymethyl)phosphonium sulfate (THPS). These compounds have mainly been used as flame retardants in cotton. The IARC evaluated the THP salts as not classifiable as to carcinogenicity in humans (IARC, 1990, 1999). This is based on the lack of epidemiological data relevant to carcinogenicity and the inadequate evidence of rodent carcinogenicity for these compounds. Data from the NTP two year bioassay of THPC and THPS showed no evidence of carcinogenicity in either sex of F344 rats or B6C3F1 mice treated by gavage with either chemical at doses up to the MTD (NTP, 1987).

Neither THPC nor THPS induced gene mutation in *S. typhimurium* in the presence or absence of metabolic activation but, in a single study, they were both positive for gene mutation in the mouse lymphoma *Tk*+/- assay without metabolic activation. THPC induced SCEs and CAs in CHO cells *in vitro*. THPS caused a marginal increase in the frequency of CAs but not MN in mouse bone marrow *in vivo* in a single study.

13.10. Discussion

The mechanisms involved in the carcinogenic process are complex, making it difficult to predict carcinogenicity using short-term biological systems or mathematical models. However, the classical concepts (Berenblum, 1941; Armuth and Berenblum, 1982) and molecular models (Vogelstein et al., 1989; Fearon and Vogelstein, 1990; Fearon et al., 1990; Vogelstein and Kinzler, 1993) indicate that at least one, and frequently several, mutagenic events are required for tumour development (Harris, 1991). The specific mutant cells that result in tumour development are themselves subject to many secondary influences (Ashby, 1992). In addition, a series of epigenetic changes may also be involved, as in the case of colorectal cancer (Fearon and Vogelstein, 1990). Although the specific mechanisms responsible for the induction and/or expression of mutant cells are not always clearly defined, it is clear that gene and/or chromosomal mutations are important events in the carcinogenic process.

There are OPs, such as cyclophosphamide and thiotepa, used as chemotherapeutic drugs that are human carcinogens. Except for the chemotherapeutic drugs, OPs evaluated by IARC have not been classified as human carcinogens nor as probable human carcinogens, generally because of the limited evidence of carcinogenicity from rodent testing and even less evidence from human epidemiology. The majority of data presented here confirms the IARC evaluations. Of the 23 OPs reviewed in this chapter, approximately half showed some evidence of mutagenicity and rodent carcinogenicity. The phosphates (dichlorvos, trimethylphosphate, and the two halogenated tris phosphates) as a group comprised the only subclass of OPs that showed convincing evidence of mutagenicity and statistically significant evidence of carcinogenicity in mice and rats. With the exception of trimethylphosphate, the phosphates induced tumours in both sexes of both species and tended to affect multiple sites. They also gave positive responses across multiple mutagenicity tests in the GAP database. These compounds are genetically active either as DNA cross-linkers or as DNA alkylators with multiple sites for potential alkylation.

Parathion, a phosphorothioate, also showed statistically significant increases in tumorigenicity in male mice and rats and equivocal evidence of tumour induction in females. Parathion was not well tested for mutagenicity, but showed some mutagenic potential *in vitro* and equivocal evidence *in vivo*. Two other OPs, HMPA, a phosphoramide, and dimethyl hydrogen phosphite, a dialkyl phosphonate, were positive for carcinogenicity in rats only. Both were mutagenic *in vitro* and HMPA was also mutagenic *in vivo*.

Of the OP pesticides reviewed here, only dichlorvos gave clear evidence of rodent carcinogenicity. Dichlorvos was positive for mutagenicity only in *in vitro* studies. Four other pesticides (acephate, glyphosate, dimethoate, and malathion) showed equivocal evidence of rodent carcinogenicity. With the exception of glyphosate, these pesticides also showed some evidence of mutagenicity *in vitro* and *in vivo*. The remaining ten pesticides were determined negative for rodent carcinogenicity. Of twelve additional OP pesticides submitted for EPA registration (not shown), only one (ethoprop) was carcinogenic in rodents (EPA, 1999). The fact that the currently regulated OP pesticides are not carcinogens may be the pragmatic result of an effective pesticide registration process under which presumptive carcinogens are eliminated through chemical and toxicological screening procedures. Such agents are seldom submitted for pesticide registration unless there is an overwhelming benefit to society that justifies the inclusion of a potential carcinogen.

Although none of the OPs reviewed here have been identified as human carcinogens, some of them have been classified as possibly carcinogenic to humans by EPA or IARC based on evidence that they are carcinogenic in rodents and mutagenic in mammalian systems. It is important to note that the chemicals which IARC has classified as human carcinogens over the past decade tend to be mutagenic across many test systems and to induce tumours at multiple sites in multiple species (Waters *et al.,* 1999). Similarly, many of the agents classified as probable human carcinogens were mutagenic in multiple test systems and were carcinogenic in at least one rodent species. Based on this observation, HMPA, dimethyl hydrogen phosphite, and the four phosphates may be potential human carcinogens. Additionally, there should be concern for the carcinogenic potential of dimethoate, malathion, and parathion-methyl because of the extensive array of mutagenicity induced by these pesticides, including *in vivo* bone marrow aberrations.

Woo *et al.* (1996) concluded in an analysis of OP structure-activity relationships that fully esterified alkyl phosphates/phosphonates and their thio derivatives should be considered to have carcinogenic potential due to alkylating activity. Since inhalation exposure provides a greater opportunity for direct acting compounds (e.g., alkylating agents) to reach the target site before being deactivated by hydrolysis, the route of exposure is an important consideration when assessing the carcinogenic potential of OP compounds. Generally there are two groups at risk to OP exposure. There is a high-risk group of pesticide applicators and workers manufacturing OPs who are exposed via inhalation or physical contact to their skin.

The general population receives some inhalation exposure to household pesticides but is primarily exposed orally through pesticide residues left on raw produce or found in the drinking water. The rapid decomposition of OPs to less toxic breakdown products reduces the potential dangers of oral exposure to the general population. Most of the *in vivo* data reported here is from feeding studies, which are more relevant to the general population than to the high-risk group. Additional inhalation studies may be required before the toxic effects of OPs can be fully assessed relative to the high-risk group.

References

Armuth, V., Berenblum I. A possible *in vivo* skin model for tumor promoter assays. *Mutation Research* 1982;**15**:343–6.

Ashby, J. Use of short-term tests in determining the genotoxicity or nongenotoxicity of chemicals. In: *Mechanisms of Carcinogenesis in Risk Identification* (IARC. Scientific Publication No. 116). Vainio, H., Magee, P.N., McGregor, D.B., McMichael, A.J. eds. International Agency for Research on Cancer; Lyon. 1992. p. 135–64.

Barrett, J.C. Mechanisms of action of known human carcinogens. In: *Mechanisms of Carcinogenesis in Risk Identification* (IARC Scientific Publication No. 116). Vainio, H., Magee, P.N., McGregor, D.B., McMichael, A.J. eds. International Agency for Research on Cancer; 1992. Lyon. p. 115–34

Berenblum, I. The carcinogenic action of cotton resin. *Cancer Research* 1941;**1**:44–8.

Brown, L.M., Blair, A., Gibson, R., *et al.* Pesticide exposures and other agricultural risk factors for leukemia among men in Iowa and Minnesota. *Cancer* 1990;**50**:6585–91.

Ecobichon, D.J. Toxic effects of pesticides. In: *Casaret and Doull's Toxicology*, 5th edition. Klassen, C.D. ed. McGraw–Hill; New York. 1996. p. 643–89.

EPA. Carcinogenicity Peer Review of Malathion. *U.S. Environmental Protection Agency*, Office of Pesticides Programs, Washington, DC; 1990.

EPA. Carcinogenicity Peer Review of Parathion. *U.S. Environmental Protection Agency*, Office of Pesticides Programs, Washington, DC; 1991a.

EPA. Carcinogenicity Peer Review of Glyphosate. *U.S. Environmental Protection Agency,* Office of Pesticides Programs, Washington, DC; 1991b.

EPA. Rfd Peer Review of Chlorpyrifos. *U.S. Environmental Protection Agency*, Office of Pesticide Programs, Washington, DC; 1993.

EPA. Dichlorvos (DDVP): Risk assessment issues for the FIFRA Science Advisory Panel, July 8, 1998. http://www.epa.gov/oscpmont/sap/1998/july/session3.pdf.

EPA. Status *Summary of organophosphate* Review Process, 1999; http://www.epa.gov/pesticides/op/status.htm (see link corresponding to chemical of interest).

Fearon, E.R., Cho, K.R., Nigro, J.M., *et al.* Identification of a chromosome 18q gene that is altered in colorectal cancers. *Science* 1990;**247**:49–56.

Fearon, E.R., Vogelstein, B. A genetic model for colorectal tumorigenesis. *Cell* 1990;**61**:759–67.

Gibel, W., Lohs, K., Wildner, G.P., *et al.* Experimental study on cancerogenic haematotoxic and hepatotoxic activity of phosphor-organic pesticides. *Archiv fur Geschwulstforschung* 1973;**41**:311–28.

Harris, C.C. Chemical and physical carcinogenesis: advances and perspective for the 1990s. *Cancer Research* 1991;(Suppl. **51**):5023–44.

IARC. International Agency for Research on Cancer. *IARC Monographs* on the evaluation of carcinogenic risks to humans, Supplement 7, Overall evaluations of carcinogenesis: an updating of IARC Monographs Volumes 1 to 42, Lyon, 1987. p. 440.

IARC. International Agency for Research on Cancer. *IARC Monographs* on the evaluation of carcinogenicity risks to humans, Vol.48, Some flame retardants and textile chemicals, and exposures in the textile manufacturing industry, Lyon, 1990. p. 345.

IARC. International Agency for Research on Cancer. *IARC Monographs* on the evaluation of carcinogenic risks to humans, Vol. 53, Occupational exposures in insecticide application, and some pesticides, Lyon, 1991. p. 612.

IARC. International Agency for Research on Cancer. *IARC Monographs* on the evaluation of carcinogenic risks to humans, Vol.71, Re-evaluation of some organic chemicals, hydrazine and hydrogen peroxide, Lyon, 1999. p. 1586.

Lee, K.P., Torchimowicz, H.J. Induction of nasal tumours in rats exposed to hexamethylphosphoramide by inhalation. *Journal National Cancer Institute* 1982;**68**:157–71.

NCI. Bioassay of Dichlorvos for Possible Carcinogenicity. *NCI Technical Report* No.10, National Cancer Institute, Bethesda, MD; 1977a.

NCI. Bioassay of Dimethoate for Possible Carcinogenicity. *NCI Technical Report* No.4, National Cancer Institute, Bethesda, MD; 1977b.

NCI. Bioassay of Tris(2,3-dibromopropyl)phosphate for Possible Carcinogenicity. *NCI Technical Report* No. 76, National Cancer Institute, Bethesda, MD; 1978a.

NCI. Bioassay of Trimethylphosphate for Possible Carcinogenicity. *NCI Technical Report* No. 81, National Cancer Institute, Bethesda, MD; 1978b.

NCI. Bioassay of Malathion for Possible Carcinogenicity. *NCI Technical Report* No.24, National Cancer Institute, Bethesda, MD; 1978c.

NCI. Bioassay of Malathion for Possible Carcinogenicity. *NCI Technical Report* No. 192, National Cancer Institute, Bethesda, MD; 1979d.

NCI. Bioassay of Parathion for Possible Carcinogenicity. *NCI Technical Report* No.70, National Cancer Institute, Bethesda, MD; 1979a.

NCI. Bioassay of Methyl Parathion for Possible Carcinogenicity. *NCI Technical Report* No.157, National Cancer Institute, Bethesda, MD; 1979b.

NCI. Bioassay of Diazinon for Possible Carcinogenicity. *NCI Technical Report* No.137, National Cancer Institute, Bethesda, MD; 1979c.

NTP. Toxicology and Carcinogenicity Studies of Dimethyl Hydrogen Phosphite in F344/N Rats and B6C3F1 Mice (Gavage Studies). *Technical Report* No. 287, *National Toxicology Program,* Research Triangle Park, NC; 1985.

NTP. Toxicology and Carcinogenicity Studies of Tetrakis(hydroxymethyl)-phosphonium Sulfate (THPS) and Tetrakis(hydroxymethyl)phosphonium chloride (THPC) in F344/N Rats and B6C3F1 Mice (Gavage Studies). *Technical Report* No. 287, *National Research Triangle Park,* NC; 1987.

NTP. Toxicology and Carcinogenicity Studies of Dichlorvos in F344/N Rats and B6C3F1 Mice (Gavage Studies). *Technical Report* No.342, *National Toxicology Program,* Research Triangle Park; 1989.

NTP. Toxicology and Carcinogenicity Studies of Tris(2-chloroethyl) phosphate in F344/N Rats and B6C3F1 Mice (Gavage Studies) *Technical Report* No. 391, *National Toxicology Program,* Research Triangle Park, NC; 1991.

Racke, K.D. Degradation of organophosphorus insecticides in environmental matrices. In: *Organophosphates.* Chambers, J.E., Levi, P.E. eds. Academic Press; San Diego.1992. p. 47–78.

Vogelstein, B., Fearon, E.R, Kern, S.E., *et al.* Allelotype of colorectal carcinomas. *Science* 1989;**224**:207–11.

Vogelstein, B., Kinzler, K.W. The multistep nature of cancer. *Trends in Genetics* 1993;**9**:138–41.

Waters, M.D., Stack, H.F., Garrett, N.E., *et al.* The genetic activity profile database. *Environmental Health Perspectives* 1991;**96**:41–5.

Waters, M.D., Stack, H.F., Jackson, M.A. Genetic toxicology data in he evaluation of potential human environmental carcinogens. *Mutation Research* 1999;**437**:21–49.

Woo, Y., Arcos, J.C., Lai, D.Y. In: *Handbook of Carcinogen Testing*. Milman, H.A., Weisburger, E.K. eds. Noyes Publications; Park Ridge, NJ.1985.

Woo, Y., Lai, D.Y., Argus, M.F., *et al.* Carcinogenicity of organophosphorous pesticides/compounds; an analysis of their structure-activity relationships. *Environmental Carcinogenesis and Ecotoxicology Reviews* 1996;**C14**:1–42.

CHAPTER 14

Organophosphorus Agents and the Environment

Elwood F Hill

14.1. Introduction

As a result of the use of organophosphorous (OP) pesticides in agriculture and for the control of vectors of diseases such as malaria, these toxic substances can enter the food chain of man and animals (Eto, 1974; Briggs, 1991; Ecobichon, 1994). OP use is a clear risk to human health as they are responsible for about 25–30% of pesticide-related hospitalisations in the United States (USA) (Hall and Rumack, 1991), and as much as 50–75% in some Asiatic countries (Ballantyne and Marrs, 1992). These are very high percentages considering that over 95% of OP is used for agriculture in areas generally removed from population centres. Domestic, industrial, and veterinary usages represent only a small portion of the OP market.

In the USA alone over 30 million hectare-treatments (i.e., hectares treated corrected for number of treatments) of OPs are applied per year to control nuisance and depredating invertebrates and vertebrates on agricultural crops, forests, and rangelands (Smith, 1987). When an OP is applied according to the label, the active ingredient is supposed to be reasonably well contained within the intended treatment area and its residual half-life is expected to be only a few days to about a month. Nonetheless, whether due to drift or runoff, OP and toxic degradates are inevitably detected in soils and water outside the treated area and often for durations well beyond the estimated residual life of the product (Ramade, 1987; Edwards and Fisher, 1991). Thus, downstream habitats, including groundwater, may be periodically contaminated with OP pesticides and potable water wells are sometimes affected. Off-site contamination may result in massive short-term mortality of aquatic organisms (US EPA, 1991). It is not yet certain what the long-term implications of such contamination may be to the ecosystem. Both on- and off-site OP exposures have caused occasional incidents of massive mortality of non-target vertebrates world-wide (e.g., Mendelssohn and Paz, 1977; Hardy et al., 1986; Smith, 1987; US EPA, 1991; Goldstein et al., 1996; Mineau et al., 1999).

Many OP pesticides are toxic to most animal species (Gaines, 1960, 1969; Johnson and Finley, 1980; Hudson *et al.*, 1984; Mayer and Ellersieck, 1986; Edwards and Fisher, 1992; Murty and Ramani, 1991), but tend to be comparatively short-lived in the natural environment (Eto, 1974). OPs are rapidly metabolised and excreted by most animals (Eto, 1974), and do not biomagnify in food chains (Stickel, 1975). These factors and broad-spectrum insecticidal efficacy favoured OP and other anticholinesterase pesticides (carbamates, CB) as replacements for the biologically persistent and problematic mercury and organochlorine pesticides (Stickel, 1975; Edwards, 1993; Osteen, 1993). For example, it is well-documented that certain organochlorine pesticides and metabolites inhibit proper eggshell formation and severely jeopardised populations of fish-eating birds such as brown pelicans (*Pelicanus occidentalis*), bald eagles (*Haliaeetus leucocephalus*), and ospreys (*Pandion haliaetus*) (Blus, 1995). It is not certain whether the high mortality of non-target vertebrates by the use of OP insecticides has critical effects on the population level. However, there is increasing evidence that mortality of raptorial birds from OP poisoning may be affecting some species at the regional level (Mineau, *et al.*, 1999).

Tolerance of terrestrial vertebrates to environmental OP exposure varies according to habitat, foraging preference, and inherent sensitivity to the pesticide (Hill, 1995). Exposure may result from direct pesticide application; contact with or ingestion of contaminated water, soil, or vegetation; or ingestion of contaminated prey or pesticide-impregnated granules. Less definitive factors also have bearing on the tolerance of an OP-contaminated environment. For example, the prey base may be altered and affect foraging success. Sublethal exposure may affect critical behaviours including reproduction and migration orientation, or proper balance between producer and consumer organisms in soil and the aquatic systems may be disrupted (Hill, 1999). Fish and other aquatic organisms also vary widely in tolerance of exposure depending on inherent sensitivity and factors of water quality, chemistry, and temperature (Rattner and Heath, 1995).

This chapter provides an overview of the environmental hazard of OP pesticides to wildlife with emphasis on terrestrial vertebrates including waterfowl, and possible implications to human health. The focus is on concepts of ecological toxicology. It is related to natural systems and their associated agricultural and community landscapes, including yards, gardens, and recreational areas. The environmental fate of representative OPs and availability to non-target wildlife are reviewed. OP toxicology as related to other factors, such as, product formulations, species and physiological status, source of exposure, and field diagnostics are considered.

14.2. General Toxicology

OP esters account for more than one-third of the registered pesticides on the world market. Thousands of OP compounds have been tested for pesticidal properties. Most registrations are for control of a large array of insect pests and disease vectors. OPs have proven effective in control of many animal pests including invertebrates and vertebrates. Of the OP products presently in production, 95–99% are used for agricultural application and mosquito control. In the USA, where about 70 OPs are registered as the active ingredient (AI) in thousands of products, about 50% of the use involves only five chemicals; parathion-methyl, parathion, terbufos, fonofos, and azinphos-methyl (Smith, 1987). Based on acute oral LD50 (tests active ingredient alone) these chemicals are among the most toxic OP pesticides to birds (e.g., mallard, *Anas platyrhynchos*, and northern bobwhite, *Colinus virginianus*; Hudson *et al.*, 1984) and laboratory rats (Gaines, 1960 and 1969). Another six chemicals, phorate, malathion, chlorpyrifos, EPN, phosalone and dimethoate, comprise more than half of the remaining field use of OP in the USA. Of these 11 chemicals nine are classed highly toxic to birds (LD50, <50 mgAI/kg body mass; Loomis and Hayes, 1996) and eight are classed highly toxic to mammals.

Only malathion is considered to be of a low order of acute toxicity to both birds and mammals (LD50, >500 mg/kg). Chlorpyrifos and phosalone are classed moderately toxic to rats (LD50, 50–500 mg/kg). In the former USSR, pesticides with a single-dose oral mammalian LD50 of less than 50 mg/kg were banned in the 1960s; a few exceptions were permitted for use of granular formulations in agriculture (Kundiev and Kagan, 1991).

The toxicity of OPs is owed primarily to disruption of the nervous system by inhibition of cholinesterase (ChE, acetylcholinesterase, EC 3.1.1.7, and nonspecific esterases) activity in the central nervous system and at neuromuscular junctions with death generally attributed to respiratory failure (O'Brien, 1967). When OP binds to ChE a relatively stable bond is formed and prevents the ChE from deactivating acetylcholine (ACh). This allows buildup of ACh and overstimulation of the cholinergic nervous system. This leads to rather predictable but non-specific, signs in birds and small mammals including lethargy, laboured-breathing, excessive bronchial secretions, vomiting, diarrhoea, tremors, convulsions and death. These toxic indicators are useful when sick animals are found near an area of recent OP application, but the signs are not uniquely different from poisoning by other neurotoxic agents. A more expansive list of toxic signs has been developed for laboratory mammals (e.g., Ecobichon, 1996) that should also apply to wildlife.

Species, such as small mammals, are seclusive and difficult to observe when poisoned in nature. Birds, especially flocking species, are commonly found in all stages of illness during episodes of acute OP poisoning (Hill and Fleming, 1982). Subacute OP poisoning of wildlife has been demonstrated in the laboratory and undoubtedly occurs in nature, but field demonstration of such effects remains elusive. Some of the postulated subacute effects involve changes in response to ambient stressors, reproductive behaviour, and migration orientation (Mineau, 1991; Hill, 1995). Acute and subacute effects of OP poisoning have been widely reported for aquatic and terrestrial invertebrates and fish, but comparatively little information is available on amphibians and reptiles (Hoffman et al., 1995).

Two other distinctive syndromes of OP insecticide toxicity have been well-documented clinically, but neither has proven to be of major importance in natural wildlife populations. The first is OP-induced delayed neurotoxicity (OPIDN) in which subacute exposure causes degeneration in the nerves and the spinal cord (Abou-Donia, 1981). This debilitating neurological toxicity leads to a stumbling gait and incoordination. OPIDN has been implicated for a few OP insecticides in humans, and has been induced in a variety of laboratory animals including chickens and mallards. However, neither mallards nor Japanese quail *(Coturnix japonica)* are as susceptible to leptophos or EPN, the classic pesticide inducers of OPIDN, as are chickens (Hoffman et al., 1984). The OPIDN syndrome has not proven to be a common manifestation of OP pesticide poisoning of wildlife, perhaps because it is not easily observed in nature. However, it is reasonable to assume that OPIDN debilitated birds and mammals would be particularly vulnerable to natural predators as well as domestic dogs and cats.

The other OP-mediated illness is referred to as the "intermediate syndrome" (Senanayake and Karalliedde, 1987, 1992). This is a potentially lethal paralytic condition of the neck, limbs, and respiratory muscles that follow an acute OP exposure by several days. This syndrome has not been reported as such in either laboratory or field studies of wildlife, but it could be an important factor in consideration of potential hazard of OPs to wildlife. For example, it is not unusual to find acutely poisoned animals in the vicinity of an OP-treated area for several days after the treatment. It has been generally assumed that they were simply new arrivals affected by residual pesticide. If the OP-mediated intermediate syndrome plays a significant role, the concern is that mortality away from the treated area could be much larger than generally believed.

14.3. OP Fate and Hazard

OP pesticides are esters of phosphoric and phosphorothioic acid and are comparatively labile in circumneutral environments. Ambient factors such as increased temperature, rain, alkalinity, and sunlight may accelerate OP degradation. Neither bioaccumulation nor biomagnification occurs to any important degree for OPs in aquatic or terrestrial food chains. Thus the main hazards of OPs to wildlife are from direct exposure to OP treatment including inhalation and percutaneous routes, and from ingestion of contaminated food or water. Classic secondary poisoning through biomagnification of highly lipid soluble pesticides such as chlorinated hydrocarbons does not happen with OPs. Instead, predators are often poisoned by feeding on prey that had been contaminated by OP application. For example, invertebrates and aquatic vertebrates absorb OP on their cutaneous or mucosal surface which is then readily dissociated and absorbed when eaten by another animal (Hill, 1995). The stomach contents of poisoned birds and mammals may also contain large concentrations of OP that have proven toxic to predators and scavengers.

OP pesticides generally have broad-spectrum toxicity to most invertebrates with cholinergic-dependent nervous system and to all vertebrates. OP products are used as stomach and contact poisons, fumigants, and as systemic poisons for nearly any type of insect control (Matsumura, 1985). They are also used as nematicides, acaricides, and bird and mammal control agents; some have herbicidal properties. In spite of their broad toxicity, OPs such as malathion and temephos are applied to wetlands and over areas of human habitation for the control of disease vectors and insect pests. Generally, however, OP use is discouraged for aquatic environments, and for many products the label specifically cautions against such use.

Nearly all OP application in the USA is on terrestrial landscapes, but whether applied to farmlands, forests, or cities, some of the pesticide and its degradates will migrate or be washed into an aquatic system. It has been theorised that all anthropogenic chemicals will eventually enter an aquatic environment and affect a much larger number of species than originally intended (Murty and Ramani, 1992). The hazard of OP to non-target life is a product of the amount, rate, and form of residual entering the aquatic system and the dynamics and chemistry of the system. For example, if the runoff from on OP application enters a stream rapid dilution and dispersal may render the contamination ecologically innocuous. In contrast, if the same runoff enters an aquatic sink such as a farm pond rich with detritus, the ecological consequences may be considerable to organisms at all levels including terrestrial species.

This type of contamination has resulted in large die-offs of waterfowl and predatory birds including golden eagles (*Aquila chrysaetos*) in the northern plains of the USA where OPs are intensively used for control of soil and foliage insects and nematodes (US EPA, 1991). In this situation, pesticides such as phorate, are incorporated into the soil and under normal farming conditions are not problematic; but if heavy rains occur, the transport of OP and degradates is facilitated and has proven lethal to aquatic and terrestrial life for as long as 2–3 weeks following the storm event.

Phorate is an example of a group of highly efficacious insecticides, including demeton and disulfoton, whose environmental degradates are more toxic and stable than the parent OP. This feature increases their potential hazard to nontarget wildlife but also increases their market appeal as broad-spectrum systemic pesticides for foliar application and incorporation into the soil. Phorate and disulfoton rank sixth and fifteenth in the market for agricultural OP pesticides in the USA. All three of these structurally similar OPs (phorate, $(EtO)_2PS.SCH_2SEt$; disulfoton, $(EtO)_2PS.SCH_2CH_2SEt$; demeton, $(EtO)_2PS.OCH_2CH_2SEt$; Corbett *et al.,* 1984) are extremely toxic to mammals (e.g., rat oral LD50, 2.3–6.8 mg/kg; Gaines, 1969) and birds (e.g., mallard oral LD50, 0.6–7.2 mg/kg; Hudson *et al.,* 1984). For comparison, the acute toxicity of parathion and parathion-methyl has been reported as 13 and 24 mg/kg for rats (Gaines, 1969) and 2.3 and 10 mg/kg for mallards (Hudson *et al.,* 1984). These pesticides are also highly toxic by the dermal route of exposure as indicated by laboratory rat LD50s of 6.2 mg/kg (phorate) to 15 mg/kg (disulfoton) as compared to 21 and 67 mg/kg for parathion and parathion-methyl (Gaines, 1969).

The primary toxicity of cholinesterase inhibition is produced by the metabolic toxication for all phosphorothioic acid pesticides such as the above examples and most other OPs. This single oxidative desulfuration step is mediated by mixed-function oxidases in the liver of vertebrates and in the fat body, Malpighian tubules, and digestive tract of invertebrates (Eto, 1974; Walker, 1978, 1980). Other anticholinesterases such as phosphoric acids and carbamates do not require metabolic transformation for maximum acute toxicity. Oxidative desulfuration also occurs in nature as mediated by microbial metabolism in soils and by phytometabolism but this process is slow compared to mixed-function oxidase metabolism in the liver of vertebrates.

14.3.1. Sulfoxides and Sulfones

For OPs such as phorate, disulfoton, and demeton, an additional oxidative pathway of toxication occurs in the environment in which the degradates are more toxic and more persistent than the parent compound (Mitchell *et al.,* 1968). This oxidative process is mediated primarily by UV irradiation in water and soil and to a lesser degree by microbial metabolism (Mitchell *et al.,* 1968), and by phytometabolism in plants (Bowman and Casida, 1958). The sulfoxide and sulfone degradates also require the oxidative desulfuration step for maximum anticholinesterase activity.

Using phorate as a model, observations on environmental fate, necessary as they are important to the ecological hazard of these unique phosphorothioic acid pesticides, gives us an insight into the problems involved. The fate of phorate in water is determined by pH, temperature, and photolysis (Eto, 1974). Phorate is stable in water at about pH 5; its half-life in pH 6 at 25°C is about 7 days (Ruzicka *et al.,* 1967). The rate of hydrolysis increases about ten-fold per pH unit under alkaline conditions. Irradiation by UV light oxidises phorate within minutes to its more potent ChE-inhibiting sulfoxide and sulfone degradates (Mitchell *et al.,* 1968). Neither aquatic invertebrates nor fish tend to bioaccumulate phorate in model ecosystems (Lichtenstein *et al.,* 1978), but phorate is highly toxic to fish. For example, in comparable standardised 96-hour LC50 tests, phorate is more than 100 times as toxic as parathion and parathion-methyl to an array of both warm and cold water game fish (Johnson and Finley, 1980).

The fate of phorate in soil is affected by pesticide formulation, the method and rate of application, soil type, pH, temperature, moisture content, irrigation and water percolation, vegetation type and abundance, and microbial populations (Getzin and Chapman, 1960; Singh and Singh, 1984). Surface application of either granular or emulsifiable phorate results in 15–20% loss due to vapourisation within 1 hour; thereafter, nearly all of the residual phorate remains bound to the soil particles, but undergoes UV irradiation and oxidation to sulfoxide and sulfone degradates within a few days. Up to 80% of these highly toxic degradates persist in various soil types for 1–2 months (Getzin and Chapman, 1960). The terrestrial dissipation half-life of phorate in irrigated soils is 2 days in sandy loam and 9–15 days in silty loam. For sulfoxide and sulfone degradates, the half-life in sandy loam is 12–18 weeks (Getzin and Shanks, 1970). Phorate movement is more rapid in summer than in winter, but it is more stable in winter, probably due to lower microbial activity (Singh and Singh, 1984). Phorate is poorly soluble in water (~50 mg/L), and residues do not migrate extensively from the treated area.

However, residues may be transported by erosion and run-off from agricultural fields into aquatic systems where they have caused major episodes of fish and bird mortality (US EPA, 1991).

Soil-incorporated phorate is readily translocated through the roots and stems of plants and provides insecticidal protection to plants for a relatively long time because of the greater persistence of the sulfoxide metabolite (Eto, 1974). The initial oxidation to sulfoxide proceeds rapidly in plants, whereas further oxidation to sulfone and desulfuration is slower. Anticholinesterase activity increases as phorate oxidation proceeds to the most toxic sufone. The oxon analogue of each form is even more potent. Therefore, the anticholinesterase activity of phorate assimilated into the plants increases over several days and only then gradually loses activity over 2–5 weeks (Eto, 1974). Because of this systemic activity, phorate clearly poses a potential hazard to herbivorous animals including wildlife and livestock, and to human health. Phorate toxicity is such that a treated field may not be entered within 48 hours of application, and 30 (corn, maize, sorghum and sugar beets) to 90 days (peanuts, potatoes) must pass prior to harvest or livestock grazing (US EPA, 1991). This restriction is comparatively long for an OP pesticide and is imposed because of its extreme dermal toxicity to mammals.

14.3.2. OPs and Wetlands

Except for a few products used for mosquito control, most OP pesticides are not permitted for use on wetlands. Nonetheless, wetlands are routinely contaminated during agricultural use of a wide array of OP products. Airborne drift, direct overspray, and runoff are the main sources of OP contamination when farmlands border natural wetlands, irrigation canals, and drainage ditches (US EPA, 1991). Ground application of OP may contaminate wetlands through vapourisation, migration, and runoff, but the technique is not as prone to drift as aerial treatment. It has been estimated that downwind drift from aerial application is conservatively four times higher than that produced by high clearance ground sprayers (Ware et al., 1969). Clearly, ground application is less contaminating to buffer zones.

Small stream and ponds are especially subject to OP contamination from overspray, drift and runoff. This is partly because they are difficult to avoid during aerial application when crops abut the wetlands. Of more importance, however, these small wetlands, often less than a hectare in size and only 1–2 meters deep, are not fully appreciated for their intrinsic value in regions dominated by expansive farmlands and monocultures.

For example: in North America's prairie pothole region of south-central Canada and north-central USA, about 65% of the original wetlands have been drained and cultivated (Dahl, 1990). The remaining wetlands contribute to more than 50% of North America's duck production (van der Valk, 1989). A very large proportion of these wetlands are near, or surrounded by, agricultural fields and are considered of high potential for excessive agricultural pesticide contamination (Sheehan *et al.*, 1987; Grue *et al.*, 1988). OP products constitute the majority of the pesticide use in the region.

Agricultural contamination of small and sometimes only seasonal wetlands are probably the most ecologically abused areas. Many of these wetlands are extremely productive in terms of biomass and wildlife dependence during critical spring and summer periods. Unfortunately, these small ponds are very shallow and contain a small volume to their surface area. They lack the dilution and buffering of toxicity compared to larger ponds and lakes. Though most OPs are acutely toxic, their hazard is clearly less than for the chemically persistent chlorinated hydrocarbon pesticides that OPs generally replaced in the early 1970s. This is because most OP products are chemically inactivated within a few hours in circumneutral aquatic environments and within a few days to 1–2 weeks in more acidic systems. This rapid degradation is ecologically advantageous because most "knocked-down" invertebrate populations seem to recover rapidly from a single operational OP treatment. However, effects of multiple applications on species diversity, balance, abundance and total biomass are not well-understood and their effects should not be underestimated among OPs, product formulations, or aquatic systems. Nor is it understood to what degree cumulative effects influence aquatic vertebrate recovery and waterbird behaviour and productivity.

In an effort to evaluate hazard of OPs and herbicides to aquatic invertebrates and waterfowl in the prairie potholes region of North America, the US Fish and Wildlife Service developed a comprehensive research plan in the mid-1980s (Grue *et al.*, 1986). The early studies focused on an array of "average" potholes of similar size and depth to determine the response of mallard and blue-winged teal (*Anas discors*) ducklings to "typical" OP treatments of ethyl and methyl parathion on wheat and sunflowers. In both studies, each of five broods was confined to a fenced pothole and permitted to roam throughout the pond and riparian zone to the edge of the treated crop which surrounded the pothole. Each pothole was believed to be of adequate size and quality to provide necessary cover, spatial, and nutritional requirements for simultaneous fledging of several mallard broods.

In the study of OP application on spring wheat, the first step was to treat all of the fields including the 10 potholes with an aerial application of the herbicide 2,4-D (0.3 kg AI/ha), which is a standard practice in the region (Tome *et al,*. 1995). One month later, one-half of the fields and ponds were treated by standard operational application of parathion (0.6 kg AI/ha), and the other fields and ponds were treated with parathion-methyl (0.3 kg AI/kg). All treatments were made from about 1.5–2 meters above the crop which resulted in a spray swath of about 18 meters. Three days prior to the insecticide treatments, 10–12 3-week-old mallards and 10–12 3-week-old teal were released on each wetland. The ducklings were sampled at 2 and 7 days after the treatment, and then at 7–8 day intervals through 30 days post-treatment. Body mass, tissue residues of OP, and brain ChE activity were evaluated at each sample period. In these wheat field studies, none of the ducklings died from OP poisoning, but within 2 days post-treatment 27% of the ducklings on parathion-treated ponds and 29% of those on the parathion-methyl treatment had significantly depressed brain ChE activity. Body mass was not affected. Behavioural and population studies did not indicate any differences in the number of wild broods or adults of either species on treated and control fields.

The next spring, an operational aerial treatment of parathion on sunflowers was evaluated (Tome *et al.,* 1991). The main differences from the above studies were the use of younger mallards (1–3 days of age), release of two broods of 10–12 ducklings with their hens in each pond, and the rate of parathion treatment was nearly double (1.12 kg AI/ha) the 0.6 kg rate used for spring wheat This was the maximum recommended treatment for sunflowers in North Dakota. One-half of the study wetlands were oversprayed to test the worst-case scenario. For the other half of the wetlands, the operator attempted to achieve complete crop coverage, while avoiding overspray of the ponds. Overall, more than 90% of the ducklings in the oversprayed ponds were dead within 3 days post-treatment. Brain ChE activity was inhibited an average of 76% compared with the norm for ducklings collected on control wetlands. In this study, parathion residues were determined in several matrices (water, vegetation, insects and snails) 1 day prior to spray and 1, 7, 14 and 29 days post-treatment. All prespray samples were clear of parathion. One day post-treatment, all samples contained parathion (mean residues: water, 0.12µg/ml; insects, 0.29 µg/g; snails, 9.04 µg/g; and vegetation, 0.42 µg/g) and by 7 days all samples were clear of detectable residues. Ground searching of the oversprayed ponds and their riparian zones yielded more than 30 dead birds with acutely inhibited brain ChE activity; i.e., OP-induced mortality (C.E. Grue, personal communication).

Over two-thirds of the dead birds were juveniles of blue-winged teal, American coot (*Fulica americana*), red-winged blackbird (*Agelaius phoeniceus*), and yellow-headed blackbird (*Xanthocephalus xanthocephalus*).

For the wetlands where reasonable effort was made to avoid direct pond overspray while providing complete crop coverage, the results were quite different (Tome, *et al.*, 1991). Parathion poisoning was not attributed to the death of any of the ducklings even though some had depressed brain ChE activity that was indicative of OP exposure. Likewise, there was no evidence of other birds having been acutely poisoned by the treatment. Wetland residues of parathion were also much less than for the oversprayed ponds. The mean residues for key wetland matrices 1 day post-treatment were: water, 0.01 μg/ml; insects, 0.13 μg/g; snails, 3.04 μg/g; and vegetation, 0.35 μg/g. Therefore, *the effort to avoid direct overspray of small wetlands was successful in elimination of OP-induced avian mortality and reduction of parathion in water (>90%) and invertebrates (34–45%)*.

14.3.3. OPs and Mosquito Control

The most serious problems in wetlands is the control of mosquitos. At present OPs are most often used for this purpose. This use is at present being supplanted by biological control agents such as *Bacillus thuringiensis israelensis* (BTI). Other agents including a variety of fungi, hormones and enzymes are in various stages of development. This transition is in response to the demand for the development of safer pesticides for application to wetlands and areas of human habitation. It is becoming necessary to overcome developing resistance, in some mosquito species, to chemical control agents.

OPs are routinely used throughout the world for suppression of mosquitos, both as a nuisance and a disease vector. For example, under the threat of encephalitis epidemics following hurricanes and floods, thousands of hectares of contiguous bottomlands and major populated areas of the USA have been aerially sprayed with undiluted OPs such as malathion at rates as small as 219 milliliters per hectare (Kilpatrick, 1967). These ultra low volume (ULV; <765 ml/ha) treatments are efficient and comparatively safe for use wherever there is a need for rapid application of OP to large or remote lands (Richter, 1992). Only a few OPs such as malathion, naled and fenthion have been used extensively for mosquito control as ULV sprays, and none have been implicated in serious health effects. This does not imply such treatments are without environmental hazard.

In May 1969, undiluted fenthion was applied by helicopter at the recommended rate of 95 milliliters per hectare to approximately 600 hectares of a portion of the Red River and residential and park areas of Grand Forks, North Dakota, USA (Seabloom *et al.,* 1973). Over the course of 2 days, more than 450 birds representing 37 species were found dead or moribund within the fenthion-treated area. Most of the dead birds were warblers and other species that feed mainly on invertebrates. The mortality was finally estimated at more than 5,000 birds in and around the city; there were no reports of OP-induced illness in the inhabitants of Grand Forks. In part, because of this extreme episode of wildlife mortality from a standard mosquito control application, many other studies have been conducted on fenthion mosquito control. Some resulted in avian mortality (Zinkl *et al.,* 1981; Smith, 1987; US EPA, 1991) while others neither affected avian survivability nor reproduction (Powell, 1984; Smith, 1987).

Mosquito control agents are normally used in areas of human activity and habitation and cannot be acutely toxic to mammals or induce serious side-effects. The oral LD50s for laboratory rats of favoured mosquito control agents in the USA such as fenthion, malathion, temephos, chlorpyrifos and naled vary from about 15 (chlorpyrifos; Hudson *et al.,* 1984) to 8,600 mg/kg (temephos; Gaines, 1969). Thus, LD50s for these OPs are considered only moderately (chlorpyrifos, fenthion and naled) to slightly (malathion and temephos) toxic according to the acute toxicity ranking of Loomis and Hayes (1996). In contrast, all of the OPs except malathion are classed highly toxic to birds (Hudson *et al.,* 1984; Smith, 1987), but only fenthion (rat oral LD50, 215 mg/kg. Gaines, 1969; mallard LD50, 5.9 mg/kg, Hudson *et al.,* 1984) has proven hazardous to birds and mammals in nature.

From a possible health-effect perspective, fenthion has been diagnosed in OP-induced intermediate syndrome in humans (Senanayake and Karalliedde, 1987, 1992).

All of the above mosquito control agents, except temephos, are broad spectrum insecticides that are widely used in agriculture. Temephos is used almost exclusively for mosquito, midge, and black fly larvae control in lakes, ponds, and wetland habitats (Smith, 1987). All of the OPs are acutely toxic to susceptible invertebrates and fish within a few minutes of exposure, but are poorly soluble and rapidly degraded in water (e.g., 2–72 h in circumneutral water) and have little potential for bioaccumulation in nature (Kenaga, 1980). Except for temephos, all of these mosquito control agents are generally more toxic to fish and aquatic invertebrates than are ethyl or methyl parathion, both restricted use pesticides in the USA, and all are extremely toxic to natural pollinators such as honey bees (*Apis mellifera*) (Briggs, 1991).

The potential hazard of these mosquito control agents to bee pollinators is greater during general aerial application for nuisance and disease vector control than when applied to wetlands for larvae control.

14.4. Comparative Toxicology: Birds and Mammals

The usual ecological consequences of OP pesticide applications are usually short-term, non-specific acute events. Some argue that this is of little importance at the population level because incidents involving several thousand birds are small compared to losses from adverse weather and infectious diseases. Nonetheless, *poisoning of large numbers of wildlife, aquatic or terrestrial, by synthetic pesticides is not only aesthetically unacceptable but such a toxic application has potential ecological ramifications that are not fully understood.* This acute hazard must not be underestimated. Other factors must be considered. Predator-prey or competitor balance among invertebrates and aquatic vertebrates may be disrupted. Daily activity patterns, energy balance, and various behaviours of many animal species may be affected. Repeated application of OP may cause cumulative physiological effects without a corresponding accumulation of chemical residues. Recovery from anti-ChE exposure may differ among pesticidal classes.

OP pesticides and product formulations are widely variable in toxicity to different aquatic and terrestrial vertebrates (Eto, 1974; Hill *et al.,* 1975; Johnson and Finley, 1980; Mayer and Ellersieck, 1986; Smith, 1987). Those pesticides that are esters of phosphoric acid (e.g., acephate, dichlorvos, dicrotophos, trichlorfon, etc.) are direct ChE inhibitors, but most OPs are esters of phosphorothioic acid (e.g., chlorpyrifos, diazinon, malathion, parathion, etc.) and must undergo an oxidative desulfuration step for maximum anti-ChE potency as described under general toxicology. This toxication step is primarily due to mixed-function oxidases (= hepatic mono oxygenase, HMO) in the liver of vertebrates. HMO activity differs widely among species within and between taxons and generally decreases among vertebrates in the following order: mammals>birds>fish (Eto, 1974; Walker, 1978, 1980). Thus, the same physiological system responsible for toxication of most OP pesticides also has a primary role in detoxication of anti-ChE. Since anti-ChE metabolism occurs primarily in the liver of vertebrates, the portal of entry into the circulation is critical to acute toxicity. Direct-acting anti-ChEs may be more hazardous through inhalation than through ingestion. Many such scenarios should be considered in hazard prediction and understanding differences of species response to different pesticidal applications.

Metabolic responses to OP pesticides are similar for birds and mammals, with any difference being more quantitative than qualitative (Pan and Fouts, 1978). Several quantitative enzymatic differences between birds and mammals are important to differential response to acute toxic exposure. Birds generally have lower levels of HMO and A-esterase activity than do mammals, which tends to make birds more sensitive to acute anti-ChE poisoning (Walker, 1978, 1980; Brealey et al., 1980). However, the majority of widely used OPs are phosphorothioic acids that must be metabolically activated to their most potent anti-ChE analogue. This oxidative desulfuration step is mediated by the same HMO pathway as is detoxication in birds and mammals (Eto, 1974). This would indicate that mammals should toxicate phosphorothioic acids more efficiently than birds, therefore be more sensitive.

But this is not so because activated OP analogues are substrates for A-esterase hydrolysis and are rapidly detoxified in the liver and blood. In a study of 14 species of birds, three species of laboratory mammals, domestic sheep, and humans, plasma A-esterase activity was at least 13 times higher in all of the mammals than in any of the avian species (Brealey et al., 1980). The importance of these enzymatic differences to birds was demonstrated with dimethoate, a phosphorothioic acid in which adult ring-necked pheasants (Phasianus colchicus) and laboratory rats were compared. The toxic oxygen analogue was rapidly formed and accumulated in pheasants, but was rapidly degrated to inactive metabolites in the rats (Sanderson and Edson, 1964). This undoubtedly contributes to the more than 10-fold difference in the acute oral sensitivity of pheasants (LD50, 20 mg/kg, Hudson et al., 1984) and rats (LD50, 215 mg/kg, Gaines, 1969).

In general, the array of domestic and wild bird species commonly studied in the laboratory are consistenty more sensitive to acute oral toxicity of OPs than are laboratory mammals and wild mice (Peromyscus spp.) and voles (Microtus spp.) (Gaines, 1960, 1969; Schafer, 1972; Schafer et al., 1983; Hudson et al., 1984; Schafer and Bowles, 1985; Smith, 1987). Though this generalisation of differential acute sensitivity is convenient for preliminary risk assessments, it is not reliable for all animal species and OP pesticides (Hill, 1999). For example, the acute toxicity of a series of phosphorothioic acid pesticides was compared for standardised LD50 tests of adult male laboratory rats (Gaines, 1969), ring-necked pheasants (Hudson et al., 1984), and red-winged blackbirds (Hudson et al., 1984). Pheasants and blackbirds were used because both species have similar general feeding habits and represent extreme body mass compared with rats (e.g., blackbirds, ~65 g; rats, ~200 g; pheasant ~1,000 g).

The rat LD50s were graded from 2.3 (phorate) to 8,600 mg/kg (temephos), with none of the successive 95% confidence intervals overlapping. By most criteria for ranking acute mammalian toxicity, phorate is classed extremely toxic, and is a restricted use chemical in the USA; tempehos is practically non-toxic (Briggs, 1991; Loomis and Hayes, 1996). At the one extreme, though phorate is also highly toxic to pheasants (LD50, 7.1 mg/kg), it is about three times more toxic to rats. At the other extreme, temephos is nearly 250 times more toxic to pheasants (LD50, 35 mg/kg) than to rats. The original premise that birds are more sensitive to OPs than mammals was borne out for red-winged blackbirds which were 2–200 times as sensitive as the laboratory rat.

This limited comparison of phosphorothioic acids has important implications for ecological risk assessment. First, avian HMO activity is inversely related to body mass, and therefore red-winged blackbirds should be more tolerant of OP poisoning than is the ring-necked pheasant, but they are not. This maybe partially explained by red-winged blackbirds (and possibly other small passerines) being particularly deficient in liver-detoxication enzymes, but also may have been influenced by small birds having a much higher metabolic rate (Walker, 1978, 1980; Pan et al., 1979). In spite of this possible detoxicating deficiency, red-winged blackbirds coexist with agrichemical treatments and are considered crop pests in many regions of the USA (Hill, 1995). Second, it was noted that OPs with rat LD50s above 200 mg/kg were usually more than 10 times as toxic to pheasants as to rats; but for OPs with LD50s less than 200 mg/kg, rats were 2–20 times more sensitive than the pheasants (Gaines, 1969; Hudson et al., 1984). This is especially important because rat LD50s are often the only acute data available for risk assessments, and LD50s above 200 mg/kg are considered only moderately toxic for wildlife (Smith, 1987). This conclusion would be critically wrong for OPs such as dimethoate, fenitrothion, and temephos; all of which are classed highly toxic with LD50s of less than 50 mg/kg for many birds (Hudson, 1984). In nature, fenitrothion applied at recommended rates on rangelands for grasshopper control resulted in bird mortality and decrease in breeding populations (Smith, 1987).

Based on the foregoing, the laboratory rat is not a good model for prediction of acute OP toxicity in birds. In contrast, laboratory rats and mice are conservative predictors of acute toxicity to wild rodents. In a study of the acute oral toxicity of a spectrum of pesticides including OPs to four species of voles and laboratory rats and mice, it was determined that laboratory rodents are generally more sensitive to acute exposure than the most sensitive of the voles, *Microtus canicaudus* (Cholakis et al., 1981).

Laboratory mice were also found to be more sensitive than deer mice (*Permyscus maniculatus*), but the relationship was erratic (Schafer and Bowles, 1985).

It follows that, acute exposure (i.e., of short course and life-threatening) is the main hazard of OP pesticides to wildlife, and standard toxicological tests, are best represented by the acute single-dose LD50 study. Response to the dose of OP is usually rapid and. if not fatal, recovery normally occurs within a few hours. This test provides a sound method for quantification of naive sensitivity to OPs and comparisons such as differences between sexes, age classes, and formulated products. The test also provides characterisation of the dose-response curve which is essential for proper hazard evaluation and risk assessment. However, the acute test is only a reference to field exposure because OP-induced mortality varies widely from repeated small doses during feeding (the degree of response depends on the level of contamination and susceptibility of the individual) to massive over-dose from rapid ingestion of highly contaminated water or a bolus of food. Therefore, a second "acute" test has also been developed to check the short-term response of birds and mammals to OP-contaminated forage. The feeding trial is designed, replicated and analyzed statistically the same as in the acute test, but provides graded levels of contaminant for 5 days. This feeding trial was developed in the 1960s as an alternative to the acute test for highly persistent pesticides that were not acutely toxic (Heath and Stickel, 1965). As for the acute test, neither does this feeding trial properly represent field exposure risks of wildlife to OPs. But in combination, the two tests provide much insight into wildlife response to OP treatments. Where the acute test provides information on inherent sensitivity to OPs, the feeding trial provides information on response to repeated chemical exposures as may be encountered in nature. These tests and their use in evaluation of ecological hazard and risk assessment have been critiqued (Hill *et al.,* 1975; Bacietto, 1985a, 1985b; Hill, 1994; Baril *et al.,* 1994; Mineau, *et al.,* 1994).

14.5. Acute Environmental Hazard

Low LD50s indicate that most common OP pesticides are highly toxic to birds and mammals. However, only a small number of these pesticides are responsible for the majority of large-scale incidents of wildlife mortality. This is probably because certain agricultural uses are more likely to bring large numbers of wildlife in contact with a few of the more commonly used pesticides. It is also likely that many incidents of wildlife mortality are not detected or reported.

Most reported incidents are of three types: (1) a few dead songbirds in a neighborhood park or backyard. (2) an unusual concentration of dead flocking birds, or (3) large conspicuous water birds or special interest species such as raptors (Hill, 1995). Sometimes large flocks of blackbird or gulls are found dead on farmlands and not reported. This is because they are often assumed to be part of an avian depradation control program. Avian depredation of crops is an international problem that has used large-scale application of pesticides including OPs since the 1950's, and though use of avicides continues in under-developed regions of the world, the recent focus has been on development of non-toxic repellents (Mason, 1997; J.O. Keith, personal communication). Small mammals may be common to abundant in many habitats routinely treated with OP pesticides, but are rarely listed in reports of even large-scale terrestrial mortality. This omission is more likely due to difficulty in detection of small secretive species (e.g., shrews, mice, voles, etc.) than to any special tolerance of OP contamination. Small mammals usually live within the treated habitat and probably retreat to their burrows upon onset of illness. There has been comparatively little documentation of reptile and amphibian mortality from OP pesticide treatments (Smith, 1987; US EPA, 1991; Hill, 1995).

Prediction of acute OP hazard to wildlife is confounded by many factors of anthropogenic and natural origin. A primary factor, and perhaps most easily addressed through limited additional testing, is the influence of pesticidal formulations on OP availability and toxicity to non-targeted wildlife. Regulatory agencies have only recently begun to consider the differential ecological hazard of finished product formulations, and then only after years of reported episodes of wildlife mortality from certain products (Hill, 1999). Some of the other factors that may affect acute OP hazard to wildlife to different degrees include the route, source and timing of exposure, and possible interactions with other chemicals, infectious diseases and weather stressors.

14.5.1. Product Formulation

OP residues on seed grains, vegetation, and formulated pesticide granules have killed large numbers of wildlife under varied environmental circumstances (Smith, 1987; US EPA, 1991). Some of the kills were due to misuse, but some of the problem was due to general lack of information on the comparative toxicology of pesticidal formulations and hazard associated with various application techniques.

Most often, potential hazard or risk to wildlife is estimated by comparison of the theoretical concentration of the active ingredient in a food item to results of standard acute tests of technical grade chemical with northern bobwhites and mallards, but without regard to the differential effects of finished product on absorption, fate, and toxicity (Hill, 1995; US EPA, 1996).

Only rarely is the technical-grade chemical actually applied in the field, and then only in very low volume as described earlier for mosquito control. Instead, OPs are normally applied as a formulated product that may differ substantially in acute toxicity compared to the technical-grade material tested. As a general rule, it has been determined that granular formulations are most often less toxic than technical-trade materials; whereas, liquid formulations are usually more toxic than technical-grade products (Hill, 1986, 1995). This conclusion was first based on a few standard feeding trials of local retail products with Japanese quail chicks and a series of acute tests of favoured granular OP products with adult northern bobwhites (Hill and Camardese, 1984 and 1986). The above relationship was confirmed with acute tests of northern bobwhites in which an emulsifiable concentrate (48% AI) of diazinon was significantly more toxic than either technical-grade (99% AI), or granular formulation (14% AI; Hill, 1992). Sometimes the LD50s among anti-ChE formulations vary as much as three- to fourfold (Hill, 1999). Comparison of liquid formulations consistently showed aqueous solutions were more toxic than oil-based solutions (Hill, 1992; E.F. Hill, unpublished data). In contrast, OP pesticides were more toxic to mallard embryos when applied to eggs in an oil vehicle than when applied in an aqueous emulsifiable concentrate (Hoffman and Eastin, 1981; Hoffman, 1990). Apparently the oil medium retarded vapourisation, increased the time of contact and facilitated the OP transport through the shell and membranes.

Though granular OPs may be less toxic in dosing studies than other formulations and are safer to handle during application; their potential environmental hazard is excessive. Thus, some granular products are presently under review in the USA by the Fish and Wildlife Service and the Environmental Protection Agency for possible restricted use status or cancellation. The hazard of granules in nature depends on whether they are haphazardly or selectively ingested. If ingestion is haphazard, then the application rate is the critical variable, but if ingestion is selective, then even the most stringent attempts to reduce granule availability may fail to reduce the hazard (Stinson et al., 1994). The colour, size, texture, and application rate of granular products are all factors for consideration in reduction of their hazard to wildlife (Best and Fischer, 1991; Gionfriddo and Best, 1996; Stafford et al., 1996; Stafford and Best, 1998).

14.5.2. Sources and Routes of Exposure

Wildlife are exposed to OP pesticides primarily through ingestion of contaminated water, soil, seeds, foliage, invertebrates, vertebrates, and formulated granular pesticide particles. All of these sources have killed large numbers of wildlife. Water is a common source of OP exposure that is poorly documented for terrestrial vertebrates. Potential OP hazard is dependent on widely variable factors of ambient water quality, movement, and the solubility and stability of the product. Water soluble formulations usually remain available longest and tend to be the most acutely toxic (Eto, 1974; Hill, 1991). How these studies relate to waterborne exposure in nature is not clear because rates of feed and water consumption vary widely among wildlife species at different ages and seasons of the year. Smaller birds and mammals have a much higher water requirement relative to body mass than do larger species under similar ambient conditions (Robbins, 1983). However, even closely related birds of similar sizes and feeding habits vary their rates of free-water consumption from about 15–40% of their body mass per day at the ambient temperature of 25°C (Bartholomew and Cade, 1963). Aquatic wildlife undoubtedly contact and ingest much more water through feeding, swimming and wading than do terrestrial species that use water primarily for hydration.

Few studies of OP pesticides in water have been reported for wildlife species. However, as previously mentioned, field applications of technical-grade of fenthion and in various formulations at 47–100 g of active ingredient per hectare over wetlands of various water depths killed a variety of passerine and wading birds (Seabloom et al., 1973; Zinkl et al., 1981; DeWeese et al., 1983). The authors concluded that contaminated insects were an important source of fenthion in the avian mortalities, but the importance of contaminated water was not dismissed. Mortality of wildlife from puddling and run-off from agricultural fields has been documented for some of the more acutely toxic OP pesticides currently registered for use in the USA (US EPA, 1991).

OP residues in foliage from topical or soil application, may be extremely hazardous to wildlife in or near to the treated area. Treatments to control insects in forests and orchards and on cultivated crops such as small grains, alfalfa, and turf grasses have all resulted in excessive mortality over the years (Smith, 1987; US EPA, 1991). Foliar treatments may be especially hazardous because they may result in exposure by inhalation, percutaneous and oral routes when animals are in the spray zone during treatment.

Turf grass treatment with OPs such as diazinon has proven particularly hazardous to waterfowl such as American wigeon (*Anas americanus*) and the Canada goose (*Branta canadensis,* Stone and Gradoni, 1985). This unique hazard to grazing waterfowl resulted in the Environmental Protection Agency issuing a cancellation notice for the use of diazinon products on golf courses and sod (turf) farms (US EPA, 1986).

Seeds, like granular pesticides, are an important sources of OP exposure to wildlife when treated with acutely toxic pesticides (Stromborg, 1977; Grue *et al.,* 1983; US EFA, 1991). In contrast to granular materials that are usually ingested haphazardly, OP-treated seeds are readily eaten by small granivorous animals in spite of being brightly coloured as a safeguard for human health. This hazard is not limited to seeds on the surface of the soil or to small animals; large-scale mortality of greylag geese (*Anser anser*) was attributed to the uprooting and ingestion of germinating OP-treated seeds (Hamilton *et al.,* 1976, 1981). It is not known whether phytometabolism of systemic OPs has been a major contribution to wildlife mortality, but a hazard to herbivores is plausible because sulfoxide and sulfone metabolites are more potent than the parent compound.

Contaminated arthropods have been proven to be lethal when eaten by wildlife after application of OP insecticides such as terbufos, monocrotophos, dimethoate, and trichlorfon (DeWeese *et al.,* 1979; Smith, 1987; Goldstein *et al.,* 1996; Mineau *et al.,* 1999). Such poisonings are most likely from OP absorbed on the cuticle of the arthropods. An absorbed chemical may be rapidly dissociated in the stomach. Recently, there was a documented incident of disulfoton-treated cotton seeds passing sufficient insecticide through the plant to grazing insects to be lethal to Swainson's hawks (Mineau *et al.,* 1999). Historically, the problem of secondary poisoning of birds eating OP-contaminated arthropods was generally associated with water birds and insectivorous passerines, but such poisoning has proved common-place for the many insectivorous accipitrid hawks (Mineau *et al.,* 1999). In a single incident, as many as 3,000 Swainson's hawks died from eating freshly-sprayed insects following monocrotophos treatment for grasshopper control. Monocrotophos is extremely toxic to birds with acute oral LD50s consistently less than 5 mg/kg, and as low as 0.76 and 0.19 mg/kg for California quail (*Callipepla californica*) and the golden eagle *(Aquila chrysaetos,* Hudson *et al.,* 1984). Approval for monocrotophos has been cancelled in the USA (Briggs, 1991).

Predatory and carrion-eating birds and mammals are known to have died from eating prey and carcasses contaminated with OPs such as monocrotophos, fenthion, mevinphos, phorate, and famphur (Henny *et al.,* 1985; US EPA, 1991; Mineau *et al.,* 1999).

These secondary poisonings were probably from unaltered chemical in the alimentary tract of the prey.

The liver and kidneys may contain some biologically available anti- ChE residues (i.e., oxons, sulfoxides, sulfones). Other post-absorptive tissues and fluids are not as hazardous as a source of secondary poisoning. For example, in an experiment with barn owls *(Tyto alba)* fed quail that had been killed with oral dosage of famphur, intact carcasses caused significant ChE inhibition in the owls; whereas, owls fed quail with the entrails removed were unaffected (Hill and Mendenhall, 1980).

The potential for secondary poisoning from aquatic vertebrates has also been demonstrated. Tadpoles exposed to as little as 1.0 mg of parathion per litre of water for 96 hours were force-fed to 14-day-old mallards at the rate of 5% of body mass. A single meal was lethal to ducklings within 30 minutes. As only parathion, and not its oxygen degredate, was found in the tadpoles and stomachs of the dead ducklings, it is likely that parathion concentrated in the protective outer mucus layer of the tadpoles was the source of the poison. The treated tadpoles appeared healthy when fed to the ducklings.

Percutaneous, ocular, and inhalation exposure undoubtedly occur when wildlife are directly oversprayed by OP pesticides, or when entering a freshly-sprayed area. The few studies conducted on these alternative routes of exposure have demonstrated that they may be important to toxicity in some circumstances, but most often ingestion is the primary source of poisoning (Driver *et al.,* 1991; Hill, 1995).

14.5.3. Toxic Interactions: Chemical and Environment

Interaction among OP pesticides and other common environmental xenobiotics has not been thoroughly studied in wildlife species. A few studies have been conducted on subchronic exposure of birds to expected field concentrations of persistent pesticides and contaminants followed by acute challenge with OP, or studies of simultaneous feeding on combinations of OPs for 5 days. Results of these studies are generally consistent with similar studies of laboratory animals, but there are some differences that may affect the ecological hazard. For example, when laboratory rodents were pretreated with chlorinated hydrocarbon pesticides that increased hepatic mixed-function oxidase activity, their sensitivity to OP insecticides was reduced (Ball *et al.,* 1954; Triolo and Coon, 1966; Menzer, 1970).

In contrast, when the chlorinated hydrocarbon DDE (a metabolite of DDT) was fed to Japanese quail for 3 months, the sensitivity to a single dose of parathion increased significantly: When the quail were pretreated with chlordane, another chlorinated hydrocarbon, acute sensitivity to parathion was decreased (Ludke, 1977). This latter relationship was also observed in similar studies with mice (Triolo and Coon, 1966).

In general, response of naive birds and rodents is additive when acutely challenged with paired OPs or OP in combination with chlorinated hydrocarbon pesticides (Hill, 1992). When more than additive effects are detected, the level of synergy is usually less than twofold, whether exposure is acute by oral dosage (DuBois, 1961; Durham, 1967), or short-term dietary presentation (Kreitzer and Spann, 1973). Little information is available on the effects of sequential exposures of wildlife, but the potential hazard may depend on the order in which the chemicals are encountered. When the initial exposure is to a carbamate, some protection from OP may occur (Gordon et al., 1978). In contrast, when the initial exposure is to an OP, toxicity of subsequent exposure to either OP or CB anti-ChE may be increased (Takahashi et al., 1987). Sequential exposure to different pesticides is a reasonable possibility in nature, especially for animals such as birds that may forage among several crops.

Temperature extremes and season of the year are natural stressors that can affect the toxicity of OPs to wildlife, but neither variable has been thoroughly investigated in nature or the laboratory. Abrupt changes in climate, particularly late cold fronts with heavy rains, may profoundly influence nesting success of birds. Whether effects of OP exposure on thermoregulation, so far demonstrated in the laboratory, would exacerbate an already dramatic physiological challenge is not known. At the other extreme, heat stress was suggested as a contributor to dimethoate toxicity in an episode of sage grouse *(Ceutrocercus urophasianus)* poisoning in Idaho, USA (Blus et al., 1989). Environmental factors affecting OP and other xenobiotic toxicity in wildlife have been reviewed (Rattner and Fairbrother, 1991; Rattner and Heath, 1995; Grue et al., 1997).

14.5.4. Diagnosis of OP Exposure

Anti-ChE pesticides have resulted in hundreds of incidents of wildlife mortality from disease vector control and agriculture throughout the world. When many dead and moribund animals of mixed-species are found in an area of known OP or carbamate treatment, the causal association may be evident but is not conclusive without biochemical and chemical confirmation.

Proper diagnosis is then contingent upon demonstration of brain ChE inhibition to a level indicative of toxicity or exposure and chemical detection of residues of the causative agent. This last step is sometimes difficult because neither OP nor carbamate residues tend to accumulate in tissues. However, a strong inferential diagnosis is possible by demonstrating depressed brain ChE activity and detection of a known anti-ChE in either ingesta or tissues (Hamilton et al., 1976; Hill and Fleming, 1982; Fairbrother, 1996).

A conservative threshold of about 50% depression in whole brain ChE activity is generally considered diagnostic of death from anti-ChE poisoning (Ludke et al., 1975), though depression of 70–95% is commonly reported for birds and mammals killed in nature by OP pesticides (Hill and Fleming, 1982). In contrast, when animals are killed in the field by carbamates, whole brain ChE activity may vary from near normal to depressions of only 60–70% (Hill and Fleming, 1982; Flickinger et al., 1986). Apparently high levels of carbamate exposure kills by systemic neuromuscular blocking before significant penetration of the central nervous system has occurred (Westlake et al., 1981a, b). Lower ChE inhibition may reflect spontaneous postmortem reactivation of carbamylated enzyme (Hill and Fleming, 1982; Hill, 1989). Brain ChE can be determined by many techniques (Fairbrother et al., 1991), but either a laboratory norm must be developed for each species or a suitable enzyme reactivation technique must be used to determine the degree of inhibition. In cases of poisoning by OP compounds, ChE activity can be reactivated in vitro by the oxime 2-PAM (pyridine - 2- aldoxime methochloride) (Fairbrother et al., 1991). Carbamylated ChE is much less stable than phosphorylated ChE, therefore simple in vitro heat reactivation will serve as a rapid indicator of carbamate exposure (Hill and Fleming, 1982). These reactivation techniques provide important guidance for analytical chemistry.

Blood plasma or serum ChE may be used as a non-destructive technique for detection of anti-ChE exposure. As for brain ChE, the species-specifc norm must be developed for diagnostic reference. If ChE depression is below the lower end of normality, i.e., more than 2 standard deviations below the baseline mean, the subject is considered to have received significant exposure to anti-ChE compound (Ludke et al., 1975). Again, heat and 2-PAM reactivation may be used as provisional indicators of carbamate and OP ChE inhibition. These concepts have been reviewed in detail for wildlife including fish (Mineau, 1991).

14.6. Sublethal Environmental Hazard

Wild birds and mammals are relatively tolerant of low-level exposure to OPs (Grue *et al.*, 1991; Hill, 1995). This is partly because the chemicals are labile and readily excreted by warm-blooded animals. Also, low-grade exposure to anti-ChE may cause changes in synaptic physiology which may include reduction of both axonal release of ACh transmitter and the density of post-synaptic ACh receptors (Silver, 1974). It is interesting to note that birds have been reported to react to increase ACh or decamethonium (C_{10}) by muscle spasms—opisthotonus, convulsions and death. Paralytic death is less common (Zaimis, 1953). Effects of small doses of OP i.e. about 5% of the LD50 (essentially non-lethal but induces significant brain ChE inhibition) may reduce the core temperature as much as 2°C in homoiothemic animals acclimatised to moderate ambient conditions of 25–30°C. However, if the ambient temperature is abruptly shifted to mimic a cold front, the core temperature may drop as much as 3–6°C from the same dose (Ahdaya *et al.*, 1976; Chattopadhyay *et al.*, 1982; Rattner and Franson, 1984). However, it has been demonstrated that even under these chilled ambient conditions, the core temperature of OP-induced hypothemic animals returns to normal within about a day (Grue *et al.*, 1997). Generally, hypothermia occurs with brain ChE inhibition of about 50%, which is the degree of inhibition often associated with general physiologic deficit and sometimes death. Hypothermia is also associated with reduced metabolic efficiency which in turn may slow metabolic degradation and excretion of OP and thereby extend OP contact at receptor sites and enhance toxicity.

Hypothermic animals are more sensitive to OP poisoning than normal (Rattner and Franson, 1984; Rattner *et al.*, 1987). Young birds may be especially susceptible to OP interference with thermoregulation because many species are not fully homoiothermic for 1–3 weeks after hatching (Shilov, 1973). Interaction between OP and ambient chilling was studied with 14-day old northern bobwhites acclimatized to 35°C and then subjected to 27.5°C for 4 hours (Maguire and Williams, 1987). Brain ChE inhibition from a single dose of chlorpyrifos in the chilled chicks was depressed by about twice as much as in chicks maintained at 35°C. Both nestling and precocial chicks could be further compromised because parental care may be affected when the female is exposed to anti-ChE (Grue *et al.*, 1982; Brewer *et al.*, 1988). Temperatures below 15°C are common throughout the breeding season of birds and small mammals in temperate climates. Mechanisms of thermoregulation and the effect of anti-ChEs have been thoroughly reviewed (Grue *et al.*, 1991, 1997; Rattner and Fairbrother, 1991).

The ability of birds and mammals to capture prey or avoid predation after subacute exposure to OP pesticides has not been properly evaluated. Controlled experiments are difficult to interpret as treatment levels were usually based on a dose that rendered the subject, predator or prey, critically ill and often immobile. The results tend to be predictable, i.e., predators will not hunt and prey cannot escape. When OP levels that do not indicate overt toxicity are tested, predators and prey seem to respond normally. Field studies are hindered by uncertainty of the subjects exposure history and inability to follow movements and observe behavior of highly mobile or reclusive species. Radio-tracking has provided some insight into effects of OP on northern bobwhite survival, but not necessarily, cause of death. One-hundred and ninety-seven wild quail were captured, equipped with a small radio transmitter, dosed once with either 0, 2, 4, or 6 mg/kg of parathion-methyl, and their movements were monitored for 14 days (Buerger et al., 1991). Quail receiving the highest dosage had lower survival than did the controls, otherwise there were no apparent treatment effects. The authors concluded that reduced survivability was due to increased OP-induced vulnerabilty to predation.

Subacute exposure of birds and mammals to various OPs has been shown to affect an array of behaviours such as activity level, alertness, aggression, foraging and drinking, learning and memory, navigation, and reproduction (Peakall, 1985; Grue et al., 1991, 1997). Though most of these behavioural studies were well planned and have important theoretical implications for survivability, laboratory studies are highly restrictive and their projection to natural populations is speculative (Benne, 1994). There are two fundamental difficulties in the use of such tests: (1) the best studied and most easily performed and quantified have the least environmental relevance; and (2) the most relevant behaviors are the most strongly conserved against change (Walker et al., 1996).

14.7. OP Hazard: Chronicity and Reproduction

The chronic toxicity of OP pesticides has not been extensively studied on wildlife because such chemicals were believed to be too labile in nature to pose a serious sublethal hazard. However, as discussed earlier, some OPs such as phorate may remain available in the soil and vegetation for several months. They may be applied to wildlife habitat several times during the growing season which may coincide with critical periods of reproduction.

Specially designed research is needed to evaluate: (1) intermittent exposure from repeated pesticide application, (2) exposure of naive animals to pesticide application at different stages in the reproductive cycle (e.g., courtship, onset of lay, incubation), and (3) exposure to systemic pesticide in plant tissue.

Chronic studies of OP pesticides with wildlife were usually some modification of the standard reproduction trial developed for pesticide registration. These tests were developed for evaluation of more persistent chlorinated hydrocarbons and heavy metals. The studies, usually of mallards or northern bobwhites, expose first-time breeders to constant rate of chemical from several weeks prior to lay through chick hatchability and 2 week survival. Effect of OPs in these studies resulted in reduced feeding, corresponding weight loss, and marked reduction in oviposition. Pharmacologic action on the endocrine system has also been demonstrated (Grue *et al.*, 1991, 1997).

Some of the most acutely toxic OPs may also pose hazards to wildlife that have gone unnoticed. Monocrotophos has been implicated in some of the largest wildlife kills, but trivial residues have also been shown to depress egg production and hatchability in northern bobwhites (Schom and Abbott, 1974; Schom *et al.*, 1979). In another study with bobwhites, to determine how reproductively active birds responded to decreasing concentrations of OP as expected from a single application in nature (Stromborg, 1986), concentrations of 0.1–1.0 of monocrotophos per kilogram of diet were provided to breeding pairs. Then at 3-day intervals the basic concentration was either continued or reduced so that at the mid-point and at end of the 15-day study, the concentrations were reduced by 50 and 75%. Finally, all birds were fed untreated diet for 2 weeks. Food consumption and egg production decreased with increased concentrations. Inhibition of oviposition was not permanent and time to recovery was dose-related. In other studies of OPs on avian reproduction, effects are mediated by anorexia, again because mildly toxic OP concentrations were fed continuously (Bennett and Bennett, 1990; Bennett *et al.*, 1991).

The most important effect of OP pesticides on avian reproduction in nature, other than killing or incapacitating the parents, is the removal of the prey base (Grue *et al.*, 1983). When prey is depleted, birds may abandon nests and leave the area, or at least have more difficulty in caring for their young. Abandonment of the first nesting attempt is especially critical to population success because subsequent attempts are usually less successful (Bennett *et al.*, 1991). Some of the subtle effects of sublethal parental poisoning have been studied for a variety of free-living birds.

Female red-winged blackbirds were captured on their nests and given a single dose of parathion-methyl (0, 2.4, or 4.2 mg/kg) and then observed for 5 hours to record behavioural responses including times spent incubating. Each nest was then monitored. Females at the highest dose showed classic signs of acute anti-ChE poisoning, but they all recovered and there was no apparent effect on nest success (Meyers et al., 1990). In a similar study, European starlings (Sturnus vulgaris) were induced to nest in artificial nest boxes. When nestlings were 10 days old, the male parent was eliminated and the female parent was dosed once with dicrotophos at 2.5 mg/kg and her activities were monitored at 2-hour intervals for the next 3 days. OP-dosed females made fewer trips in search of food for their young and stayed away from their nests longer than did the controls. Nestlings of treated females lost significant amounts of weight, which could have affected their post-fledging success (Stromborg et al., 1988).

Though the potential for reduced prey availability may affect avian reproduction, neither decreased nestling growth nor fledgling success was detected for free-living passerines in spite of 50–70% depletion of primary insect prey due to aerial application of fenthion or trichlorfon (DeWeese et al., 1979; Powell, 1984). The importance of relative depletion of insect prey probably varies widely depending on prey abundance at the time of pesticide application and the size, mobility, and energy demands of the insectivore.

Studies of nest attentiveness or other breeding behavior in wild birds gave mixed results when subjects were dosed with OPs at rates producing 10–50% brain ChE inhibition, but without causing observable signs of toxicity. Sharp-tailed grouse (Tympanuchus phasianellus) given a single dose of malathion at 200 mg/kg were less effective in defending breeding territories on lakes (McEwen and Brown, 1966). One member per pair of incubating laughing gulls (Larus atricilla) was dosed once with parathion at 6 mg/kg and incubation behaviour was observed for 10-minute intervals throughout the day for 3 days. No effects on incubation were detected on the day of dosing, but parents dosed with parathion spent less time incubating on day 2 and the morning of day 3; activities appeared normal thereafter (White et al., 1983). This study was motivated by a natural event in which adult laughing gulls gathered parathion-poisoned insects in nearby cotton fields and either died leaving chicks to starve, or returned and poisoned the chicks through presentation of parathion-contaminated insects (White et al., 1979).

OP pesticides are not passed through the mother to the egg in biologically important amounts, but such pesticides may be deposited on the egg from parents feathers during incubation or from direct contamination by pesticide application.

Effects of such topical exposures have been studied extensively with northern bobwhite and mallard eggs at day 3 of incubation. Eggs were immersed for 30 seconds in aqueous emulsion or were dosed with a single topical application in nontoxic oil. OPs were shown to be as much as 18 times more toxic when applied to the shell in oil than when immersed in water (Hoffman and Albers, 1983).

14.8. Conclusions

Toxic OP esters enter anthropogenic and natural environments during pesticidal treatment for control of insect pests and disease vectors. About 200 OPs have been formulated into thousands of products in the world's marketplace for application to wetlands, rangelands, forests, cultivated crops, cities, and towns. OP use is a clear risk to human health as they are responsible for an inordinately large proportion of pesticide-related hospitalisations throughout the world.

Though most of the OP applications target cropland and other terrestrial habitats, the chemicals and toxic degradates are inevitably detected in aquatic systems and affect a much larger number of species than originally intended. Significant concentrations of OP residues are sometimes detected in ground water including well water for human consumption. Most OP pesticides are acutely toxic to invertebrates with a cholinergic-dependent nervous system and all vertebrates, but OPs are comparatively labile in nature and the effects of even multiple applications on species diversity, abundance, and total biomass are not well-understood.

The more extensively used OPs require only brief exposure to kill or incapacitate most animals. Thus, the environmental effect most often reported is episodes of acute exposure and large-scale mortality of fish or other vertebrate wildlife. Little attention has been given to evaluation of sublethal effects of OP on the reproduction or behaviour of wildlife or on the effects of chemical interactions and formulated end-use products on toxicity. It may be of particular importance that a large proportion of agricultural applications of OPs coincides with avian reproduction. Birds may be differentially susceptible to OP exposure at various times during the reproduction cycle.

OPs are comparatively labile and are efficiently metabolised by most vertebrates, but their environmental presence may be extended in acidic medium such as soils, sediments, and water common to regions prone to acid precipitation. Persistence of such pesticides is also enhanced when incorporated in soils or when applied as granular products.

Continued hazard in both aquatic and terrestrial systems is documented for months after application in association with storm events leading to puddling or run-off into streams and ponds. There is also a potential hazard to grazing vertebrates.

Classic secondary poisoning of birds and mammals such as occurs with stable lipophilic chlorinated hydrocarbons does not occur with OP pesticides. Instead, the prey or carrion is simply the conduit for exposure to unaltered chemical. That is, OP in the gastrointestinal tract of birds and mammals, mucus covering of aquatic animals, and mucus or cuticle of invertebrates is the more likely source of exposure than active anti-ChE in post-absorptive tissues.

Prevention of OP hazards to wildlife requires evaluation of each pesticidal product, the rate and method of application, the stability and fate in the target habitat, and the likely entrance into wetlands and other aquatic systems. OP hazard is most often after acute exposure and the cause of localised mortality to both aquatic and terrestrial animals, but the potential effects of sublethal exposure should not be trivialized.

Regulations protecting human and livestock health from OP exposure undoubtedly benefit wildlife. But human and livestock activities can be controlled to reduce the likelihood of exposure, whereas wildlife activities cannot. The question is whether uncontrollable incidental exposure constitutes an unacceptable hazard to the wildlife populations. There is no doubt that protection of aquatic and terrestrial ecosystems and wildlife from OP hazard will also benefit humans directly and indirectly from the perspective of aesthetics and quality of the environment.

References

Abou-Donia, M.B. Organophosphous ester-induced delayed neurotoxicity. *Annual Review of Pharmacology and Toxicology* 1981;**21**:511–48.

Ahdaya, S.M., Shar, F.V., Guthrie, F.E. Thermoregulation in mice treated with parathion, carbaryl, or DDT. *Toxicology and Applied Toxicology* 1976;**35**:575–80.

Ball, W.I., Sinclair, I.W., Crevier, M., *et al.* Modification of parathion's toxicity for rats by pretreatment with chlorinated hydrocarbon insecticides. *Canadian Journal of Biochemistry and Physiology* 1954;**32**:440–5.

Ballantyne, B., Marrs, T.C. Clinical toxicology by geographical regions. In: *Clinical and Experimental Toxicology of Organophosphates and Carbamates.* Ballantyne, B., Marrs, T.C. eds.Oxford: Butterworth–Heinemann Ltd; 1992. p. 461–510.

Baril, A., Jobin, B., Mineau, F., *et al.* A Consideration of Inter-Species Variability in the Use of the Median Lethal Dose (LD50) in Avian Risk Assessment. *Technical Report Series 216. Headquarters, Canadian Wildlife Service*: Hill, Quebec .1994.

Bartholomew, G.A., Cade, T.I. The water economy of land birds. *Auk* 1963;**80**:504–39.

Bascietto, I. Hazard Evaluation Division Standard Evaluation Procedure: Avian Single-dose Oral LD50. EPA-540/9-85-007- *U.S. Environmental Protection Agency.* Washington, D.C. 1985a.

Bascietto, I. Hazard Evaluation Division Standard Evaluation Procedure: Avian Dietary LC50 Test. EPA-540/9-85-008. *U.S. Environmental Protection Agency:* Washington, D.C. 1985b.

Bennett, J.K., Bennett, RS. Effects of dietary methyl parathion on northern bobwhite egg production and eggshell quality. *Environmental Toxicology and Chemistry* 1990;**9**:1481–5.

Bennett, R.S. Do behavioral responses to pesticide exposure effect wildlife population parameters? In: *Wildlife Toxicology and Population Modeling: Integrated Studies of Agroecosystems.* Kendall, R.I., Lacher, T.E., Jr. eds.,: Lewis Publishers; Boca Raton Florida 1994. p. 241–50.

Bennett, R.S., Williams, B.A., Schmedding, D.W., *et al.* Effects of dietary exposure to methyl parathion on egg laying and incubation in mallards. *Environmental Toxicology and Chemistry* 1991;**10**:501–7.

Best, L.B., Fischer, D.L. Granular insecticides and birds: Factors to be considered in understanding exposure and reducing risk. Environmental Toxicology and Chemistry 1991;**11**:1495–508.

Blus, L.I. Organochlorine pesticides. In: *Handbook of Ecotoxicology.* Hoffman, D.I., Rattner, B.A., Burton, G.A., Jr., Cairns, I., Jr. eds. CRC Press, Inc; Boca Raton, Florida. 1995. p. 275–300.

Blus, L.I., Staley, C.S., Henny, C.I., *et al.* Effects of organophosphorus insecticides on sage grouse in southeastern Idaho. *Journal of Wildlife Management* 1989;**53**:1139–46.

Bowman, I.S., Casida, I.E. Further studies on the metabolism of Thimet by plants, insects, and mammals. *Journal of Economic Entomology* 1958;**51**:838–43.

Brealey, C.J., Walker, C.H., Baldwin, B.C. A-esterase activities in relation to the differential toxicity of pirimiphos-methyl to birds and mammals. *Pesticide Science* 1980;**11**:546–54.

Brewer, L.W., Driver, C.J., Kendall, R.J., *et al.* Effects of methyl parathion in ducks and duck broods. *Environmental Toxicology and Chemistry* 1988;7:375–9.

Briggs, S.A.   *Basic Guide to Pesticides: Their Characteristics and Hazards.* Washington, D.C: Taylor and Francis; 1992.

Buerger, T.T., Kendall, R.J., Mueller, B.S., *et al.* Effects of methyl parathion on northern bobwhite survivability. *Environmental Toxicology and Chemistry* 1991;**10**:527–32.

Chattopadhyay, D.P., Dighe, S.K., Dube, D.K., *et al.* Changes in toxicity of DDVP, DFP, and parathion in rats under cold environment. *Bulletin of Environmental Contamination and Toxicology* 1982;**29**:605–10.

Cholakis, J.M., McKee, M.J., Wong, L.C.K., *et al.* Acute and subacute toxicity of pesticides in microtine rodents. In: *Avian and Mammalian Wildlife Toxicology: Second Conference, ASTM STP757.* Lamb, D.W., Kenaga, E.E. eds. American Society for Testing and Materials; Philadelphia. 1981. p. 143–54.

Corbett, J.R, Wright, K., Baillie, A.C.   *The Biochemical Mode of Action of Pesticides.* Academic Press Inc: London; 1984.

Dahl, T.   *Wetland Lasses in the United States-1780s to 1980s.* Washington, D.C.: U.S. Fish and Wildlife Service; 1990.

DeWeese, L.R, Henny, C.J., Floyd, R.L., *et al. Response of Breeding Birds to Aerial Sprays of Trichlorfon (Dylox) and Carbaryl (Sevin-4-Oil) in Montana Forests. Fish and Wildlife Service Special Scientific Report Wildlife 224.* Washington, D.C.: U.S. Fish and Wildlife Service; 1979.

DeWeese, L.R. McEwen, L.C., Settinri. L.A., *et al.* Effects on birds of fenthion aerial application for mosquito control. *Journal of Economic Entomology* 1983;**76**:906–11.

Driver, C.J., Ligotke. M.W., Van Voris, P., *et al.* Routes of uptake and their relative contribution to the toxicological response of northern bobwhite (Colinus virginianus) to an organophosphate pesticide. *Environmental Toxicology and Chemistry* 1991;**10**:21–33.

DuBois, K.P.   Potentiation of the toxicity of organophosphorus compounds. *Advances in Pest Control Research* 1961;**4**:117–51.

Durham, W.F. The interaction of pesticides with other factors. *Residue Reviews,* 1967;**18**:21–103.

Ecobichon, D.J. Organophosphorus ester insecticides. In: *Pesticides and Neurological Diseases*, 2nd ed Ecobichon, D.J., Joy, R.M. eds. CRC Press, Inc; Boca Raton, Florida. 1994. p. 171–249.

Ecobichon, D.J. Toxic effects of pesticides. In: *Casarett and Doull's Toxicology: The Basic Science of Poisons*, 5th edition. Klaassen, C.D., Amdur, M.O., Doull, J. eds.: McGraw-Hill; New York. 1996. p. 643–89.

Edwards, C.A., Fisher, S.W. The use of cholinesterase measurements in assessing the impacts of pesticides on terrestrial and aquatic invertebrates. In: *Cholinesterase-inhibiting Insecticides: Their Impact on Wildlife and the Environment.* Mineau, P. ed.Amsterdam: Elsevier; 1991. p. 255–75.

Edwards. C.A. The impact of pesticides in the environment. In: *The Pesticide Question: Environment, Economics, and Ethics.* Pimentel, D., Lehman, H. eds. Routledge, Chapman & Hall, Inc; New York. 1993. p. 1346.

Eto, M. *Organophosphorus Pesticides: Organic and Biological Chemistry.* Cleveland, Ohio: CRC Press, Inc; 1974.

Fairbrother, A. Cholinesterase-inhibiting pesticides. In: *Noninfectious Diseases of Wildlife.* 2nd ed. Fairbrother, A., Locke, L.N., Holf, G.L., eds. Ames, University Press; Iowa. 1996. p. 52–60.

Fairbrother, A., Mardin, B.T., Bennett, J.K., *et al.* Methods used in determination of cholinesterase activity. In: Mineau, P. ed. *Cholinesterase-inhibiting Insecticides: Their Impact on Wildlife and the Environment.* Amsterdam: Elsevier; 1991. p. 35–71.

Flickinger, E.L., Mitchell, C.A., White, D.H., *et al.* Bird poisoning from misuse of the carbamate Furadan in a Texas rice field. *Wildlife Society, Bulletin* 1986;**14**:59–62.

Gaines, T.B. Acute toxicity of pesticides. *Toxicology and Applied Pharmacology,* 1969;**14**:515–34.

Gaines, T.B. The acute toxicity of pesticides to rats. *Toxicology and Applied Pharmacology* 1960;**2**:88–99.

Getzin, L.W., Chapman, R.K. The fate of phorate in soils. *Journal of Economic Entomology* 1960;**53**:47–51.

Getzin, L.W., Shanks, C.H. Persistence, degradation, and bioactivity of phorate and its oxidative analogues in soil. *Journal of Economic Entomology* 1970;**63**:52–8.

Gionfriddo. J.P., Best, L.B. Grit color selection by house sparrows and northern bobwhite. *Journal of Wildlife Management* 1996;**60**:836–42.

Goldstein M.I., Woodbridge, B., Zaccagnini, M.E., *et al.* An assessment of mortality of Swainson's Hawks on wintering grounds in Argentina. *Raptor Research* 1996;**30**:106–7.

Gordon, J.J., Leadbeater, L., Maidment, M.P. The protection of animals against organophosphate poisoning by pretreatment with a carbamate. *Toxicology and Applied Pharmacology* 1978;**43**:207–16.

Grue, C.E., De Weese, L.R, Mineau, P., *et al.* Potential impacts of agricultural chemicals on waterfowl and other wildlife inhabiting prairie wetlands: An evaluation of research needs and approaches. *Transactions of the North American Wildlife and Natural Resources Conference* 1986;**51**:357–83.

Grue, C.E., Fleming, W.J., Busby, D.G., *et al.* Assessing hazards of organophosphatae pesticides to wildlife. *Transactions of the North American Wildlife and Natural Resources Conference* 1983;**48**:200–20.

Grue, C.E., Gibert, P.L., Seeley, M.E. Neurophysiological and behavioural changes in non-target wildlife exposed to organophosphate and carbamate pesticides: Thermoregulation, food consumption, and reproduction. *American Zoologist*, 1997;**37**:369–88.

Grue, C.E., Hart, A.D.M., Mineau, P. Biological consequences of depressed brain cholinesterase in wildlife. In: *Cholinesterase-inhibiting Insecticides: Their Impact on Wildlife and the Environment.* Mineau, P. ed. Elsevier Science Publishers; 1991. Amsterdam. p. 151–209.

Grue, C.E., Powell, G.V.N., McChesney, M.J. Care of nestlings by wild female starlings exposed to an organophosphate pesticide. *Journal of Applied Ecology*, 1982;**19**:327–35.

Grue, C.E., Tome, M. W-., Swanson, G.A., *et al.* Agricultural chemicals and the quality of prairie pothole wetlands for adult and juvenile waterfowl—what are the concerns? In Proceedings of the National Symposium on Protection of Wetlands from Agricultural Impacts, (P.J. Stuber), Biological Report 88 (16). U.S. Fish and Wildlife Service: Washington, D.C. 1988. p. 55–64.

Hall, A.H., Rumack, B.H. Incidence, presentation and therapeutic attitudes to anticholinesterase poisoning in the USA. In: *Clinical and Experimental Toxicology of Organophosphates and Carbamates.* Ballantyne, B., Marrs, T.C. eds. Butterworth–Heinemann Ltd; Oxford.1992. p. 471–81.

Hamilton, A.D., Ruthven, D.A., Findlay, E., *et al.* Wildlife deaths in Scotland resulting from misuse of agricultural chemicals. *Biological Conservation* 1981;**21**:315–26.

Hamilton, G.A., Hunter, K., Ritchie, A.S., *et al.* Wild geese by carbophenothion-treated winter wheat. *Pesticide Science* 1976;**7**:175–83.

Hardy, A.R., Fletcher, M.R, Stanley, P.I. Pesticides and wildlife: Twenty years of vertebrate wildlife investigations by MAFF. *State Veterinary Journal* 1986;**40**:182–92.

Heath, R.G., Stickel, L.F. Protocol for testing the acute and relative toxicity of pesticides to penned birds. In: *The Effects of Pesticides on Wildlife.* U.S. Department of Interior: Washington, D.C. 1965. p. 18–24.

Henny, C.J., Blus, L.J., Kolbe, E.J., *et al.* Organophosphate insecticide (famphur) topically applied to cattle kills magpies and hawks. *Journal of Wildlife Management* 1985;**49**:648–58.

Henny, C.J., Kolbe, E.J., Hill, E.F., *et al.* Case histories of bald eagles and other raptors killed by organophosphorus insecticides applied to livestock. *Journal of Wildlife Diseases* 1987;**23**:292–5.

Hill, E.F. Acute and subacute toxicology in evaluation of pesticide hazard to avian wildlife. In: *Wildlife Toxicology and Population Modeling: Integrated Studies of Agroecosystems.* Kendall, R.J., Lacher, T.E. Jr. eds. Lewis Publishers; 1994. Boca Raton, Florida. p. 207–26.

Hill, E.F. Caution: Standardized Acute Toxicity Data May Mislead. *Research Information Bulletin, U.S. Fish and Wildlife Service*: Washington, D.C. 1986.

Hill, E.F. Divergent effects of postmortem ambient temperature on organophosphorus- and carbamate- inhibited brain cholinesterase activity in birds. *Pesticide Biochemistry and Physiology* 1989;**33**:264–75.

Hill, E.F. Organophosphorus and carbamate pesticides. In: *Handbook of Ecotoxicology..* Hoffman, D.J., Rattner, B.A., Burton, G.A., Jr., Cairns, J., Jr. eds. CRC Press, Inc; 1995 Boca Raton, Florida. p. 243–74.

Hill, E.F. Wildlife toxicology. In: *General and Applied Toxicology.* Vol. 2, 2nd ed. Ballantyne, B., Marrs, T.C., Syversen, T. eds. Macmillan Reference Ltd; London: 1999. p. 1327–63.

Hill, E.F. Avian toxicology of anticholinesterases. In: *Clinical and Experimental Toxicology of Organophosphates and Carbamates.* Ballantyne, B., Marrs, T.C. eds. Butterworth–Heinemann Ltd; Oxford.1992. p. 272–94.

Hill, E.F., Fleming, W.L. Anticholinesterase poisoning of birds: Field monitoring and diagnosis of acute poisoning. *Environmental Toxicology and Chemistry* 1982;**1**:27–38.

Hill, E.F., Camardese, M.B. Lethal Dietary Toxicities of Environmental Contaminants and Pesticides to Coturnix. *Fish and Wildlife Technical Report 2. U.S. Fish and Wildlife Service:* Washington, D.C. 1986.

Hill, E.F., Camardese, M.B. Toxicity of anticholinesterase insecticides to birds: technical grade versus granular formulations. *Ecotoxicology and Environmental Safety* 1984;**8**:551–63.

Hill, E.F., Heath, R.G., Spann, J. W., *et al.* Lethal Dietary Toxicities of Environmental Pollutants to Birds. *Fish and Wildlife Service Special Scientific Report Wildlife 191. U.S. Fish and Wildlife Service:* Washington, D.C. 1975.

Hill, E.F., Mendenhall, V.M. Secondary poisoning of barn owls with famphur, an organophosphate insecticide. *Journal of Wildlife Management* 1980;**44**:676–81.

Hoffman, D.J. Embryotoxicity and teratogenicity of environmental contaminants to bird eggs. *Reviews of Environmental Contamination and Toxicology*, 1990;**115**:40–89.

Hoffman, D.J., Albers, P.H. Evaluation of potential embryotoxicity and teratogenicity of 42 herbicides, insecticides, and petroleum contaminants to mallard eggs. *Archives of Environmental Contamination and Toxicology* 1983;**13**:15–27.

Hoffman, D.J., Eastin, W.C., Jr. Effects of malathion, diazinon, and parathion on mallard embryo development and cholinesterase activity. *Environmental Research*, 1981;**26**:472–85.

Hoffman, D.J., Rattner, B.A, Burton, G.A, Jr, *et al.* Introduction. In: *Handbook of Ecotoxicology.* Hoffman, D.J., Rattner, B., Burton, G.A., Jr., Cairns, J. Jr. eds. CRC Press, Inc; 1995. Boca Raton, Florida. p. 1–10.

Hoffman, D.J., Sileo, L., Murray. H.C. Subchronic organophosphorus ester-induced delayed neurotoxicity in mallards. *Toxicology and Applied Pharmacology* 1984;**75**:128–36.

Hudson, R.H., Tucker, RK., Haegele, M.A *Handbook of Toxicity of Pesticides to Wildlife*, 2nd ed. Resource Publication 137. U.S. Fish and Wildlife Services: Washington, D.C. 1984.

Johnson, W.W., Finley, M.T. *Handbook of Toxicity of Pesticides to Wildlife.* Resource Publication 153. U.S. Fish and Wildlife Service: Washington, D.C. 1980.

Kenaga, E.E. Predicted bioconcentration factors and soil sorption coefficients ofpesticides and other chemicals. *Ecotoxicology and Environmental Safety* 1980;**4**:26–38.

Kilpatrick, J.W. Performance specifications for ultra low volume aerial application ofinsecticides for mosquito control. *Pest Control* 1967;**35**:80–4.

Kreitzer, J.F., Spann, J.W. Tests of pesticidal synergism with young pheasants and Japanese quail. *Bulletin of Environmental Contamination and Toxicology* 1973;**9**:250–6.

Kundiev, Y.I., Kagan, Y.S. Anticholinesterase used in the USSR: poisoning, treatment and preventable measures. In: *Clinical and Experimental Toxicology of Organophophates and Carbamates.* Ballantyne, B., Marrs, T.C. eds. Butterworth–Heinemann Ltd; Oxford: 1992. p. 494–501.

Lichtenstein, E.P., Liang, T.T., Fuhrman, T.W. A compartmentalized microcosm for studying the fate of chemicals in the environment. *Journal of Agriculture and Food Chemistry*, 1978;**26**:948–78.

Organophosphates and Health

Loomis, T.A., Hayes, A.W. *Essentials of Toxicology*, 4th ed. San Diego, California: Academic Press Inc; 1996.

Ludke, J.L. DDE increases the toxicity of parathion to coturnix quail. *Pesticide Biochemistry and Physiology* 1977;7:28–33.

Ludke, J.L., Hill, E.F., Dieter, M.P. Cholinesterase (ChE) response and related mortality among birds fed ChE inhibitors. *Archives of Environmental Contamination and Toxicology* 1975;3:1–21.

Maguire, C.C., Williams, B.A. Cold stress and acute organophosphorus exposure: interaction effects in juvenile northern bobwhites. *Archives of Environmental Contamination and Toxicology* 1987;16:477–81.

Mason, J.R. Repellents in Wildlife Management: Proceedings of a Symposium. U.S. Department of Agriculture: Fort Collins, Colorado. 1997.

Matsumura, F. *Toxicology of Insecticides*. Plenum: New York.

Mayer, F.L., Jr., Ellersieck, M.R. *Manual of Acute Toxicity: Interpretation and Data Base for 410 Chemicals and 66 Species of Freshwater Animals*. Resource Publication 160. U.S. Fish and Wildlife Service: Washington, D.C. 1985.

McEwen, L.C., Brown, R.L. Acute toxicity of dieldrin and malathion. *Journal of Wildlife Management,* 1966;30:604–11.

Mendelssohn, H., Paz, U. Mass mortality of birds of prey by Azodrin, an organophosphorus insecticide. *Biological Conservation,* 1977;11:163–70.

Menzer, RE. Effect of chlorinated hydrocarbons in the diet on the toxicity of several organophosphorus insecticides. *Toxicology and Applied Pharmacology* 1970;16:446–52.

Meyers, S.M., Cummings, J.L., Bennett, RS. Effects of methyl parathion on red-winged blackbird (*Agelaius phoeniceus*) incubation behavior and nesting success. *Environmental Toxicology and Chemistry* 1990;9:807–13.

Mineau, P. *Cholinesterase-inhibiting Insecticides: Their Impact on Wildlife and the Environment*. Amsterdam: Elsevier Science Publishers; 1991.

Mineau, P., Fletcher, M.R, Glaser, L.C., *et al.* Poisoning of raptors with organophosphorus and carbamte pesticides with emphasis on Canada. *U.S. and U.K. Journal of Raptor Research* 1999;30:1–37.

Mineau, P., Jobin, B., Baril, A. A Critique of the Avian 5-Day Dietary Test (LD50) as the Basis of Avian Risk Assessment. *Technical Report Series 215. Headquarters, Canadian Wildlife Service*: Hull, Quebec. 1994.

Mitchell, T.H., Ruzicka, J.R, Thomson, J., *et al.* The chromatographic determination of organophosphorus pesticides. *Journal of Chromatography,* 1968;32:17–32.

Murty, A.S., Ramani, A.V. Toxicity of anticholinesterases to aquatic organisms. In: *Clinical and Experimental Toxicology of Organophosphates and Carbamates.* Ballantyne, B., Marrs, T.C. eds. Butterworth–Heinemann Ltd; 1992. Oxford. p. 305–17

O'Brien, R.D. *Insecticides: Action and Metabolism.* New York: Academic Press; 1967.

Osteen, C. Pesticide use trends and issues in the United States. In: *The Pesticide Question: Environment, Economics, and Ethics.* Pimentel, D., Lehman, H. eds. Routledge, Chapman & Hall, Inc; 1993. New York. p. 307–36.

Pan, H.P., Fouts, J.R. Drug metabolism in birds. *Drug Metabolism Reviews* 1978;**7**:1–253.

Pan, H.P., Fouts, J.R., Devereux, T.R. Hepatic microsomal N-hydroxylation of p-chloraniline and p-chloro-N-methylaniline in red-winged blackbirds compared with rat. *Xenobiotica* 1979;**9**:441–6.

Peakall, D.B. Behavioural responses of birds to pesticides and other contaminants. *Residue Reviews* 1985;**96**:45–77.

Powell, G.V.N. Reproduction by an altricial songbird, the red-winged blackbird, in fields treated with the organophosphate insecticide fenthion. *Journal of Applied Ecology* 1984;**21**:83–95.

Ramade, F. *Ecotoxicology.* New York: John Wiley & Sons; 1987.

Rattner, B.A, Becker, J.M., Nakatsugaway, T. Enhancement of parathion toxicity to quail by heat and cold exposure. *Pesticide Biochemistry and Physiology* 1987;**27**:330–9.

Rattner, B.A., Fairbrother, A. Biological variability and the influence of stress on cholinesterase activity. In: *Cholinesterase-inhibiting Insecticides: Their Impact on Wildlife and the Environment.* Mineau, P. ed. Elsevier Science Publishers; 1991. Amsterdam. p. 107.

Rattner, B.A., Franson, J.C. Methyl parathion and fenvalerate toxicity in American kestrels: acute physiological responses and effects of cold. *Canadian Journal of Physiology and Pharmacology* 1984;**62**:787–92.

Rattner, B.A., Heath, A.B. Environmental factors affecting contaminant toxicity in aquatic and terrestrial vertebrates. In: *Handbook of Ecotoxicology.* Hoffman, D.J., Rattner, B.A., Burton, G.A., Jr., Cairns. J. Jr. eds. CRC Press, Inc; 1995. Boca Raton, Florida. p. 519–35.

Richter, E.D. Aerial application and spray drift of anticholinesterases: protective measures. In: *Clinical and Experimental Toxicity of Organophosphates and Carbamates.* Ballantyne, B., Marrs, T.C. eds. Butterworth–Heinemann Ltd; 1992. Oxford. p. 623–31.

Robbins, C.T. *Wildlife Feeding and Nutrition.* Academic Press; New York:1983.

Ruzicka, J.H., Thomson, J., Wheals, B.B. The gas chronatographic determination of organophosphorus pesticides. II. A comparative study of hydrolysis rates. *Journal of Chromatography* 1967;**31**:37–47.

Sanderson, D.M., Edson, E.F. Toxicological properties of the organophosphorus insecticide dimethoate. *British Journal of Medicine,* 1964;**21**:52–64.

Schafer, E.W. The acute oral toxicity of 369 pesticidal, pharmaceutical, and other chemicals to wild birds. *Toxicology and Applied Pharmacology,* 1972;**21**:315–30.

Schafer, E.W., Bowles, W.A, Jr. Acute oral toxicity and repellancy of 933 chemicals to house and deer mice. *Archives of Environmental Contamination and Toxicology,* 1985;**14**:11–29.

Schafer, E.W., Bowles, W.A, Jr., Hurlbut, I. The acute oral toxicity, repellancy, and hazard potential of 998 chemicals to one or more species of wild and domestic birds. *Archives of Environmental Contamination and Toxicology* 1983;**12**:355–82.

Schom, C.B., Abbot, U.K. Studies with bobwhite quail: reproduction characteristics. *Poultry Science,* 1974;**53**:1860–5.

Schom, C.B., Abbot, U.K., Welker, N.E. Adult and embryo responses to organophosphate pesticide: Azodrin. *Poultry Science,* 1979;**58**:60–6.

Seabloom, R.W., Pearson, G.L., Oring, L.W., *et al.* An incident of fenthion mosquito control and subsequent avian mortality. *Journal of Wildlife Diseases,* 1973;**9**:18–20.

Senanayake, N., Karalliedde, L. Neurotoxic effects of organophosphorus insecticides. *New England Journal of Medicine,* 1987;**316**:761–3.

Senanayake, N., Karalliedde, L. Intermediate syndrome in anticholinesterase neurotoxicity. In: *Clinical and Experimental Toxicity of Organophosphates and Carbamates.* Ballantyne, B., Marrs, T.C. eds. Butterworth–Heinemann Ltd; 1992. Oxford. p. 126–31.

Sheehan, P.I., Baril, A., Mineau, P., *et al.* The Impact of Pesticides on the Ecology of Prairie Nesting Ducks. *Technical Report Series Number 19. Canadian Wildlife Service:* Ottawa. 1987.

Shilov, L.A. *Heat Regulation in Birds.* Anlerind Publishing; New Delhi: 1973.

Silver, A. The biology of cholinesterases. *Frontiers of Biology* 1974;**36**:1–449.

Singh, G., Singh, Z. Persistence and movement of phorate at high concentrations in soil. *Ecotoxicology and Environmental Safety* 1984;**8**:540–8.

Smith, G.L.   Pesticide Use and Toxicology in Relation to Wildlife: Organophosphorus and Carbamate Compounds. *Resource Publication 170. U.S. Fish and Wildlife Service*: Washington, D.C. 1987.

Stafford, T.R, Best, L.B., Fischer, D.L.   Effects of different formulations of granular pesticides on birds. *Environmental Toxicology and Chemistry*, 1996;**15**:1606–11.

Stafford, T.R., Best, L.B.   Effects of application rate on avian risk from granular pesticides. *Environmental Toxicology and Chemistry*, 1998;**3**:526–9.

Stickel, W.H.   Some effects of pollutants in terrestrial ecosystems. In: *Ecological Toxicology Research*. McIntyre, A.D., Mills, C.F. eds. Plenum Publishing Company; 1975. New York. p. 25–74.

Stinsen, E.R., Bromely, P.T.   Pesticides and Wildlife: A Guide to Reducing Impacts on Animals and Their Habitats. Publication 420-004. *Virginia Department of Game and Inland Fisheries:* Richmond, Virginia. 1991.

Stinsen. E.R., Hayes, L.E., Bush, P.B., *et al.*   Carbofuran affects wildlife on Virginia corn fields. *Wildlife Society Bulletin*, 1994;**22**:566–75.

Stone, W.B., Gradoni, P.B.   Wildlife mortality related to use of the pesticide diazinon. *Northeastern Environmental Science*, 1985;**4**:30–8.

Stromborg, K.L.   Reproductive toxicity by monocrotophos to bobwhite quail. *Poultry Science* 1986;**65**:51–7.

Stromborg, K.L.   Seed treatment pesticide effects on pheasant reproduction at sublethal doses. *Journal of Wildlife Management* 1977;**41**:632–42.

Stromborg, K.L., Grue, C.E., Nichols, I.D., *et al.*   Post-fledging survival of European starlings exposed as nestlings to an organophosphorus insecticide. *Ecology* 1988;**69**:590–601.

Takahashi, H., Kato, A, Yamashita, E., *et al.*   Potentiations of N-methylcarbamate toxicities by organophosphorus insecticides in male mice. *Fundamental and Applied Toxicology* 1987;**8**:139–46.

Tome, M.W., Grue, C.E., DeWeese, L.R.   Ethyl parathion in wetlands following aerial application to sunflowers in North Dakota. *Wildlife Society Bulletin* 1991;**19**:450–7.

Tome, M.W., Grue, C.E., Henry, M.G.   Case studies: Effects of agricultural pesticides on waterfowl and prairie pothole wetlands. In: *Handbook of Ecotoxicology*. Hoffman, D.J., Rattner, B.A., Burton, G.A., Jr., Cairns, J., Jr. eds. CRC Press, Inc.; 1995. Boca Raton, Florida. p. 565–76.

Triolo, A.I., Coon, J.M.   Toxicological interactions of chlorinated hydrocarbon and organophosphate insecticides. *Journal of Agricultural and Food Chemistry* 1966;**14**:549–54.

US EPA (1986). Intent to cancel registrations on denial of applications for registration of pesticide products containing diazinon; Conclusion of special review. Federal Register, 51, 35034-35046. US EPA (1991). Formal Request for Endangered Species Act Section 7 Consultation on 3 Pesticides for All Uses, On All Listed Species. *Office of Pesticides and Toxic Substances. U.S. Environmental Protection Agency.* Washington, D.C.

US EPA. Ecological Effects Test Guidelines. EPA-712-C-96-139. *U.S. Environmental Protection Agency.* Washington, D.C. 1996.

Van der Valk, A. *Northern Prairie Wetlands.* Iowa State University Press. 1989.

Walker, C.H. Species differences in microsonal monooxygenase, and their relationship to biological half lives. *Drug Metabolism Reviews,* 1978;**7**:295–323.

Walker, C.H. Species variation in some hepatic microsonal enzymes. *Progress in Drug Metabolism* 1980;**9**:211–26.

Walker, C.H., Hopkins, S.P., Sibly, R.M., *et al. Principals of Ecotoxicology.* London: Taylor and Francis, Ltd; 1996.

Ware, G.W., Estesen, B.I., Cahill, W.B. Pesticide drift: 1. High clearance versus aerial application of sprays. *Journal of Economic Entomology* 1969;**62**:840–3.

Westlake, G.E., Bun. van, P.I., Martin, A.D., *et al.* Organophosphate poisoning. Effects of selected organophosphate pesticides on plasma enzymes and brain esterases of Japanese quail (*Coturnix coturnix japonica*). *Journal of Agriculture and Food Chemistry,* 1981a;**29**:772–8.

Westlake, G.E., Bunyan, P.I., Martin, A.D., *et al.* Carbamate poisoning. Effects of selected carbamate pesticides on plasma enzymes and brain esterases of Japanese quail (*Coturnix coturnix japonica*). *Journal of Agriculture and Food Chemistry,* 1981b;**29**:779–85.

White, D.H., Mitchell, C.A., Kolbe, E.I., *et al.* Parathion alters incubation behavior of laughing gulls. *Bulletin of Environmental Contamination and Toxicology,* 1983;**31**:93–7.

White, D-H., King, K.A, Mitchell, C.L, *et al.* Parathion causes secondary poisoning in a laughing gull breeding colony. *Bulletin of Environmental Contamination and Toxicology,* 1979;**23**:281–4.

Zaimis, E.I. Motor end plate differences as a determining factors in the mode of action of neuromuscular blocking substances. *Journal of Physiology* 1953;**22**:238–51

Zinkl , J.G., Jessup. D.A., Bischoff, A.I., *et al.* Fenthion poisoning of wading birds. *Journal of Wildlife Diseases* 1981;**17**:117–9.

CHAPTER 15

Biochemical and Toxicological Investigations Related to OP Compounds

R. Swaminathan and Brian Widdop

SECTION A- Biochemical Investigations

15.1. Introduction

Exposure to organophosphorous (OP) compounds can be diagnosed either by detecting the compounds, their metabolites in biological specimens (blood, urine etc) (see below) or by their effects. Organophosphorous compounds produce their effect by covalently binding to cholinesterases at their anionic binding site for acetylcholine, changing the cholinesterases to enzymatically inactive proteins. This inhibition is irreversible and leads to accumulation of acetylcholine at synapses causing overstimulation and subsequent disruption of nerve impulses in both peripheral and central nervous systems (Bardin *et al.,* 1994; O'Malley, 1997). Exposure to OP compounds could be diagnosed by measuring the activity of the enzyme cholinesterase.

15.2. Cholinesterase

15.2.1. Introduction

Cholinesterases (ChE) are a group of enzymes that hydrolyse choline esters faster than other esters under optimal conditions. There are two types of ChE in the body. Acetylcholinesterase (AChE) or acetylcholine acetylhydrolase (EC3.1.1.7) also known as true, specific, genuine or type 1 ChE, is found in all excitable tissues, both peripheral and central, spleen, placenta and erythrocytes. AChE, a membrane bound glycoprotein of molecular weight of 80,000, exists in several molecular forms. The major physiological role of AChE is to hydrolyse the neurotransmitter acetylcholine (ACh) at cholinergic nerve endings in synapses and in effector organs. The second ChE is called Pseudo-cholinesterase (BuChE) or acylcholineacylhydrolase (EC 3.1.1.8) and is also known as plasma/serum, benzoyl, false, butyryl, non specific or type II ChE.

In addition to plasma it is also present widely: in liver, smooth muscle, intestinal mucosa, pancreas, heart and peripheral and central nervous system (Davis *et al.,* 1997). BuChE in plasma is synthesised by the liver. The true physiological function of BuChE is not known (Brown *et al.,* 1981). Postulated functions of BuChE include a role in the transmission of slow nerve impulses, in lipid metabolism, a regulatory role in choline homeostasis, role in permeability of membranes, in the protection of foetus from toxic compounds, a role in the degradation of acetylcholine (Norel *et al.,* 1993) and in tumourigenesis (Soreq *et al.,* 1991).

BuChE is made up of four identical subunits, the molecular weight of each subunit being 85,000. The two enzymes AChE and BuChE show different biochemical properties (Table 15.1). AChE shows high affinity for ACh and low affinity for non choline esters, whereas BuChE has low affinity for ACh.

Table 15.1. Differences between two subgroups of cholinesterase

	AChE	BuChE
Heterogeneity	One enzyme, may be a variant	Many enzymes and isoenzymes
Molecular weight	80,000—monomer	340,000 Tetramer—held together by disulphide bond
Natural Substrates	Acetylcholine, Acetyl-β-methylcholine	Fatty acyl ester and aromatic ester
Test Substrates	Acetylcholine, Acetyl-β-methylcholine	Benzoylcholine Butyrylthiocholine
Substrate kinetics	Acetylcholine, >propionylcholine> very low rate for butyrylcholine	Butyrylcholine> propionylcholine>low rate for acetylcholine
Assay advantages	Better reflection of synaptic inhibition	Easier to assay, declines fast
Use of assay	Acute exposure, response to treatment, unsuspected prior exposure	Acute exposure
Major tissue disturbance	CNS, erythyrocyte, lung, spleen	Heart, liver, pancreas, white matter of brain
Optimum substrate	Acetylcholine	Aliphatic choline esters e.g. butyrylcholine

15.3. Serum/plasma cholinesterase

15.3.1. Methods

15.3.1.1. Laboratory methods

Available methods for the determination of BuChE in plasma or serum include the following categories: biological assays, assays based on the enzyme activity where a product or the substrate left is measured and measurement of the mass of the protein by immunoassay.

In the **biological assays**, the physiological functions of the ACh is measured. Such assays include the degree of shortening in a physostigmine-paralysed animal muscle, and effects on perfused heart. Biological assays are difficult to standardise, have poor precision and require relatively large volume of sample.

BuChE can also be measured by **immunoassay** (Jones *et al.,* 1991) where the mass of the protein is measured but this method has not been investigated in OP toxications where activity rather than mass is likely to be reduced.

All other methods are based on the enzyme activity of BuChE and measure either the product or the substrate by one of many ways.

The general reaction for these methods is

$$\text{X-choline} + H_2O \xrightarrow{\text{ChE}} \text{choline} + X^- + H^- \tag{15.1}$$

The rate of this reaction (and thus the enzyme activity) can be measured by determining the appearance of one of the products or disappearance of substrate.

a) Measurement of acid

Hydrogen ions formed during the hydrolysis of choline esters are followed by manometric, titrimetric or electrometric methods (Silk *et al.,* 1979). In the manometric method the H^+ reacts with bicarbonate in the reaction mixture to release CO_2 which is measured using a manometric apparatus.

In titrimetric methods, the amount of H^+ released is quantitated by continuous titration with a standardised alkali solution at constant pH using an indicator. The H^+ released can also be measured by monitoring pH changes (Writter et al., 1966; Barenghi et al., 1986). In the electrometric procedure, highly automated titration instrumentation is used to add base continuously to neutralise the H^+ released.

These instruments maintain the reaction at constant pH and the amount of base added is related to the enzyme activity (Ellin and Vicario, 1975). Hydrogen ions released can also be measured by a spectrophotometric method using indicator such as Phenol red (Caraway, 1956). The major disadvantage of this type of method is that the method is linear only over a limited pH range (7.2–7.7).

b) Measurement of unreacted ester (substrate)

The quantity of unreacted acetylcholine or other substrate remaining at the end of 60 min at 37°C can be measured using hydroxylamine and ferric ions. When benzylcholine is used as substrate, the decrease in absorbance of the substrate at 240 nm is monitored (De La Huerga et al., 1952; Silk et al., 1979). Although the maximum absorbance difference between the substrate (benzylcholine chloride) and product (benzoate) is at 235 nm, measurements are made at 240 nm to avoid interference from plasma (Whittaker, 1977).

c) Measurement of product
    (i) Chromogenic procedure

This is the most commonly used group of methods. In this group of methods acetylcholine or another choline ester is coupled to colour reagents and the formation or disappearance of colour is measured. Most popular of the methods is that described by Ellman et al. (1961) in which acetylthiocholine or another acetylcholine ester is used as a substrate and the rate of hydrolysis is monitored by coupling the thiocholine liberated with 5,5'-dithiobis (2-nitrobenzoic acid) (DTNB) to form a coloured compound, 5 thio-2-nitrobenzoate which has an absorbance maxima in the region of 412 nm.

$$\begin{array}{l} \qquad\qquad\quad \text{ChE} \\ \text{Acetylthiocholine} \quad \rightarrow \quad \text{thiocholine + acetic acid} \qquad\qquad (15.2) \\ \text{Thiocholine + DTNB} \quad \rightarrow \quad \text{coloured product} \end{array}$$

The disadvantage of the DTNB method is that the absorbance maxima of the coloured product is 412 nm which is close to that of haemoglobin and therefore in haemoglobin-containing samples the sensitivity would be reduced. In order to overcome this problem an alternative substrate 6,6'dithiodinicotinic acid (DTNA) has been used. The absorbance of the coloured product in the DTNA method can be measured at 340 nm thus avoiding interference from haemoglobin (Wellig et al., 1996). Interference from haemoglobin can also be reduced by measuring the absorbance at 436 nm when using DTNB (Worek et al., 1999) or by using other compounds such as 2,2'dithiodipyridine (Ceron et al., 1996) or 4,4'dithiopyridone (Augustinsson et al., 1978).

In a modification of the Ellman method butyrylthiocholine has been used as a substrate (Das and Liddell, 1970). This substrate is more specific for BuChE and it is not hydrolysed by the erythrocyte AChE. Propionyl thiocholine has also been used (Dietz et al., 1973).

(ii) Couple enzyme assay

BuChE can be measured by a coupled enzyme using choline oxidase and peroxidase (Abernethy et al., 1988; George et al., 1988). In this procedure choline liberated by ChE is oxidised by choline oxidase in the presence of peroxidase, 4 aminophenozone and phenol, to yield a chromogen which is read at absorbance 500 nm. This method can be easily automated (Brock, 1988; Ratnaike et al., 1987). This method has been adopted as an enzyme sensor (Morelis et al., 1991; Palleschi et al., 1990) where the choline oxidase is immobilised onto a membrane. This enzyme sensor technique has been used for the detection of ChE inhibitors such as OP (Campanella et al., 1992; Salamoun and Remieu, 1992). The choline oxidase method has also been linked to fluorogenic substrate and this fluorimetric assay has been reported to be more sensitive (Kusu et al., 1990).

Method for BuChE (Whittaker, 1977)

The method is based on that described by Ellman et al. (1961) who measured the rate of enzymic hydrolysis of acetylthiocholine by coupling the liberated thiocholine with DTNB.

In the method described here butyrylthiocholine is used as substrate, this is more specific for BuChE as this substrate is not hydrolysed by erythrocyte acetylcholinesterase (Das and Liddell, 1970). This method can easily be adapted for automated analysers.

Reagents:

Phosphate buffer (0.067 mmol/L) pH 7.4: Dissolve 7.6 g anhydrous Na_2HPO_4 and 1.8 g anhydrous KH_2PO_4 in 1 L distilled water.

DTNB (0.27 mmol/L): Dissolve 10.7 mg DTNB in 100 ml buffer. Store in dark bottle in refrigerator (stable for about 4 weeks).

Butyrylthiocholine iodide (90 mmol/L): Dissolve 29.8 g in 1 ml distilled water. Store in dark bottle in refrigerator (stable for 4 weeks).

Wavelength 408 nm. Glass cuvette 1 cm light path. Temperature 25°C. Incubate DTNB solution at 25°C.

To 2.9 ml of DTNB, add 20 µl plasma and 100 µl butyrylthiocholine iodide solution mix by inversion. Read the increase in absorbance at 408 nm at intervals of half a minute, at 25°C for 5 minutes. The rate of change in absorbance is calculated. The spontaneous hydrolysis of butyrylthiocholine under these conditions is usually negligible but can be checked by substituting buffer for the plasma and repeating the assay.

Calculation

The cholinesterase activity is expressed as micromoles of substrate hydrolysed in 1 minute at 25°C by 1 ml of plasma or serum.

The molar absorbance of the product of the chemical reaction, 5-thio-2-nitrobenzoic acid is 13,600 (Ellman, 1959) and the cholinesterase activity expressed in µmol/min/ml is calculated as follows:

The cholinesterase activity is

$$\text{Units/ml} = \Delta A/\text{min} \times \frac{TV}{SV} \times \frac{1}{E} \times \frac{10^6}{1} \times \frac{1}{10^3}$$

$$= \Delta A/\text{min} \times \frac{3.02}{0.02} \times \frac{1}{13,600} \times \frac{10^6}{1} \times \frac{1}{10^3} \quad (15.3)$$

$$= \Delta A/\text{min} \times 11.1$$

ΔA min is the rate of increase in absorbance corrected for any blank reaction, TV is the total volume of reaction, SV is the sample volume (in ml), and E is the molar absorbance of the product.

If the measuring temperature is different from 25°C a temperature correction can be made by adding or subtracting 9% for each 1°C variation of the reaction mixture from 25°C (Das and Liddell, 1970). Normal values are 2.5–6.7 μmol of butyrylthiocholine hydrolysed/min/ml serum plasma.

15.3.2. Specimens

For the measurement of BuChE serum is the preferred sample. Serum samples can be stored at room temperature or at 4°C for several weeks. Enzyme activity in serum is stable at room temperature for up to 80 days and for 3 years at -20°C (Wilding et al., 1977). Moderate haemolysis does not interfere with the assay as long as the samples are centrifuged to remove red cell ghosts/membranes which contain the erythrocyte enzyme.

Plasma samples collected into EDTA or heparin tubes can also be used for analysis. Fluoride oxalate and citrate should be avoided as anticoagulants as they inhibit the enzyme activity (Brown et al., 1981). If samples are to be transported to a distant site it is preferable to send them cold to avoid extremes of temperature. It is preferable to separate the serum/plasma as soon as possible after collection.

Lipaemia and high bilirubin leads to no significant effect (Young, 1993). Freezing and thawing up to 9 cycles over 9 weeks had no effect (Turner et al., 1984; Huizenga et al., 1985). However some atypical enzymes (see below under genetic variation) are not stable after freezing (Primo-Parmo et al., 1997).

15.3.3. Reference range

Reference values reported in the literature vary according to the method. Each method uses different units and thus it is difficult to compare values between methods. One approach to this problem is to express the results of any patient as a percentage of mean reference value for that method. Different assay results can also be compared by referring each method to a standardised reference method. Several factors such as age, sex and pregnancy influence BuChE activity.

The range in a 'healthy population' can vary 3 fold. However within an individual, variation is fairly small. The intraindividual variation has been estimated to be 4.3% (Chu, 1985). Thus in a given subject changes in serum ChE are highly significant.

Plasma/serum ChE activity in neonates and infants less than 6 months has been reported to be up to 50% lower than in adults with some methods (Karlsen et al., 1981; Zsigmond et al., 1971). In a recent study using acetylthiocholine as substrate plasma ChE in foetal cord blood was found to be only 16% lower than adult non pregnant females (de Peyster et al., 1994). In preterm infants there is a transient low value which rises within 2 weeks (Strausse and Modanlou, 1986). Activity increases rapidly for 2 months after birth reaching values higher than in adults. Thereafter there is a slower rise reaching a peak at 6 yrs from which there is a gradual decrease to adult values at puberty (Hutchinson and Widdowson, 1952). Young adult females between the ages of 18 to 35 y have lower values than corresponding males (Laine-Cessac et al., 1989; Huizenga et al., 1985). During pregnancy serum BuChE decreases (Howard et al., 1978). BuChE decreases throughout pregnancy and lowest values are seen at 3rd trimester when it was 19% lower than in non-pregnant women (de Peyster et al., 1994). The activity returned to non-pregnant values by the 6th week post partum. Although the 3rd trimester value was significantly lower than non-pregnant group, 98% of the pregnant values were within the conventional reference range.

In a longitudinal study of BuChE during pregnancy Evans et al. (1988) noted 3 patterns of change: a decrease in activity which returned to preconception levels after delivery, a decrease in activity which returned partially or completely to preconception values before delivery and no change in activity during pregnancy. The pattern of change appears to be related to age—no change is seen in older women and most change is seen in younger women.

Serum BuChE also increases with increasing body weight (Brock and Brock, 1993; Young, 1993; Lepage, 1985). BuChE concentration decreases after strenuous exercise (Nagel et al., 1990; Soeder et al., 1989).

There appear to be racial differences in serum ChE. For example, BuChE activity in Irish subjects was reported to be higher than in Iranian subjects (Hosseini et al., 1997), subjects of Asian origin had higher BuChE than in African origin (Pinto Pereira et al., 1996) and Malaysians had higher values than Chinese or Asians (Chan et al., 1994).

15.3.4. Factors affecting serum BuChE

15.3.4.1. Factors which decrease serum BuChE (Table 15.2.)

BuChE is synthesised by the liver and it has been used as a sensitive marker of synthetic capacity of liver. In acute and chronic hepatitis serum ChE can be 30–50% lower. 50–70% decrease is seen in cirrhosis and in patients with liver metastases (Brown et al., 1981).

BuChE is lower in patients with malignancy and the degree of depression is related to the extent of malignancy and the site of the primary tumour (Kaniaris et al., 1979)—lowest activity is seen in patients with hepatic metastases. In carcinoma of the breast the decrease in BuChE is not marked (Khan et al., 1991).

BuChE is decreased in malnutrition (Umeki, 1993) and hypothyroidism (Davis et al., 1997). In renal failure there is about 20% reduction and this is not related to dialysis (Phillips and Hunter, 1992). Oral contraceptives reduce BuChE by about 20% after 3 months of use (Robertson, 1967).

Serum ChE is decreased in burns patients and it is related to severity of burns (Brown et al., 1981). The initial decline seen in the first 24 h is probably due to movement out of the circulation (cf albumin) and to fluid therapy. The changes seen later are probably due to derangement of liver function (Viby-Morgensen et al., 1975).

BuChE decreases rapidly on plasmaphoresis and during cardiopulmonary bypass (Jackson et al., 1982) which lasts for 7 days.

15.3.4.2. Effect of drugs and chemicals

A number of drugs and chemicals can inhibit BuChE - some competitively and others non-competitively. OP compounds are classic examples of non competitive inhibition and are discussed later.

Cyclophosphamide reduces BuChE by 50–60% (Dillman, 1987). Ecothiopate, a drug used in the treatment of glaucoma, is an irreversible organophosphate inhibitor. When used as eye drops most patients show no effect or small decrease in BuChE whereas in some patients serum BuChE is almost completely inhibited (Pantuck, 1966; Messer et al., 1992).

Table 15.2. Factors causing a decrease in serum BuChE

Physiological
    Pregnancy
    Low calorie diet
    Neonates
Pathological
    Prematurity
    Liver diseases
        Acute hepatitis
        Chronic hepatitis
        Cirrhosis
        Carcinoma-
        Secondaries in liver
        Malnutrition

    Acute Diseases
        Acute infection
        Myocardial
        Infarction
        Burns

    Collagen diseases
        Progressive muscular dystrophy
        Congential myotonia
        Dermatomyositis

    Other diseases
        Tuberculosis
        Chronic anaemia
        Myxodema
        Chronic debilitating disease
        Carcinoma
        Shock

Chemical and Drug Induced
Ambenonium
Antimalarial drugs
Asparaginase
Bambuterol
Contraceptive pill
Cyclophosphamide
Danazol
Demecarium
Distigmine
Ecothiophate
Edrophonium
Glucocorticoid
Iodipamide
Iopanoic Acid
Metoclopramide
Metrifonate
Neostigmine
Opium alkaloids
Organophosphorous poisoni
Paracetamol
Physostigmine
Procainamide
Pyridostigmine
Ranitidine
Streptokinase

Inherited
Genetic variants

Competitive or reversible inhibitors of BuChE include drugs such as ambenonium, demecarium, neostigmine, physostigmine, pyridostigmine, distigmine and edrophonium (Baraka, 1977, 1992). Bambuterol, a prodrug of terbutaline causes a reversible inhibition of ChE (Turnek and Svensson, 1988). Ranitidine in therapeutic dose inhibits BuChE (Kirch et al., 1984).

Pancuronium causes a 40% reduction in ChE (Stovner et al., 1975). Metoclopramide inhibits ChE at therapeutic concentrations (Chemnitius et al., 1996) and in patients treated with this drug the action of suxamethonium is prolonged (Kao and Turner, 1989; Dao et al., 1990). Antimalarial drugs such mefloquine and chloroquine (Lim and Go, 1985) and opioids are non-competitive inhibitors of BuChE.

Procainamide has been shown to inhibit BuChE in vitro at therapeutic concentrations (Kamban et al., 1987). Asparaginase (Cucuianu et al., 1972), danazol (Laurell and Rannevik, 1979) and glucocorticoids decrease BuChE probably by inhibiting hepatic synthesis (Verjee et al., 1977). Iodipamide, a radio contrast media is a powerful inhibitor of BuChE (Lasser and Lang, 1966). Metrifonate, an antiparasitic agent is a powerful inhibitor of BuChE and the enzyme activity can be reduced by as much as 70% after a single dose (Nhachi et al., 1991). Streptokinase may cause a reduction in BuChE by hypoxic or toxic liver damage (Schmidt et al., 1972).

15.3.4.3. Factors which increase BuChE (Table 15.3.)

Hyperthyroidism increases BuChE by about 20% (Thompson and Whittaker, 1965) and in nephrotic syndrome a high BuChE and low albumin is seen (Davis et al., 1997). Increased BuChE activity due to an inherited variation has also been reported. Antiepileptic drugs carbamazepine, valproate and phenytoin cause significant increase in BuChE probably by inducing the hepatic synthesis (Puche et al., 1989).

15.3.4.4. Genetic variation

One of the important factors determining the serum BuChE activity is genetic variation. Inheritance of BuChE is controlled by a locus located in the long arm of chromosome 3 (Gaugham et al., 1991).

Enzyme variations arise from a mutation at this locus. Some of the common variants and their relative enzyme activity are given in Table 15.4. The mutation that gives rise to the atypical gene involves change in the structure of the active centre. The atypical gene is almost absent is sub-Saharan Africans, Orientals (Japan and Korea) and parts of Central and South America.

The incidence of atypical gene is high in Egypt, North-West India and Turkey and the highest frequency is seen in Jewish populations of Iran, Iraq with a frequency of 0.075 and 0.047.

The fluoride resistant gene (F) is rare. Higher frequency for this gene is seen in Punjab, Malawi, Zimbabwe, Zambia, Iceland and the Orkney Isles - places where the frequency of atypical gene is lower. The silent gene is even rarer but it is more frequent in certain populations such as Eskimos of Alaska, some tribes in Andra Pradesh (India) where a frequency of 2% has been reported (Whittaker, 1986). The frequency of K alleles has also been reported to be similar in Whites and Brazilian populations (Souza *et al.*, 1998).

Table 15.3. Factors causing an increase in serum BuChE

Physiological	Pathological	Drugs
Obesity	Nephrotic syndrome	Carbamazepine
	Haemachromatosis	Phenytoin
	Obese diabetics	
	Thyrotoxicosis	

Table 15.4. Some of the common inherited variants in the BuChE gene

Name	Allele frequency	Plasma activity
Usual-U	0.98	Normal
Atypical-A	0.02	Decreased by 70%
Silent-S	0.0003	No activity
Fluoride-F	0.003	Activity decreased by 60%
H-type	Not known	Activity decreased by 90%
K-type	0.13	Activity decreased by 30%
J-type	Not known	Activity decreased by 66%

(adapted from Davis *et al.*, 1997).

15.3.5. Red cell ChE

Sample

For the measurement of erythrocyte ChE (AChE) whole blood sample collected into heparin, EDTA or acid-citrate-dextrose (ACD) can be used.

Whole blood specimens in ACD are stable at 4°C for 20 days and heparinised samples are stable for 6 days at 0°C (Beutler *et al.*, 1977).

Method

Method for AChE in red cells is similar to that of plasma except that acetylcholine is used as substrate. There is confusion as to the best method for expressing the results. Methods used are U/10⁶ RBC U/L of RBC and U/G Hb. Each of these have advantages and disadvantages and no method is best.

15.3.5.1. Factors affecting red cell AChE (Table 15.5.)

Red cell AChE is higher in young red cells compared to older cells (Prall *et al.*, 1998, Galbraith and Watts, 1981). It is lower in neonates by about 50% (de Peyster *et al.*, 1994). Activity increases gradually and reaches adult value by the age of 1 y (Kaplan and Tildon, 1963). There is no difference between males and females (Garcia-Lopez and Monteoliva, 1988). During pregnancy RBC AChE activity is increased and reaches a peak during the 3rd trimester when the values are 13% higher than in non pregnant values with 87% outside the reference range for non pregnant subjects. The values return to non pregnant values by 6 weeks after pregnancy (de Peyster *et al.*, 1994). Like the serum enzyme RBC AChE between people (interindividual variation) varies over a wide range (Sawhney and Loth, 1986, Lotti, 1995). The intraindividual variation is small so that in an individual a 15% change in enzyme activity is significant (Lotti, 1995; Mutch *et al.*, 1992).

In patients with Alzheimer's disease RBC AChE has been reported to be lower in some studies (Inestrosa *et al.*, 1994) but not in others (Sirvio *et al.*, 1989). In victims of smoke inhalation AChE in red cells was significantly lower (Houeto *et al.*, 1999).

As the activity of AChE is higher in young red cells, high RBC AChE has been reported in individuals who have an increased turnover of red cells (Eluwa *et al.*, 1990; Streichman *et al.*, 1983).

Neostigmine reduces the activity by 10–25% (Sakuma *et al.*, 1992). Edrophonium had no significant effect (Sakuma *et al.*, 1992).

Ecothiopate (Young, 1999), and metoclopramide (Chemnitius *et al.*, 1996) cause inhibition of RBC AChE. Galanthamine, a drug with potential for use in the treatment of Alzheimer's disease inhibits RBC AChE (Fulton and Benfield, 1996).

Table 15.5. Factors affecting red cell AChE

Haemoglobinopathies
Diseases with reduced red cell survival
Alzheimer's disease
Organophosphorous poisoning
Smoke inhalation

Drugs	Metoclopramide
	Galanthamine
	Neostigmine

15.3.6. Field methods

Based on the laboratory method described earlier several field kits are available. This includes a test paper to measure serum BuChE but it is not reliable enough (Oudart and Holmstedt, 1970). Furthermore centrifugation is required in the field to obtain plasma/serum and a modified micro-centrifuge has been developed for this purpose (Ryhanen and Hanninen, 1987).

One of the field kits is the tintometric field kit which uses a colour comparator for semi-quantitative measurement of the enzyme activity in whole blood (Edson, 1950) from exposed individuals as a percentage of activity in blood from an unexposed control. This method depends on subjective assessment. In an evaluation of this method the sensitivity varied from 58 to 92% while the specificity varied from 98% to 63% —depending on the 'cut off' value (McConnell and Magnotti, 1994) and the authors conclude that the result using this kit should be interpreted with caution.

The classical Ellman method has been used as a field method. One such kit is the Lovibond cholinesterase kit where the colour produced is assessed using a disc with different colours. In order to improve the performance of this kit, a set of standard solutions has been suggested (da Silva *et al.*, 1994). Improvements to this method have been introduced with the use of stable premixed inexpensive reagents and a battery operated colorimeter (Magnotti et al., 1987;1988).

Evaluation of a battery-operated colorimeter kit under field conditions has shown satisfactory results (McConnell *et al.*, 1992). In this method haemoglobin is measured in addition to AChE to adjust results. Adjusting the results to haemoglobin reduce the coefficient variation (McConnell *et al.*, 1992). A commercial kit based on the spectrophotometric method (Test-Mate-OP) has been evaluated under field conditions and compared to a laboratory method (London *et al.*, 1995). In this kit BuChE as well as red cell AChE are measured. An inhibitor is used to prevent interference from serum BuChE when whole blood (RBC) ChE is measured. The precision for BuChE was poor but that of the red cell method was better, but still poorer than the laboratory method. The sensitivity and specificity were 89% and 100% respectively. It was concluded that this kit is adequate for surveillance studies. An alternative approach to field method is to freeze the blood sample and send it to a laboratory for analysis (Oliverira-Silva *et al.*, 2000).

15.4. Interpretation

15.4.1. Acute poisoning

OP compounds and carbamates act by inhibiting AChE at nerve endings. In addition these compounds inhibit AChE at other sites including red cell AChE and serum BuChE. Although serum BuChE is inhibited effectively by OP and carbamates this has no relation to inhibition of red cell or neuronal AChE. Thus inhibition of BuChE can be regarded as a marker of exposure to OP but not an index of toxicity (Lotti, 1995). Inhibition of RBC AChE on the other hand reflects somewhat the inhibition at synapses. Thus inhibition of RBC AChE can be regarded as a biomarker of toxicity (Midtling *et al.*, 1985).

However, for a given compound, the relationship between inhibition of RBC AChE and that in the nervous system is not known. As OP and carbamate can reach the circulation easier than the nervous system, inhibition of RBC AChE probably overestimates the inhibition of AChE in the brain (Lotti, 1995).

The recovery of RBC AChE in circulation depends on the appearance of new red cells from the bone marrow, as the inhibition is irreversible and red cells in circulation cannot synthesise new enzyme. The recovery rate of RBC AChE has been estimated to be 1% whereas the half-life of AChE resynthesis in the nervous system has been reported to be 5–7 days (Lotti, 1995). Thus AChE in brain will recover before that in red cells. The recovery of BuChE is more rapid than the red cell AChE.

There is general correlation between the degree of inhibition of red cell AChE and severity of symptoms (Table 15.6). However, it must be remembered that there are many other factors which may cause a decrease in red cell AChE and serum BuChE and therefore a low value does not necessarily indicate OP exposure.

Furthermore a value within the reference range does not exclude exposure to OP or carbamate as the variation between people is large (wide reference range). As the enzyme activity within an individual does not vary much (<10%), if the value of AChE is known before exposure even minor degree of exposure could be easily detected.

Table 15.6. Relationship between inhibition of red cell AChE and severity of symptoms

Severity of poisoning	Degree of inhibition	Muscarinic effects	Nicotinic effects	CNS effects
Mild	<60%	Nausea, vomiting, diarrhoea, salivation, lacrimation, bronchoconstriction. Increased bronchial secretion. Bradycardia		Headache, dizziness
Moderate	60-80%	As before and miosis urinary/faecal incontinence	Muscle fasciculations	As before and dysarthia ataxia
Severe	80%		As before and fasciculations of diaphragm and respiratory muscle	As before and coma, convulsion

(adapted from Lotti, 1991; Lotti, 1995)

The correlation between severity of symptoms of poisoning and the magnitude of the decrease in enzyme activity is not always good (Wykoff *et al.*, 1968). Near total inhibition of serum ChE and 60–70% inhibition of red cell AChE has been reported with absence of any overt signs of poisoning (Porter, 1999). Furthermore patients who have recovered fully from organophosphorous poisoning may still have undetectable or low AChE. This inhibition of AChE is irreversible and therefore the rate of return of the enzyme values depends on the turnover of the enzyme. As the red cells have a long half life it takes longer - 13–17 weeks - for the red cell AChE to return to normal compared to the serum enzyme which returns to normal within 3–6 weeks (Brown *et al.*, 1981). Another factor complicating the interpretation of serum BuChE is genetic variation. It has been reported that the risk of poisoning is higher in subjects with unusual types of BuChE (Fontoura-da-Silva and Chautard-Freire-Maria, 1996).

A red cell and/or serum ChE result within the reference range does not exclude organophosphorous poisoning for reasons mentioned earlier. If pre exposure values are known it is easier to arrive at a diagnosis. If pre exposure values are not available serial samples or estimating the regeneration of the enzyme in vitro by treating with pralidoxime may give a clue. The degree of inhibition of ChE required to produce symptoms is not known. It is believed that the variation in the degree of inhibition required to produce symptoms is related to the rate of inhibition rather than the degree of inhibition (Midtling *et al.*, 1985; O'Malley *et al.*, 1990).

15.4.2. Chronic poisoning

In chronic organophosphorous poisoning ChE activity may gradually decrease to very low values without any symptoms or with minimal symptoms. Because of the wide reference values it is best to have a baseline value in workers likely to be exposed to OPs chronically (Guidance Note MS17 HSE). As the half life of the enzyme in red cells and serum vary, measurement of both may help. If only serum ChE is inhibited it is likely to be due to brief or early chronic low exposure. If both enzymes are low it indicates moderate exposure. If red cell AChE is only low it is likely to indicate recovery from exposure to OPs.

The significance of a given percentage inhibition of AChE may be difficult to assess. Practical guidelines for interpreting red cell AChE measurements given by WHO (Lotti, 1995) is 20–30% inhibition indicate evidence of exposure a 30-50% inhibition indicates hazard and >50% would suggest poisoning.

SECTION B-. Toxicological Investigation of OP Agents

Toxicological Assays

In an acute clinical situation it is most important to gauge the severity of OP poisoning and the efficacy of treatment by measurements of cholinesterase activity as described above. Detecting and identifying the particular agent responsible has little bearing on immediate treatment. The organophosphate insecticides are diverse in their chemical and physical properties and, therefore, a variety of analytical techniques can be applied to their detection and analysis as part of a toxicological investigation. Most are poorly soluble in water, but all are degraded in aqueous solution by hydrolysis to polar water-soluble products. Some compounds, such as dichlorvos (a dimethyl phosphate) and omethoate (a dimethyl phosphorothioate), are quickly detoxified in the body by hydrolysis and de-esterification. However, some of the lipophilic diethyl phosphorothioates can be sequestered in the tissues for several days and patients who appear to have recovered may suffer a recurrence of toxic effects. Identification of the agent involved can alert clinicians to this possibility.

It is often much easier to detect and identify poisonous substances first by examining suspect materials where the concentrations are likely to be quite high and relatively simple analytical procedures can be applied to, for example, liquids, food, clothing, water and soil. Nevertheless, if evidence for the presence of an OP compound *in vivo* can also be established, the diagnosis can be made on much firmer ground. Some of the simple tests can be used on stomach contents with some success provided the sample has been collected soon after ingestion. For tissue samples, the results tend to be far less clear-cut except in cases of very severe poisoning. As previously stated, most OP compounds undergo both chemical and enzymatic degradation in biological material. The only reliable way in which to halt or slow down these processes is immediate freezing of the samples and this is not usually a feasible option except under experimental conditions. Adding the common preservative sodium fluoride to blood samples can have the effect of accelerating chemical breakdown and should be avoided altogether (Moriya et al, 1999).

In general, the concentrations of insecticides in biological fluids during intoxication are very low. This, coupled with their instability in tissues and other aqueous materials, has led analysts to give attention to the detection and measurement not only of the parent substances, but also of the more stable breakdown products. In recent years there has been a resurgence of interest in hair analysis for drugs and other substances such as trace elements. Substances circulating in the blood are incorporated into the hair shaft and, since no metabolic or excretory processes take place, they remain there until the hair falls out or is removed by cutting. They may also be removed by washing, although this is generally a slow process. Hair collection is non-invasive and the sample can be used to detect either continuing exposure to drugs and chemicals or a single exposure that took place weeks or even months previously. Hair analysis would therefore offer a means of monitoring occupational and environmental exposure to OP insecticides and work has already begun to test its validity in this context (Tsatsakis *et al* 1998, Cirimele *et al* 1999)..

For many years there has been increasing public concern about the release of OP insecticides into the environment and this has led to the development of numerous methods to monitor their concentrations in soil, water supplies, rivers, lakes and in foodstuffs. In some countries, legislative control of permissible levels has been in force for many years. Another catalyst of method development has been the use of OP nerve agents in warfare and terrorist attacks and the potential for this to become more widespread. In these areas, as in those of biological fluid and tissue analysis, complex modern analytical techniques such as gas liquid chromatography, high performance liquid chromatography, mass spectrometry, biosensor technology and immunoassay have been deployed by scientists based in medical, industrial and military establishments.

Group detection tests

Bioassay

One of the oldest tests for pesticides was to expose fruit flies (*Drosophila melanogaster*) either to the suspect substance, stomach contents or the dried organic solvent extracts of samples and to count the mortality 24 hours later (Needham, 1960). This was first applied in agricultural research institutes and in government laboratories concerned with the control of pesticide contamination in food and was adopted subsequently by forensic scientists. Claims of high sensitivity have been made (Geldmacher von Mallinckdrodt and Machbert, 1997) as shown in Table 15.7.

Table 15.7. Detection limits for OP compounds using the *Drosophila melanogaster* bioassay.

Compound	Detection Limit (μg)
Dimethoate	10
Disyston	25
Metasystox	50
Metasystox R	100
Parathion	1
Thiometon	10

The test is non-specific in that any pesticide is likely to increase the mortality count. Moreover, the development of resistance to various pesticides by insects makes the inclusion of a control group of *Drosophila* essential. Nevertheless, in laboratories with only the most rudimentary equipment a simple bioassay of this kind can be an useful tool.

Colorimetric tests

Tests on stomach contents and suspect materials

The simplest method uses strips of filter paper which have been impregnated with buffered acetylcholine solution containing phenol red indicator and 1,2-propylene glycol as a wetting agent (Fishl et al 1968).

The suspect material is transferred to the paper and a drop of normal serum is added. If the acetylcholinesterase activity is unaffected, acetic acid is released and the indicator changes to yellow. In the presence of an acetylcholinesterase inhibitor, the indicator turns a red/ violet colour. A limit of detection for parathion of 1.2µg/l and 0.8 to 2.2µg/l for a range of other OPs has been claimed. The method can also be applied to examination of serum from a suspected poisoned patient, i.e. if the paper turns red after adding a drop of serum a cholinesterase inhibitor may have been taken. These strips are not easy to prepare or to store and are not viable for more than a day. There is, therefore, a danger of both false negative and false positive results and they cannot be recommended as field test kits unless nothing else is available.

Ellman Test on serum

This test is also suitable for laboratories with basic equipment and was adapted from the well-known Ellman method (Ellman et al, 1961). The stomach contents are filtered and the procedure is as follows:

To each of two test-tubes add 3mls of dithiobisnitrobenzoic acid solution (100mg/l in pH 7.4 phosphate buffer), 0.1 ml of acetylthiocholine iodide solution (5% w/v) and 20µl of normal serum. To one tube add 200µl of water and to the other the same volume of filtered sample. Allow to stand for 2 minutes and note any significant change in colour between the tubes.

If the control tube contents are a deeper yellow than those in the sample tube, this is an indication that a cholinesterase inhibitor is present. The test can also be carried out on a serum sample and, for further evidence, a third tube can be incorporated to which 200µl of the test serum and the same volume of aqueous pralidoxime chloride solution (200g/l) has been added. A lighter yellow colour in the test serum tube and the pralidoxime tube than that in the control tube suggests cholinesterase inhibition, although not necessarily by an OP compound.

Direct colorimetric method on urine

Recently a quantitative method has been developed (Namera *et al.*, 2000) that is based on the reaction of OP compounds with 4-(4-nitrobenzyl)pyridine (NBP). The reaction mechanism is shown in Fig. 15.1.

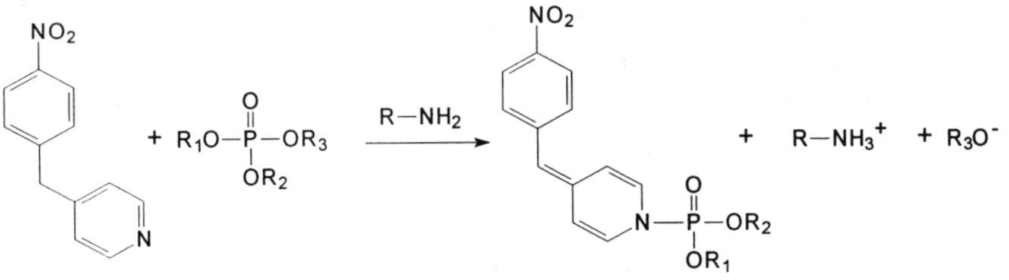

Figure 15.1. Reaction of OPs with 4-(4-nitrobenzyl)pyridine.

The method involves adding 0.1ml of the NBP reagent (45% in acetone) to 1ml of urine and heating the mixture to 100°C for 20 minutes. The mixture is then cooled to room temperature and 0.1ml of tetraethylenepentamine is added. In the presence of an organophosphate, a purple/blue colour develops. The colour is stable for several hours and therefore the method can be made quantitative by use of spectrophototometry. Detection limits are quoted as 0.10–10µg/ml in urine. These limits varied according to the molar absorptivity of a particular organophosphate pesticide, but for 17 out of 27 tested, the values were found to be 0.3µg/ml or less.

The method was evaluated by using urine samples from 12 cases of pesticide poisoning where assays were also carried out by gas chromatography linked to mass-spectrometry (GC-MS). An OP compound had been reputedly ingested in 8 of these cases and the method gave positive results in 7 of these. These results were confirmed by GC-MS. No reaction occurred with samples from other cases where non-OP compounds (paraquat, propanil and carbaryl) were present.

Gas detection tubes

It is possible to test suspect substances and stomach contents for vapourised OP compounds by gas-detector technology, which exploits the biochemical mechanism of OP toxicity.

The hand-held Drager device is the most familiar and consists of a pump connected to a tube containing chemically reactive material. Operation of the pump draws air and any vapours into the tube and through the reactive zone. For detecting OP compounds, the zone is impregnated with cholinesterase and a substrate of this enzyme (butyrylthiocholine). Suppression of enzyme activity by the presence of OP pesticides results in a colour change. Other volatile cholinesterase inhibitors such as carbamates give positive results.

Detection and measurement of urinary metabolites

Nitro-phenol test on urine

The substances listed in Table 15.8 give rise to derivatives of 4-nitrophenol in urine and measurement of these breakdown products can be used as an index of exposure.

The nitrophenols can be detected by hydrolysing the urine sample, extracting with an organic solvent and back-extracting the compounds into an alkaline solution. Phenolates are indicated by a yellow colour and, by reacting the alkaline solution with O-cresol in the presence of titanium trichloride to form the corresponding indophenol dye (blue). The method can be made quantitative by spectrophotometric measurement of the absorbance (Elliot et al., 1960; Geldmacher von Mallinkdrodt and Hermann, 1969).

Table 15.8. OP compounds metabolised to 4-nitrophenol derivatives

Compound	Nitrophenol derivative
Parathion-ethyl	4-nitrophenol
Parathion-methyl	
Paraoxon	
EPN (O-ethyl-O-p-nitrophenyl-phenyl-thionophosphonate)	
Dicapthon	2-chloro-4-nitrophenol
Chlorthion	3-chloro-4-nitrophenol
Folithion	3-methyl-4-nitrophenol

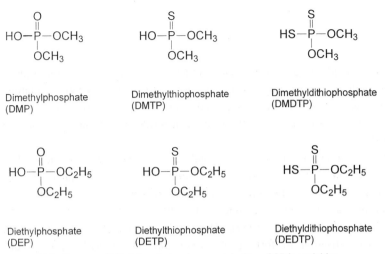

Figure 15.2. Common dialkylphosphate urinary metabolites of OP insecticides

This conversion step is advisable as a number of other nitrophenol pesticides such as DNOC (dinitro-o-cresol) and dinoseb (2-sec-butyl-4,6-dinitrophenol) are excreted into the urine as yellow phenolates, but do not form indophenol dyes. The colorimetric method has a detection limit range of 2-10mg/L for the nitrophenol metabolites and is considered sufficiently sensitive to detect moderate to severe poisoning.

For lower levels of exposure to these compounds, for example when monitoring occupational intake, more refined methods are essential such as high performance liquid chromatography (HPLC) (Diamond and Quebbemann, 1979; Ott, 1979). This technique is capable of automation (Diamond and Quebbemann, 1979) and has a sensitivity of detection of 0.05 to 0.10mg/l. Liquid chromatography with mass spectrophotometric detection (LC-MS) has also been applied to the analysis of the insecticides and their hydrolysis products (Farran, De Pablo, Barcelo, 1988).

Measurement of alkyl phosphate metabolites in urine

With the continued need to monitor human exposure to organophosphate insecticides, both in those occupationally exposed and in the general population, highly sensitive methods have evolved for the detection of urinary dialkylphosphates. These appear in the urine as a result of enzymatic cleavage of OP insecticides

It is not possible to link the urine analyses to exposure to an individual insecticide, since the majority are degraded to only six common metabolites (Fig. 15.2.). However, this makes the task of monitoring decidedly simpler.

Over recent years, methods of extreme sensitivity have evolved (Aprea, Sciarra, Lunghini, 1996; Moate *et al.,* 1999). These rely on solvent extraction using acetonitrile, derivatisation to form pentafluorobenzyl ethers and capillary gas-chromatography with detection by phosphorus specific flame photometry. The procedures involve numerous intricate purification stages and are therefore slow and laborious. Nevertheless, they achieve their objective of monitoring low level exposure and this is borne out by the fact that in supposedly blank urine samples, i.e. from non-exposed individuals, it is rare not to detect low concentrations of alkylphosphates derived from food residues.

Chromatographic tests for individual OPs

Thin layer chromatography (TLC)

OP compounds are quite amenable to detection and identification by this relatively simple and inexpensive technique and a considerable number of methods have been published (Antoine and Mees, 1971; Tewari and Harpalani, 1977; Bakry and Abou-Donia, 1980; Kurhekar, Pundik, Meghal, 1980; Ziminski and Manning, 1981; Erdman, Brose, Schultz, 1990; Sevalkar, Patil, Katkar, 1991; Futagami *et al.,* 1997).

The method proposed by Antoine and Mees (1971) was designed to detect and identify upwards of 25 compounds and two types of adsorbent for the chromatography (silica gel and polyamide), seven developing solvent systems and seven visualisation techniques were examined.   As a result of this thorough investigation, they were able to recommend a procedure that used a maximum of four consecutive chromatograms with the OP compounds detected by UV absorption and spraying the plates with either nitropyridine or palladium chloride. Tewari and Harpalani (1977) were concerned with tissue analysis and developed a complicated technique of extracting macerated samples of liver, kidney, intestine, spleen, heart, lung and brain by refluxing with hexane and then re-extracting the compounds into acetonitrile.   This was then diluted 10 times with water, saturated with sodium sulphate and re-extracted with hexane. The evaporated hexane extract was reconstituted in acetone prior to chromatography. A second procedure using minced tissues, refluxing with a mixture of sodium sulphate, dilute sulphuric acid and acetone, and final extraction with chloroform is also described.   Thin-layer chromatography data in 25 different solvent systems is listed and location is by ultraviolet light, ammoniacal silver nitrate and palladium chloride reagent. Reactions towards a further 7 chromogenic reagents are also described. The authors also introduced quantification via densitometry.   The paper contains data on the tissue concentrations of OP pesticides detected in 5 cases of poisoning. A detection sensitivity of $0.2\mu g$ of the insecticides is claimed. Bakry and Abou-Donia (1980) concentrated on phosfolan (0,0-diethyl 1,3-dithiolan-2-ylidenephosphoramidate), mephosfolan (0,0-diethyl 4-methyl-1, 3-dithiolan-2-ylidenephosphoramidate) and some of their breakdown products. The technique chosen was sequential thin-layer chromatography (STLC) using glass fibre sheets impregnated with silicic acid. STLC was invoked because of the difficulty in separating the two compounds when using single developing solvent systems. The authors were able to select two systems from 14 that they examined. The primary solvent (2-butanone-1-butanol-water) was allowed to travel 6 cm and the plate was then developed further in the secondary solvent (acetonitrile-hexane-benzene-acetic acid) to 16cm.   The spots were visualised by exposure to iodine vapour.

This gave a good separation of the two parent insecticides together with several related compounds. Kurhekar *et al.* (1980) produced a method for confirming the presence of OP compounds containing a nitro group (parathion, parathion methyl, fentrothion). Small quantities of each insecticide (5μg) were spotted onto a thin-layer plate and covered with 2–3 drops of a derivatising agent (zinc chloride in concentrated sulphuric acid and ethanol) and heated at 100°C for 10 minutes. This reduced each compound to its amino derivative. Spots of the parent insecticides were then added to the same plate and this was developed in a mixture of hexane, acetone and ethanol. Both the parent substances and their amino derivatives were made visible by spraying with mercuric nitrate followed by diphenylcarbazone. The Rf values for the amino compounds were approximately half those of the untreated insecticides. Additional confirmation was gained by eluting the amino derivatives from the plate and subjecting them to a standard diazotisation procedure for confirmation of an amine. Ziminski and Manning (1981) were conscious of the need for rapid identification of insecticides in an emergency clinical situation and used a combination of conventional thin-layer chromatography and reversed phase thin-layer chromatography (RPTLC). Urine or gastric contents were extracted with diethyl ether at pH 8.5 and the organic extract was allowed to evaporate to dryness at room temperature. The extracts were spotted onto a normal silica gel TLC plate alongside pure insecticide standards. A RPTLC plate was made by dipping a normal plate in a mixture of paraffin oil and petroleum ether and allowing it to dry. This was then spotted with the extracts and standard insecticide solutions. The conventional plate was developed in a mixture of isooctane and ethyl acetate and separated compounds were visualised by spraying with silver nitrate solution followed by brief exposure to high intensity UV light. The plate was then re-sprayed with bromophenol blue reagent. The RPTLC plate was developed in a mixture of ethanol, acetonitrile and water and the same spray reagents applied. The conventional TLC gave a good separation of organophosphate, organochlorine and carbamate insecticides. RPTLC also gave a good separation, but the order of separation between the compounds was reversed. RPTLC was therefore a means of confirming the results of the conventional TLC method. Erdman *et al.* (1990) published a huge compilation of TLC corrected retention time data for 170 common insecticides including the OPs. The data were presented for three developing solvents systems selected on the basis of their discriminating power. Sevalkar *et al.* (1991) examined the value of a zinc chloride-diphenylamine reagent that had previously been used for detecting organochlorine insecticides.

The reagent is prepared by dissolving 1 gram of zinc chloride and 0.5 gram of diphenylamine in 100ml of acetone. After spraying, the TLC plate is heated at 110°C and the authors found that the chlorine containing OPs, phorate, phosphamidon, DDVP and phosphalone gave intense blue-green spots identical to those produced by organochlorine compounds. OPs that contain a nitro group (parathion, parathion methyl and fenitrothion) give an intense blue colour with this reagent.

High-performance thin layer chromatography (HPTLC) is a rapid and simple means of identifying OPs and Futagami *et al.* (1997) showed that this could be applied to their detection in human serum. Both solid phase and liquid-liquid extraction techniques were devised and applied to spiked serum samples. The extracts and a standard solution of insecticides were chromatographed in three different developing solvent systems and the OPs were visualised by examination under ultra violet light and by treating the plates either with a 4-(4-nitrobenzyl) pyridine-tetraethylenepentamine reagent, that gave mainly blue colours, or with a palladium chloride reagent that gave brown colours. The authors evaluated 25 common organophosphate insecticides with the method and were confident that the detection limits would allow it to be used to detect the compounds in the serum of acutely poisoned patients and thereby provide useful information to clinicians during pralidoxime therapy. Finally, it is worth taking note of one of the earlier publications (Geike, 1970) that used enzymatic detection based on the inhibition of acetylcholinesterase. The plates were sprayed first with a solution containing cholinesterase prepared from bovine liver and then incubated for an hour at 37°C. The substrate (a mixture of β-naphthylacetate and Fast Blue B Salt BB) was then sprayed onto the plate and produced a red background due to the release of naphthol from the ester by the action of cholinesterase. OPs and other inhibitors of cholinesterase appear as white spots. This is a sensitive and universal system for detecting cholinesterase inhibitors that may well come back into fashion as ready-made commercial cholinesterase preparations become cheaper and more widely available.

Gas-Liquid Chromatography (GLC).

Gas chromatographic methods have been applied to the detection and quantification of OPs in drinking and ground water (Zapf et al, 1995; Sega and Tomkins Baand Griest, 1997), plants and tissues (Holstege *et al.* 1991; Holstege *et al.* 1994; Abbas and Hayton, 1996) and in urine (Brealey and Lawrence, 1979; Abou-Donia and Abou-Donia, 1982). Prior to analysis, the compounds are purified away from the sample matrix into organic solvents and the choice of extraction technique depends on the nature of the sample being analysed. For example, drinking water is relatively pure and a simple liquid-liquid procedure can suffice. Zapf *et al.* (1995) took large volumes of tap-water (400mls) and extracted these once only with a very small volume of toluene (500µl). No further purification was necessary and by using gas-chromatography with electron capture and nitrogen phosphorus detection the authors claimed recovery values of at least 50% of added pesticides. Ground water contains many more impurities and Sega and Tomkins Baand Griest (1997) were concerned with the detection of trace levels of hydrolysis products of the nerve agents VX (S-2-diisopropylaminoethyl O-ethyl methylphosphonothiolate) and Sarin (isopropylmethylphosphonofluoridate). Solid phase extraction using silica bonded with a quaternary ammonium phase was applied to 50ml samples of water and the eluents were derivatised with methanolic trimethylphenylammonium hydroxide before capillary chromatography and detection by flame photometry. The detection limits for the three hydrolysis products were quoted as between 3 and 9 µg/l. Plant and animal tissues need special extraction and purification steps. Holstege *et al.* (1991) homogenised the tissues and extracted the homogenate with 5% w/v ethanol in ethyl acetate. Samples that had a high lipid content were passed through an automated system of silica gel permeation columns and any highly pigmented extract received a further cleanup with solid phase extraction columns. By this stage the concentrated extracts were fit for analysis by gas-chromatography.

High Performance Liquid Chromatography (HPLC)

As a general analytical technique HPLC offers considerable advantages over gas liquid chromatography, not least in its ability to deal with compounds that are thermally labile, polar and non-volatile.

Many OP insecticides and their metabolites have these characteristics and a variety of HPLC methods have appeared over the years (Brealey and Lawrence, 1979; Abou-Donia and Abou-Donia, 1982; Priebe and Howell, 1985; Unni et al 1992; Ramsteiner and Hormann, 1975; Clark et al, 1985; Szalontai, 1976, Martinez *et al.,* 1992; Thapar et al, 1994). Sample preparation can be quite simple. For instance, Brealey and Lawrence (1979) diluted plasma 5 times with buffer, added 0.2 ml of this to 0.1ml of ice cold methanol to precipitate proteins, centrifuged the tubes and injected the supernatant straight onto the HPLC column. Others have preferred solvent extraction with, for example, ethyl acetate (Abou-Donia and Abou-Donia, 1982), chloroform (Unni et al, 1992) or solid phase extraction (Martinez *et al.,* 1992). Because of the chemical diversity of the OP insecticides, it is usually necessary to employ both isocratic and gradient elution to gain adequate separation on the LC column. UV detection has proved quite effective in most applications, although of course this is limited to those compounds with suitable chromophoric constituents. Moreover, without an effective cleanup procedure, UV detection is open to interference from a multitude of other substances that are present in biological matrices. This led to a search for more selective and sensitive detectors for use with HPLC. One of the first used cholinesterase inhibition (Ramsteiner and Hörmann, 1975). The liquid chromatograph effluent was led into an AutoAnalyzer and cholinesterase inhibition was measured by a modification of the Ellman method. The method was said to have adequate sensitivity for residue analyses, but there were problems in maintaining the long-term operation of the technique and it was suitable only for polar compounds. Szalontai (1976) used a liquid chromatograph with a transport wire flame ionisation detector to examine the adsorption properties and normal phase separation of 23 OP insecticides on silica gel columns, but there is no record of this method ever being applied to residues or biological materials. One of the most complex means of detection was that invented by Priebe and Howell (1985). This was based on the photodegradation of OP compounds to orthophosphate in the presence of ammonium peroxydisulphate. A further chemical reaction then took place to form reduced heteropolymolybdate, a substance with an absorbance maximum at 885nm, i.e. a region where other materials in the sample matrix would be unlikely to interfere. The authors produced good evidence for the applicability of the method to residue analysis in food and analysis of dialkylphosphates in urine, but the technique was rather limited.

It could deal only with polar OPs and, for urine, it was necessary first to remove large amounts of interfering orthophosphates derived from dietary sources by an iron precipitation step. Electrochemical detection has been used with some success in analysing residues in waters and food and has the advantage over UV detection in not being so prone to interference from plant materials (Clark, Goodwin, Smiley, 1985)

Mass-spectrometry

In recent years there has been growing interest in being able to identify and monitor extremely low levels of OP compounds and their breakdown products in the environment. Advances in mass-spectrometric techniques have made this possible and minute quantities of these compounds can be detected, identified and measured in soil, water supplies, foodstuffs and biological samples. The technique is versatile in that the analyst has a choice of chromatographic systems, either gas-chromatography or liquid chromatography, to perform the initial separation. In due course, capillary electrophoresis will be another option. Some workers have chosen gas-chromatography (GC-MS) on the grounds of greater sensitivity of detection, particularly if the compounds are derivatised prior to the detection stage (Singh *et al.*, 1986; Schacterle and Feigel, 1996; Nagao *et al.*, 1997; Miki *et al.*, 1999).

Others favour liquid chromatography (LC-MS), since this is amenable to the separation and detection of polar (water-soluble) substances and, if the sample under analysis is reasonably clean, (e.g. ground water), samples can be analysed directly without any extra need for extraction or other purification process (Spliid and Koppen, 1996; Lacorte and Barcelo, 1996; Aguilar et al, 1998; Chiron et al, 1998; D'Agostino et al, 1999). The mass spectrometer configuration itself can be varied both in respect to the mechanism by which the molecules are ionised and the means of deriving and analysing the fragmentation patterns.

It is fair to say that LC-MS is the most versatile system at present and this view was supported by the work of Chiron *et al.* (1998) who were interested in detecting pirimiphos methyl degradation products in industrial water. They evaluated a GC-MS method with either electron impact or chemical ionisation modes and an LC-MS method using either an ionspray or atomic pressure chemical ionisation interface.

It was found that the LC-MS method successfully identified six of the degradation products and that two of these remained undetected by GC-MS even after a derivatisation procedure. Ideally, both techniques should be available so that whichever is the most appropriate can be brought to bear on a particular analytical problem.

Other techniques

Biosensors

Sensors with a biological coating have been devised for various medical applications over the last 5 years and the prospect of having a simple, relatively cheap and mobile system for the early detection of contamination with OP compounds is appealing. Some of the most recent methods have been developed by Mulchandani *et al.* (1998a and 1998b). This group modified a pH electrode by coating with a layer of *Escherichia coli* cells that expressed OP hydrolase (OPH) onto the cell surface. OP compounds are hydrolysed by OPH to release protons and thus generate a signal that is proportional to the concentration of the substrate. The authors claimed that the device could detect as low as 2μmol of paraoxon, methyl parathion and diazinon. In addition, the device was stable with multiple use and could be stored for long periods without losing efficacy. In their later publication they describe the adaption of the microbial sensor to a fibre optic device whereby the enzyme reaction gave rise to chromophoric products. These products absorb light at specific wavelengths and the back-scattered radiation was measured using a photomultiplier tube and correlated with the OP concentration. Detection limits for parathion and paraoxon of 3μmol were reported and the whole test took about 10 minutes. Again, the device was stable and lost no sensitivity with multiple use.

The development of OP compounds as chemical warfare agents has stimulated a huge investment in sophisticated early warning systems by the defence industry. One of these, known as the Nerve Agent Immobilised System (NAIAD), contains the enzyme butyrylthiocholine esterase, which has been immobilised by binding it to an amberlite exchange resin.

The immobilised enzyme is incorporated into a temperature controlled paper pad irrigated with a solution of butyrylthiocholine methane sulphonate in aqueous phosphate buffer. The enzyme catalyses the hydrolysis of the ester to produce butyrylthiocholine and the concentration of this product is monitored using an electrochemical cell. This in turn is adapted so that the reaction produces an oxidation potential the size of which depends on the concentration of thiocholine at the surface of a pyrolytic graphite anode. The supply of butyrylthiocholine is maintained at a pre-selected oxidation potential referenced to a standard silver-silver chloride electrode. Any nerve agent drawn through the enzyme pad by a diaphragm pump inhibits the catalytic activity of the butyrylcholinesterase and therefore affects the rate of production of butyrylthiocholine at the surface of the graphite electrode. The rate and extent by which the anode potential increases is monitored and an alarm is triggered once a preset condition is reached. The instrument is portable, has high sensitivity and is said to be very reliable.

Immunoassay

A technique that is sensitive, rapid, requires no expensive equipment and can be used on a sample with very little prior purification is clearly attractive as a tool for detecting and measuring pesticides in food, water and biological fluids. Immunoassay technology has all these qualities and methods have been developed both to quantify pesticide residues in food and crops as well as to provide rapid screening for contaminants in field samples. For OP compounds the techniques of Radioimmunoassay (RIA) and Enzyme Linked Immunoabsorbant Assay (ELISA) have received the most attention. The latter is particularly favoured in view of its long-term stability and simplicity in use. RIA is usually more sensitive, but carries the perceived health risks associated with using radioactive chemicals. In the simplest form of the ELISA technique, antibodies raised against the antigen (in this case an organophosphate) are bound to the plastic wells of an assay plate. The sample is added and any organophosphate molecules present become bound to the immobilized antibodies. The plate is washed to remove unreacted components and then a solution of labelled antibodies is added to the wells. These also attach to the bound antigen and after a short incubation time, the wells are washed to remove excess labelled antibodies.

The label can be, for example, a fluorescent chemical so that the intensity of fluorescence is proportional to the quantity of bound antibody and, by extrapolation, to the quantity of the organophosphate in the sample. Monoclonal antibodies raised in mice appear to offer greater sensitivity than rabbit polyclonal antibodies and methods using this source have been successful in detecting fenitrothion in methanol extracts of commercially treated grain (McAdam et al 1992, Hill et al 1992). An assay sensitivity as low as 100ng/ml was reported. At about the same time these workers also developed grain assays for fenitrothion and also for chlorpyrifos-methyl, and pirimiphosmethyl using rabbit antisera (Skerritt et al 1992). The cross-reactivity characteristics of the different antisera were very low and this allowed these workers to design a multi-assay plate system by coating the wells with a mixture of antibodies, adding the sample extract and then the appropriate labelled antibodies. There was a good correlation between the assay and those derived by a gas chromatographic method and the assay took only 60 minutes to complete. There has been less success in producing reliable immunoassays for use on biological samples. As long ago as 1982, Vallejo et al (1982) were concerned with devising an assay for parathion. As with all immunoassays for small molecules, the first step was to generate antibodies against the analyte by linking a parathion analogue chemically to a carrier protein, in this case bovine serum albumin (BSA). They successfully generated rabbit antisera that could recognise the immunising BSA-hapten, but there was no reaction with native parathion. The authors drew the conclusion, after several attempts to improve matters by varying the type of BSA-hapten link, that the parathion molecule was too small to produce a good immunogenic antigen and this is likely to be the case with several of the other organophosphate insecticides. Szurdoki et al (1995) produced ELISA assays for methyl and ethyl parathion, fenitrothion and 4-nitrophenol metabolites in urine samples that are said to be applicable to environmental monitoring. Finally, promising results have been reported by scientists working in the area of military defence where sensitive ELISA assays for the OP soman that are capable of measuring this agent in biological samples at around 200µg/l (Erhard et al., 1989; Erhard et al., 1990).

Conclusion

Biochemical evaluations are a necessity in the prevention, monitoring and confirmation of exposure to OP agents. Furthermore, serial measurements have become useful in assessing the response to therapeutic regimens, including treatment with the oximes.

An obvious gap in the literature concerning many of the clinical reports associated with OP exposure is the lack of biochemical evidence to indicate not only the severity of intoxication, but also the physio-pathological derangements associated with particular exposures.

Technology associated with biochemical investigations may be beyond the reach of many health services. However, such information is valuable in improving our understanding of the toxicity of OP compounds in man. Thus, it is necessary to consider developing regional or national centres of excellence for laboratory support particularly in the countries where OP associated ill-health is a major concern.

References

Abbas, R., Hayton, W.L. Gas chromatographic determination of parathion and paraoxon in fish plasma and tissues. *Journal of Analytical Toxicology* 1996;**20**:151–4.

Abernethy, M.H., Fitzgerald, H.P., Ahern, K.M. An enzymatic method for erythrocyte acetylcholinesterase. *Clinical Chemistry* 1988;**34**:1055–7.

Abou-Donia, S.A., Abou-Donia, M.B. High-performance liquid chromatography of phospholan, mephospholan and related compounds. *Journal of Chromatography* 1982;**240**:532–8.

Aguilar, C., Borrull, F., Marce, R.M. Identification of pesticides by liquid-liquid chromatography-particle beam mass spectrometry using electron ionisation and chemical ionisation. *Journal of Chromatography A* 1998;**805**:127–35.

Alkondon, M., Ray, A., Sen, P. Effect of beta-adrenergic blocking agents and some related drugs on plasma and RBC cholinesterase enzyme in vitro. *Indian Journal of Experimental Biology* 1983;**21**:519–21.

Antoine, O., Mees, G. Test de routine pour la determination des insecticides organo-phosphorés par la chromatographie en couche mince. *Journal of Chromatography* 1971;**58**:247–56.

Aprea, C., Sciarra, G., Lunghini, L. Analytical method for the determination of urinary alkylphosphates in subjects occupationally exposed to OP pesticides and in the general population. *Journal of Analytical Toxicolology* 1996;**20**:559–63.

Artiss, J.D., McGowan, M.W., Strandbergh, D.R et al. A procedure for the kinetic colorimetric determination of serum cholinesterase activity. *Clinica Chemica Acta* 1982;**124**:141–8.

Augustinsson, K.B., Eriksson, H., Faijersson, Y. A new approach to determining cholinesterase activities in samples of whole blood. *Clinica Chimica Acta* 1978;**89**:239–52.

Bakry, N.M., Abou-Donia, M.B. Sequential thin-layer chromatography of phosfolan, mephosfolan and related compounds. *Journal of Analytical Toxicology* 1980;**4**:212–5.

Baraka, A. Suxamethonium block in the myasthenic patient. *Anaesthesia* 1992;**47**:217–9.

Baraka, A. Suxamethonium-neostigmine interaction in patients with normal or atypical cholinesterase. *British Journal of Anaesthesia* 1977;**49**:479–83.

Bardin, P.G., Van Endens, S.F., Moolman, J.A. et al. Organophosphate and carbamate poisoning. *Archives of Internal Medicine* 1994;**154**:1433–41.

Barenghi, L., Ceriotti, F., Luzzana, M. et al. Measurement of erythrocyte acetylcholinesterase and plasma cholinesterase activity by a differential pH technique. *Annals of Clinical Biochemistry* 1986;**23**:538–45.

Beutler, E., Blume, K.G., Kaplan, J.C. *et al.* International Committee for Standardisation in Haematology: Recommended methods for red-cell enzyme analysis. *British Journal of Haematology* 1977;**35**:331–40.

Brealey, C.J., Lawrence, D.K. High-performance liquid chromatography of pirimiphos methyl and five metabolites. *Journal of Chromatography* 1979;**168**:461–9.

Brock, A, Brock, V. Factors affecting inter-individual variation in human plasma cholinesterase activity: body weight, height, sex, genetic polymorphism and age. *Archives of Environmental Contamination and Toxicology.* 1993;**24**:93–9.

Brock, A. Plasma cholinesterase genetic variants phenotyped using a Cobas-Fara centrifugal analyser. *Journal of Clinical Chemistry and Clinical Biochemistry* 1988;**26**:873–5.

Brown, S.S., Kalow, W., Pilz, M. et al. The plasma cholinesterases: a new perspective. *Advances in Clinical Chemistry* 1981;**22**:1–123.

Campanella, L., Cocco, R., Tomassetti, M. Determination of compounds with anticholinesterase activity in commercial drugs by a new enzyme sensor. *Journal of Pharmaceutical and Biomedical Analysis* 1992;**10**:741–9.

Caraway, W.T. Photometric determination of serum cholinesterase activity. *American Journal of Clinical Pathology* 1956;**26**:945–55.

Ceron, J.J., Fernadex del Palacio, M.J., Bernal, L.J., Gutierrez, C. Automated spectrophotometric method using 2,2'-dithiodipyridine acid for determination of cholinesterase in whole blood. *Journal of Association of Official Analytical Chemists* 1996;**79**:757–63.

Chan, L., Balabaskaran, S., Delilkan, A.E. et al. Blood cholinesterase levels in a group of Malaysian blood donors. *Malay Journal of Pathology* 1994;**16**:161–4.

Chemnitius, J.M., Haselmeyer, K.H., Gonska, B.D. et al. Indirect parasympathomimetic activity of metoclopramide; reversible inhibition of cholinesterases from human central nervous system and blood. *Pharmacological Research Communications* 1996;**34**:65–72.

Chiron, S., Rodrigez, A., Fernandez-Alba, A. Application of gas and liquid chromatography-mass-spectrometry to the evaluation of pirimiphos methyl degradation products in industrial water under ozone treatment. *Journal of Chromatography A* 1998;**823**:97–107.

Chu, S.Y. Depression of serum cholinesterase activity as an indicator for insecticide exposure-consideration of the analytical and biological variations. *Clinical Biochemistry* 1985;**18**:323–6.

Cirimele, V., Kintz,P., Ludes,B. Evidence of pesticides exposure by hair analysis. *Acta Clin Belg* 1999 :**Suppl 1**:59-63.

Clark, G.J., Goodin, R.R., Smiley, J.W. Comparison of ultraviolet and reductive amperometric detection for determination of ethyl and methyl parathion in green vegetables and surface water using high performance liquid chromatography. *Analytical Chemistry* 1985;**57**:2223-8

Cucuianu, M., Bornuz, F., Macava, I. Effects of L-asparaginase therapy upon serum pseudocholinesterase and caeruloplasmin levels in patients. *Clinica Chimica Acta* 1972;**38**:97.

D'Agostino, P.A., Hancock, J.R., Provost, L.R. Packed capillary liquid chromatography-electrospray mass spectrometry analysis of OP chemical warfare agents. *Journal of Chromatography A* 1999;**840**:289–94.

Da Silva, E.S., Midio, A.F., Garcia, E.G. A field method for the determination of whole blood cholinesterase. *Medicina del Lavoro* 1994:**85**:249–54.

Dao, Y.J., Tellez, J., Turner, D.R.   Dose-dependent effect of metoclopramide on cholinesterases and suxamethonium metabolism. *British Journal of Anaesthesia* 1990;**65**:220–4.

Das, P.K., Liddell, J.   Value of butyrylthiocholine assay for identification of cholinesterase variants. *Journal of Medical Genetics* 1970;**7**:351–5.

Davis, L., Britten, J.J., Morgan, M.   Cholinesterase. *Anaesthesia* 1997;**52**:244–60.

De la Huerga, J., Yesiniki, C., Popper, H.   Colorimetric method for the determination of serum cholinesterase. *American Journal of Clinical Pathology* 1952;**22**:1126–33.

de Peyster, A., Willis, W.O., Liebhaber, M.   Cholinesterase activity in pregnant women and newborns. *Clinical Toxicology* 1994;**32**:683–96.

Diamond, G., Quebbemann, A.J.   Rapid separation of p-nitrophenol and its glucuronide and sulphate conjugates by reversed phase high-performance liquid chromatography. *Journal of Chromatography* 1979;**177**:368–71.

Dietz, A.A., Rubinstein, H.M., Lubrano, T.   Colorimetric determination of serum cholinesterase and its genetic variants by the propionylthiocholine-dithiobis (nitrobenzoic acid) procedure. *Clinical Chemistry* 1973;**19**:1309–13.

Dillman, J.B.   Safe use of succinylcholine during repeated anaesthestics in a patient treated with cyclophosphamide. *Anaesthesia and Analgesia* 1987;**66**:351–3.

Edson, E.F.   Blood tests for users of OP pesticides. *World Crops* 1950;**10**:49–51.

Ellin, R.I., Vicario, P.   A pH method for measuring blood cholinesterase. *Archives of Environmental Health* 1975;**30**:263–5.

Elliot, J. W., Walker, K.C., Penick, A.E. et al.   A sensitive procedure for urinary p-nitrophenol determination as a measure of exposure to parathion. *Journal of Agriculture and Food Chemistry*;**8**:111–7.

Ellman,G. L. Tissue sulfhydryl groups. *Archives of Biochemistry and Biophysics* 1959;**82**:70

Ellman, G.L., Courtney, K.D., Andres, V. et al.   A new and rapid colorimetric determination of acetylcholinesterase. *Biochemical Pharmacology* 1961;**7**:88–95.

Eluwa, E.O., Obidoa, O., Ogan, A.U. et al.   Erythrocyte membrane enzymes in sickle cell anaemia. Acetylcholinesterase and ATPase actvities. *Biochemical Medicine and Metabolic Biology* 1990;**44**:234–7.

Erdman, F., Brose, C., Schültz, H.   A TLC screening program for 170 commonly used pesticides using the corrected R_f value (R_f^c value). *International Journal of Legal Medicine* 1990;**104**:25–31.

Erhard, M.H., Schmidt, P., Kühlmann, R.et al. Detection of the OP nerve agent soman by an ELISA using monoclonal antibodies. *Archives of Toxicology* 1990;**64**:580–5.

Erhard, M.H., Schmidt, P., Kühlmann, R. et al. Development of an ELISA for detection of an OP compound using monoclonal antibodies. *Archives of Toxicology* 1989;**63**:462–8.

Evans, R.T., O'Callagham, J., Norman, A. A longitudinal study of cholinesterase changes in pregnancy. *Clinical Chemistry* 1988;**34**:2249–52.

Farran, A., De Pablo, J., Barcelo, D. Identification of OP insecticides and their hydrolysis products by liquid chromatography in combination with UV and thermospray-mass-spectrometric detection. *Journal of Chromatography* 1988;**455**:163–72.

Fischl, J., Pinto, N., Gordon, C. Rapid detection of OP poisons. *Clinical Chemistry* 1968;**14**:371–3.

Fontoura-da-Silva, S.E., Chautard-Freire-Maia, E.A. Butyrylcholinesterase variants (BUCHE and CHE2 loci) associated with erythrocyte acetylcholinesterase inhibition in farmers exposed to pesticides. *Human Heredity* 1996;**46**:142–7.

Fulton, B., Benfield, P. Galanthamine. *Drugs and Aging* 1996;**9**:60–5.

Futagami, K., Narazaki, C., Kataoka, Y. et al. Application of high-performance thin-layer chromatography for the detection of OP insecticides in human serum after acute poisoning. *Journal of Chromatography B* 1997;**704**:369–73.

Galbraith, D.A., Watts, D.C. Human erythrocyte acetylcholinesterase in relation to cell age. *Biochemical Journal* 1981:**195**:221–8.

Garcia-Lopez, J.A., Monteoliva, M. Physiological changes in human erythrocyte cholinesterase as measured with the 'pH-stat'. *Clinical Chemistry* 1988;**34**:2133–5.

Gaugham, G., Park, H., Priddle, J. et al. Refinement of the localisation of human butyrylcholinesterase to chromosone 3q26.1-q26.2 using a PCR-derived probe. *Genomics* 1991;**11**:455–8.

Geike, F. Dünnschichtchromatographisch-enzymatscher nachwiess von carbamaten. I. Nachwiess insektizider carbamate mit rinderleber-esterase. *Journal of Chromatography* 1970;**53**:269–77.

Geldmacher-v. Mallinckrodt, M., Machbert, G. Pesticides. In:. *Analytical Toxicology for Clinical, Forensic and Pharmaceutical Chemists*. Brandenburger, H. and Maes, R.A.A. eds. Walter de Gruyter: Berlin, New York. 1997. p. 215–63

Geldmacher-v. Mallinckrodt, M., Herrman, A. Gruppenreaktion zur Erfassung von p-Nitrophenolen, p-Aminophenolen and p-Phenylendiaminen im Harn. *Zeitschrift Kliniche un Cheme Kliniche Biochemie* 1969;7:34–7.

George, P.M., Joyce, S.L., Abernety, M.H. Screening for plasma cholinesterase deficiency: an automated succinylcholine based assay. *Clinical Biochemistry* 1988;**21**:159–62.

Gruss, R., Scheller, F. Amperometric method for the determination of the activity of cholinesterases and detection of the inhibitors of the enzymes. *Analytical Chemistry* 1989;**333**:29–32.

Guidance Note MS 17 from the *Health and Safety Executive*. Biological monitoring of workers exposed to OP pesticides. *HMSO* 1987. ISBN 0 11 8839519.

Hill, A.S., Beasley, H.L., McAdam, D.P. et al. Mono- and polyclonal antibodies to the organophosphate fenitrothion. 2. Antibody specificity and assay performance. *Journal of Ariculture and Food Chemistry* 1992:**40**:1471-4

Holstege, D.M., Scharberg, D.L., Tor, E.R. et al. A rapid multiresidue screen for OP, organochlorine and N-methyl carbamate insecticides in plant and animal tissues. *Journal of AOAC International* 1994;**77**:1263–74.

Holstege, D.M., Scharnberg, D.L., Richardson, E.R. et al. Multi-residue screen for OP insecticides using gel permeation chromatography-silica gel cleanup. *Journal of Association of Official Analytical Chemists* 1991;**74**:394–9.

Hosseini, J., Firuzian, F., Feely, J. Ethnic differences in the frequency distribution of serum cholinesterase activity. *Irish Journal of Medical Sciences* 1997;**166**:10–2.

Houeto, P., Borron, S.W., Baud, F.J. et al. Assessment of erythrocyte cholinesterase activity in victims of smoke inhalation. *Journal of Toxicology Clinical Toxicology* 1999;**37**:321–6.

Howard, J., East, M., Chaney, J. Plasma cholinesterase activity in early pregnancy. *Archives of Environmental Health* 1978;**33**:277–9.

Huizenga, J.R., Van Der Belt, K., Grips, G.H. The effect of storage at different temperatures on cholinesterase activity in human serum. *Journal of Clinical Chemistry and Clinical Biochemistry* 1985;**23**:283–5.

Hutchinson, A.O., Widdowson, E.M. Cholinesterase levels in the serum of healthy British children. *Nature* 1952:**169**:284–5.

Inestrosa, N.C., Alarcon, R., Arriagada, J. et al. Blood markers in Alzheimer disease: subnormal acetylcholinesterase and butyrylcholinesterase in lymphocytes and erythrocytes. *Journal of Neurological Sciences* 1994;**122**:1–5.

Jackson, S.H., Bailey, G.W.H., Stevens, G. Reduced plasma cholinesterase following haemodilutional cardiopulmonary bypass. *Anaesthesia* 1982;**37**:319–20.

Jones, J.W., Whittaker, M., Braven, J. Immunological assay of erythrocyte acetylcholinesterase. *Clinicia Chimica Acta* 1991;**200**:175–81.

Kamban, J.R., Naukam, R.J., Sastry, B.V.R. The effect of procainamide on plasma cholinesterase activity. *Canadian Journal of Anaesthesia* 1987;**34**:579–81.

Kaniaris, P., Fassoulaki, A., Liarmakopoulo, K. et al. Serum cholinesterase in patients with cancer. *Anaesthesia and Analgesia* 1979;**58**:82–4.

Kao, Y.J., Turner, D.R. Prolongation of succinylcholine block by metoclopramide. *Anaesthesiology* 1989;**70**:905–8.

Kaplan, E., Tildon, J.T. Changes in red cell enzyme activity in relation to red cell survival in infancy. *Pediatrics* 1963;**32**:371–5.

Karlsen, R.L., Sterri, S., Lyngaas, S. et al. Reference values for erythrocyte acetylcholinesterase and plasma cholinesterase activities, implications for organophosphate intoxication. *Scandinavian Journal of Clinical and Laboratory Investigation* 1981;**41**:301–2.

Khan, N., Tyagi, S.P., Salahddin, A. Diagnostic and prognostic significance of serum cholinesterase and lactate dehydrogenase in breast cancer. *Indian Journal of Pathology and Microbiology* 1991;**34**:126–30.

Kirch, W., Hoensch, H., Janisch, H.D. Interactions and non-interactions with ranitidine. *Clinical Pharmacokinetics* 1984;**8**:493–510.

Krause, A., Lane, A.B., Jenkins, T., et al. Pseudocholinesterase variation in Southern African populations *South African Medical Journal* 1987;**71** 298–301.

Kurhekar, M.P., Pundik, M.D., Meghal, S.K. Confirmation of parathion, methyl parathion and fenitrothion in biological material on thin-layer plates. *Journal of Analytical Toxicology* 1980;**4**:322–3.

Kusu, F., Tsuneta, T., Takamura, K. Fluorometric determination of pseudocholinesterase activity in postmortem blood samples. *Journal of Forensic Sciences* 1990;**35**:1330–4.

Lacorte, S., Barcelo, D. Determination of parts per trillion levels of OP pesticides in groundwater by automated on-line liquid-solid extraction followed by liquid chromatography/atmospheric pressure chemical ionisation mass spectrometry using positive and negative ion modes of operation. *Analytical Chemistry* 1996;**68**:2464–70.

Laine-Cessac, P., Turcant, A., Allain, P. Automated determination of cholinesterase activity in plasma and erythrocytes by flow injection analyses and application to identify subjects sensitive to succinyl choline. *Clinical Chemistry* 1989;**35**:77–80.

Lasser, E.G., Lang, J.H. Inhibition of acetylchinesterases by some organic contract media. *Investigative Radiology* 1966;**1**:237.

Laurell, C-B., Rannevik, G. A comparison of plasma protein changes induced by danazol, pregnancy and oestrogens. *Journal of Clinical Endocrinology and Metabolism* 1979;**49**:719–25.

Lepage, L., Schiele, F., Guaquen, R.,et al. Total cholinesterase in plasma: biological variations and references limits. *Clinical Chemistry* 1985;**31**;546–50.

Lim, L.Y., Go, M.L. The anticholinesterase activity of mefloquine. *Clinical and Experimental Pharmacology and Physiology* 1985;**12**:527–31.

London, L., Thompson, M.L., Sacks, S. et al. Repeatability and validity of a field kit for estimation of cholinesterase in whole blood. *Occupational and Environmental Medicine* 1995;**52**:57–64.

Lotti, M. Treatment of acute organophosphate poisoning. *Medical Journal of Australia* 1991;**154**:51–5.

Lotti, M. Cholinesterase inhibition: Complexities in interpretation. *Clinical Chemistry* 1995;**41**:1814–8.

Magnotti, R.A. Jr, Eberly, J.P., Quarm, D.E. et al. Measurement of acetylcholinesterase in erythrocytes in the field. *Clinical Chemistry* 1987;**33**:1731–5.

Magnotti, R.A., Dowling, K., Eberly, J.P. et al. Field measurement of plasma and erythrocyte cholinesterases. *Clinica Chimica Acta* 1988;**315**:315–32.

Martinez, R.C., Gonzalo, R., Moran, M.J.A. et al. Sensitive method for the determination of OP pesticides in fruits and surface waters by high performance liquid chromatography with ultra violet detection. *Journal of Chromatography* 1992;**607**:37–45.

McAdam, D.P., Hill, A.S., Beasley, H.L. et al. Mono- and polyclonal antibodies to the organophosphate fenitrothion.1. Approaches to hapten-protein conjugation. *Journal of Ariculture and Food Chemistry* 1992:**40**:1466-70

McConnell, R., Cedillo, L., Keifer, M. et al. Monitoring organophosphate insecticide-exposed workers for cholinesterase depression. New technology for office or field use. *Journal of Occupational Medicine* 1992;**34**:34–7.

McConnell, R., Magnotti, R. Screening for insecticide overexposure under field conditions: a re-evaluation of the tintometric cholinesterase kit. *American Journal of Public Health* 1994;**84**:479–81.

Messer, G.J., Stoudemire, A., Knos, G. et al. Electroconvulsive therapy and the chronic use of pseudocholinesterase-inhitor (ecothiopate iodide) eye-drops for glaucoma. *General Hospital Psychiatry* 1992;**14**:56–60.

Midtling, J.E., Barnett, P.G., Coye, M.J. *et al.* Clinical management of field worker organophosphate poisoning. *Western Journal of Medicine* 1985;**142**:514–8

Miki, A., Katagi, M., Tsuchihashi, H. et al. Determination of alkylmethylphosphoric acids, the main metabolites of OP nerve agents in biofluids by gas-chromatography-mass spectrometry and liquid-liquid -solid – phase- transfer -catalysed pentafluorobenzylation. *Journal of Analytical Toxicology* 1999;**23**:86–93.

Moate, T.F., Lu, C., Fenske, R.A. et al. Improved cleanup and determination of dialkyl phosphates in the urine of children exposed to OP insecticides. *Journal of Analytical Toxicology* 1999;**23**:230–6.

Morelis, R.M., Coulet, P.R., Simplot, A.et al. Rapid and sensitive discriminating determination of acetylcholinesterase activity in amniotic fluid with a choline sensor. *Clinica Chimica Acta* 1991;**203**:295–303.

Moriya, F., Hashimoto, Y., Kuo Tsung-Li. Pitfalls when determining tissue distributions of OP chemicals: sodium fluoride accelerates chemical degradation. *Journal of Analytical Toxicology* 1999;**23**:210–5.

Mulchandani, A., Kaneva, I., Chen, W. Biosensor for direct determination of OP nerve agents using recombinant *Escherichia coli* with surface expressed OP hydrolase. 2. Fibre-optic microbial biosensor. *Anaytical Chemistry* 1998;**70**:5042–6.

Mulchandani, A., Mulchandani, P.O., Kaneva, I. et al. Biosensor for direct determination of OP nerve agents using recombinant Escherichia coli with surface coated OP hydrolase. 1. Potentiometric microbial electrode. *Analytical Chemistry* 1998;**70**:4140–5.

Mutch, E., Blain, P.G., Williams, F.M. Interindividual variation in enzymes controlling organophosphatase toxicity in man. *Human and Experimental Toxicity* 1992;**11**:430–2.

Nagao, M., Takatori, T., Matsuda, Y. *et al.* Detection of sarin hydrolysis products from sarin–like OP agent-exposed human erythrocytes. *Journal of Chromatography B* 1997;**701**:9–17.

Nagel, D., Seiler, D., Franz, H. et al. Ultra-long-distance running and the liver. *International Journal of Sports Medical* 1990;**11**:441–5.

Namera, A., Utsumi, Y., Yashiki, M. et al. Direct colorimetric method for determination of OPs in human urine. *Clinica Chimica Acta* 2000;**291**:9–18.

Needham, P.H. An investigation into the use of bioassay for pesticide residues in foodstuffs. *Analyst* 1960;**85**:792–809.

Nhachi, C.F.B., Marabiwa, W., Kasilo, O.J. *et al.* Effect of a single oral dose of metrifonate on human plasma cholinesterase levels. *Bulletin of Environmental Contamination and Toxicology* 1991;**47**:641–5.

Norel, X., Angrisani, M., Labat, C., et al. Degradation of acetylcholine in human airways: role of butyrylcholinesterase. *British Journal of Pharmacology* 1993;**108**:914–10.

O'Malley, M. Clinical evaluation of pesticide exposure and poisoning. *Lancet* 1997;**349**:1161–6.

O'Malley, M., McCrdy, S. Subacute poisoning with the organophosphate insecticide phosalone. *Western Journal of Medicine* 1990;**153**:619–24.

Oliveira-Silva, J.J., Alves, S.R., Inacio, A.F. et al. Cholinesterase activities determination in frozen blood samples: an improvement to the occupational monitoring in developing countries. *Human and Experimental Toxicology* 2000;**19**:173–7.

Ott, D.E. Mechanized system for liquid chromatographic determination of 4-nitrophenol and some other phenolic pesticide metabolites in urine. *Journal of Association of Official Analytical Chemists* 1979;**62**:93–9.

Oudart, J.L., Holmstedt, B. Determination of plasma cholinesterase activity by means of a test paper and its use in the field. *Archives of Toxicology* 1970;**27**:1–12.

Palleschi, G., Lavagnini, M.G., Moscone, D. et al. Determination of serum cholinesterase activity and dibucaine numbers by an amperometric choline sensor. *Biosensor and Bioelectronica* 1990;**5**:27–35.

Pantuck, E.J. Ecothipate iodide eye drops and prolonged response to suxamethonim. *British Journal of Anaesthesia* 1966;**38**:406–7.

Phillips, B.J., Hunter, J.M. Use of mivacrium chloride by constant infusion in the anephric patient. *British Journal of Anaesthesia* 1992;**68**:492–8.

Pinto Pereira, L.M., Clement, Y., Telang, B.V. Distribution of cholinesterase activity in the population of Trinidad. *Canadian Journal of Physiology and Pharmacology* 1996;**74**:286–9.

Porter, W.H. In: *Tietz Textbook of Clinical Chemistry.* Burtis, C.A. and Ashwood, E.R. eds 3rd edition. 1999; p 906–81.

Prall, Y.G., Gambhir, K.K., Ampy, F.R. Acetylcholinesterase: an enzymatic marker of human red blood cell ageing. *Life Sciences* 1998;**63**:177–84.

Price, E.M., Brows, S.S. Scope and limitations of propionylthiocholinesterase in the characterisation of cholinesterase variants. *Clinical Biochemistry* 1975;**8**:384–90.

Priebe, S.R., Howell, J.A. Post-column reaction detection system for the determination of OP compounds by liquid chromatography. *Journal of Chromatography* 1985;**324**:53–63.

Primo-Parmo, S.L., Lightstone, H., La Du, B.N. Characterization of an unstable variant (BuChE115D) of human butyrylcholinesterase. *Pharmacogenetics* 1997;7:27–34.

Puche, E., Garcia Morillas, M., Garcia de la Serranna, H. et al. Probable pseudocholinesterase induction by valproic acid, carbamazepine and phenytoin leading to increased serum aspirin-esterase activity in epileptics. *International Journal of Clinical Pharmacology Research* 1989;**9**:309–11

Ramsteiner, K.A. Hörmann, W.D. Coupling high-pressure liquid chromatography with a cholinesterase inhibition AutoAnalyzer for the determination of organophosphate and carbamate insecticide residues. *Journal of Chromatography* 1975;**104**:438–42.

Ratnaike, S., Gray, F., Deam, D. Cholinesterase assay automated in the Cobas-Bio centrifugal analyser. *Clinical Chemistry* 1987;**33**:1460–2.

Robertson, G.S. Serum protein and cholinesterase changes in association with contraceptive pills. *Lancet* 1967;**i**:232–5.

Ryhanen, R., Hanninen, O. A simple method for the measurement of blood cholinesterase activities under field conditions. *General Pharmacology* 1987;**18**:189–91.

Sakuma, N., Hasimoto, Y., Iwatsaki, N. Effects of neostigmine and edrophonium on human hydroxylacetyl cholinesterase activity. *British Journal of Anaesthesia* 1992;**68**:316–7.

Salamoun, J., Remien, J. Indirect detection of anti-acetylcholinesterase compounds in microcolumn liquid chromatography using packed bed reactor with immobilised human red blood cell acetylcholinesterase and choline oxidase. *Journal of Pharmaceutical and Biomedical Analysis* 1992;**20**:931–6.

Sanz, P., Rodriguex-Vicente, M.C., Diaz, D. et al. Red blood cell and total blood acetylcholinesterase and plasma pseudocholinesterase in humans: observed variances. *Journal of Toxicology Clinical Toxicology* 1991;**29**:81–90.

Sawhney, A.C., Loth, J.A. Acetylcholinesterase and cholinesterase. In: *Clinical Enzymology*. Loth, J.A. and Wolf, P.L eds. Fied, Rich and Associates Inc New York. 1986. p. 1–26.

Schacterle, S., Feigel, C. Pesticide residue analysis in fresh produce by gas chromatography-tandem mass spectrometry. *Journal of Chromatography A* 1996;**754**:411–22.

Schmidt, E., Poliwoda, H., Bhl, V. *et al.* Observations of enzyme elevations in the serum during streptokinase treatment. *Journal of Clinical Pathology* 1972;**25**:650.

Sega, G.A., Tomkins Baand Griest, W.H. Analysis of methylphosphonic acid, ethyl methylphosphonic acid and isopropyl methyl phosphonic acid at low microgram per litre levels in ground water. *Journal of Chromatography A*, 1997;**990**:143–52.

Sevalkar, M.T., Patil, V.B., Katkar, H.N. Zinc-chloride-diphenylamine reagent for thin layer chromatographic detection of some OP and carbamate insecticides. *Journal of Association of Official Analytical Chemists* 1994:**74**;545-6

Silk, E., King, J., Whittaker, M. Assay of cholinesterase in clinical chemistry. *Annals of Clinical Biochemistry* 1979;**16**:57–75.

Singh, A.K., Hewetson, D.W., Jordon, K.C. et al. Analysis of OP insecticides in biological samples by selective ion monitoring gas chromatography-mass-spectrometry. *Journal of Chromatography* 1986;**369**:83–96

Sirvio, J., Kutvonen, R., Soininen, H. et al. Cholinesterase in the cerebrospinal fluid, plasma and erythrocytes of patients with Alzheimer's disease. *Journal of Neural Transmission* 1989;**75**:119–27.

Skerritt, J.H., Hill, A.S., Beasley, H.L. et al. Enzyme-linked immunoabsorbent assay for quantitation of organophosphate pesticides:fenitrothion, chlorpyrifos-methyl and pirimiphos-methyl in wheat grain and flour milling fractions. *Journal of AOAC International* 1992:**75**:519-27

Soeder, G., Golf, S.W., Graef, V. et al. Enzyme catalytic concentrations in human plasma after a marathon. *Clinical Biochemistry* 1989;**22**:155–9.

Sommariva, D., Territo, M., Ottomanco, C. *et al.* Serum lipoprotein subfractions before and during low calorie diet in obese women. *Ricerca in Clinica e in Laboratorio* 1985;**15**:258–66.

Soreq, H., Lapidot-Lifson, Y., Zakut, H.   A role for cholinesterases in tumourigenesis? *Cancer Cells* 1991;**3**:511–6.

Souza, R.L., Castro, R.M., Pereira, L. et al.   Frequencies of the butyrylcholinesterase K mutation in Brazilian population of European and African origins.   *Human Biology* 1998;**70**:965–70

Spliid, N.H., Koppen, B.   Determination of polar pesticides in ground water using liquid chromatography-mass spectrometry with atmospheric pressure chemical ionisation. *Journal of Chromatography A* 1996;**736**:105–14.

Stovner, J., Oftedal, N., Holmboe, J.   The inhbition of cholinesterases by pancuronium. *British Journal of Anaesthesia* 1975;**47**:949–53.

Strausse, A.A., Modanlou, H.D.   Transient plasma cholinesterase deficiency in preterm infants. *Developmental Pharmacology and Therapeutics* 1986;**9**:82–7.

Streichman, S., Klin, A., Tatarsky, I.et al.   Unique profile for erythrocyte membrane acetylcholinesterase in hereditary spherocytosis. *Biochimica et Biophysica Acta* 1983;**757**:168–75.

Szalontai, G.   High-performance liquid chromatography of OP insecticides. *Journal of Chromatography* 1976;**124**:9–16.

Szurdoki, F., Jaeger, L., Harris, A. et al.   Rapid assays for environmental and biological monitoring. *Journal of Environment Science and Health* 1995:**B31**:451-8

Tewari, S.N., Harpalani, S.P.   Detection and determination of OP insecticides in tissue by thin-layer chromatography.   *Journal of Chromatography* 1977;**130**:229–36.

Thapar, S., Bhushan, R., Mathur, R.P.   Simultaneous determination of a mixture of OP and carbamate pesticides by high performance liquid chromatography. *Biomedical Chromatography* 1994;**8**:153–7.

Thompson, J.C., Whittaker, M.   Pseudocholinesterase activity in thyroid disease. *Journal of Clinical Pathology* 1965;**18**:811–2.

Tsatsakis, A.M., Tutudaki, M.I., Tzatzarakis, M.N. et al. Pesticide deposition in hair: preliminary results of a model study of methomyl incorporation into rabbit hair. *Veterinary Human Toxicology* 1998:**40**:200-3.

Tunek, A., Svensson, L.A.   Bambuterol, a carbamate ester pro-drug of terbutaline, as inhibitor of cholinesterases in human blood. *Drug Metabolism and Disposition* 1988;**16**:759–64.

Turner, J.M., Hall, R.A., Whittaker, M. et al.   Effects of storage and repeated freezing and thawing on plasma cholinesterase activity. *Annals of Clinical Biochemistry* 1984;**22**:363–5.

Umeki, S. Biochemical abnormalities of the serum in anorexia nervosa. *Journal of Nervous and Mental Disease* 1993;**176**:503–6.

Unni, L.K., Hannant, M.E., Becker, R.E. High-performance liquid chromatographic method using ultraviolet detection for measuring metrifonate and dichlorvos levels in human plasma. *Journal of Chromatography* 1992;**573**:99–103.

Vallejo, R.P., Bogus, E.R., Mumma, R.O. Effects of hapten structure and bridging groups on antisera specificity in parathion immunoassay development. *Journal Agriculture and Food Chemistry* 1982;**30**:572–80.

Verjee, Z.H., Behal, R., Ayim, E.M. Effect of glucocorticoids on liver and blood cholinesterase. *Clinica Chimica Acta* 1977;**81**:41–6.

Viby-Morgensen, J., Hamel, H.K., Hansen, H.E. *et al*. Serum cholinesterase activity in burned patients. I. Biological findings. *Acta Anaesthesiologica Scandinavica* 1975;**19**:159–68.

Wellig Hunter, D.L., Pam, P.D., Padilla, S. Validation of the use of 6,6' dithiodinicotinic acid as a chromogen in the Ellman method for cholinesterase determination. *Veterinary and Human Toxicology* 1996;**38**:249–53.

Whittaker, M. Estimation of plasma cholinesterase activity and the use of inhibitors for the determination of phenotypes. *Association of Clinical Pathologists, Broadsheet 87*, 1977. BMA publication, London.

Whittaker, M. Ethnic distribution. In: *Monographs in Human Genetics*. Vol 11: cholinesterase. Beckman L. ed. Basel: Karger, 1986. p. 45–64.

Wilding, P., Zilva, J.F., Wilde, C.E. Transport of specimens for clinical chemistry analysis. *Annals of Clinical Biochemistry* 1977;**14**:301–6.

Worek, F., Mast, U., Kiderlen, D.et al. Improved determination of acetylcholinesterase activity in whole blood. *Clinica Chimica Acta* 1999;**288**:73–90.

Writter, R.F., Grubbs, L.M., Farrior, W.L. A simplified version of the Michel method for plasma and red cell cholinesterase. *Clinica Chimica Acta* 1966;**13**:76–81.

Wykoff, D.W., Davies, J.E., Banquet, A. et al. Diagnostic and therapeutic problems of parathion poisoning. *Annals of Internal Medicine* 1968;**68**:875–81.

Young, D. Effects of preanalytical variables on clinical laboratory tests. AACC Press, New York 1993.

Zapf, A., Heyer, R., Stan, H.J. Rapid micro liquid-liquid extraction method for trace element analysis of organic contaminants in drinking water. *Journal of Chromatography A* 1995;**694**:453–61.

Ziminski, K.R., Manning, T.J.   Separation of organophosphate, chlorinated and
    carbamate insecticides using conventional and reverse phase thin-layer
    chromatography. *Clinical Toxicology* 1981;**18**:731–5.
Zsigmond, E.K., Downs, J.R.   Plasma cholinesterase activity in newborns and
    infants. *Canadian Anaesthestists Society Journal* 1971;**18**:278–83.

CHAPTER 16

Monitoring Occupational Exposures to Organophosphorus Compounds

Angelo Moretto and Marcello Lotti

16.1. Monitoring Environmental Exposure

16.1.1. Types of Exposures

16.1.1.1. Anticholinesterase Organophosphates

Organophosphates (OPs) having anticholinesterase properties are mainly insecticides. Both industrial workers and farmers (field workers) may be exposed but the characteristics of the exposures differ.

1. Industrial workers; they are usually exposed to few specific substances (the active ingredients, their precursors and the co-formulants) during manufacturing and formulating and exposure conditions do not vary significantly over time. Both personal hygienic practices and adequacy of personal and environmental protective equipment can easily be controlled.

2. Field workers: the characteristics of exposure in the field vary. Moreover, differences occur between agricultural workers and professional pesticide applicators. In the latter case, workers are exposed to many different formulations and active ingredients, possibly during the same working day or week. They are usually better trained than most agricultural workers and more conscious in the use of the protective equipment. Agricultural workers are generally exposed to fewer compounds and for lesser time; they may have little or no training and the use of protective equipment is generally less frequent or inadequate. Training of workers is essential not only for the adoption of the appropriate hygienic measures while using pesticides, but also for their proper storage.

The literature reports examples of unexpected poisonings by OPs stored in anonymous containers or in inappropriate temperature conditions with the consequent formation of more toxic impurities (Soliman *et al.*, 1982; Baker *et al.*, 1978). This appears to be particularly relevant in tropical countries (Jeyaratnam, 1985; Clarke *et al.*, 1997; Tinoco-Ojanguren and Halperin, 1998) where the use of protective equipment may also be problematic due to climate (Chester *et al.*, 1990; Van Sittert and Dumas, 1990). Different tasks potentially expose the field worker to pesticides:

a. Mixing and loading: operators dilute the formulation and fill the device to be used for application. Splashes and spills might occur. The operations generally last few minutes and are repeated several times during the day.

b. Application: many different devices are used to apply the pesticides according to the type and amount of crop to be treated. Exposures might derive from hand-held devices (such as sprayers and aerosol generators) to knapsacks or vehicle mounted mistblowers. By-standers and flagmen might also be heavily exposed. During sheep dipping, the plunger submerges the sheep with his hands or, more recently, with a stick or paddle, and dermal exposure maybe significant. The pesticide might be sprayed on trees or might be applied to low crops: in the latter case, dispersion in air of the compound is less significant. Use of ultra-low volume systems may pose additional risks (Gun *et al.*, 1988).

c. Cleaning of equipment and protective devices: exposure is generally short-lasting and can be significant only if accidents occur. Sometimes, certain maintenance or repair procedures cannot be easily performed while wearing gloves. Therefore, dermal exposures become relevant (Gun *et al.*, 1988).

d. Re-entry in the field: farmers re-entering treated fields to perform tasks other than pesticide application are exposed to residual environmental levels of the applied pesticide. Levels vary according to the amount sprayed and the degradation rate of the active ingredient. This in turn depends on both the crop and the atmospheric conditions (Popendorf and Leffingwell, 1982). It has been shown that certain thiophosphates might be oxidized to oxygen analog (e.g. parathion to paraoxon) which is more toxic than the parent compound (Spear *et al.*, 1977; Popendorf and Leffingwell, 1982). Models to calculate re-entry times have been developed (Popendorf, 1992).

In conclusion, occupational exposure is generally dermal; inhalation is less significant because the sprayed particles are too large to be inhaled. Oral exposure might occur only following inadequate hygienic behaviour such as eating or smoking in the workplace.

16.1.1.2. Non Anticholinesterase OPs

Certain OPs are used as herbicides (e.g. anilifos, butamifos, piperophos) or fungicides (e.g. edifenfos, iprobenfos, pyrazophos, tolclofos-methyl). They are not cholinesterase inhibitors and are generally of low toxicity.

Certain triarylphosphates, mainly tricresyl phosphate (TCP) are used in the formulation of lubricants as an antiwear additive to enhance load-carrying capacity and tolerance to increase speed of rotating or sliding motion (Mackerer *et al.*, 1999). These properties are unique to this class of compounds which in certain situations cannot be replaced by less toxic compounds. Commercial TCPs contain tri-ortho-cresyl phosphate (TOCP) which causes organophosphate-induced delayed polyneuropathy (OPIDP). Negligible exposures occur during formulation of these products. The record of their use by mechanics and maintenance workers is safe, since almost all cases of poisoning, resulting in OPIDP, were caused by contamination of food or the inadvertent use of TOCP itself as a cooking oil (Inoue *et al.*, 1988). Recent technological improvements have led to the production of lubricants containing very low amounts of TOCP: percentages of ortho-substitutes in TCPs added to lubricants declined from about 25% in 1940s–1950s to <1% in more recent products. Accidental poisoning with these more recent products are unlikely to result in OPIDP even if the dose is massive (Mackerer *et al.*, 1999).

16.2. Measuring Exposure

Environmental monitoring provides a measurement of the amount of substance reaching the body barrier(s) and available for absorption (exposure). Patch monitoring, air sampling and hand washing are examples of environmental monitoring methods routinely used in the assessment of pesticide exposure.

A number of exposure models have been proposed for risk assessment (Popendorf, 1990; Krieger *et al.*, 1992; Fenske and Teschke, 1995; Kreiger, 1995; Nielsen *et al.*, 1995; Van Hemmen *et al.*, 1995; EUROPOEM, 1996) requiring default assumptions and extrapolations which are not applicable for the assessment of a single applicator's exposure.

16.3. Monitoring of Dermal Exposure

Dermal exposure to OPs can occur by:

1. Immersion: worker's skin comes into contact with the formulation/ mixture of the pesticide. This is most common during mixing and loading and unless accidental, can be prevented or reduced by wearing appropriate protective equipment: e.g. gloves, boots, masks. Monitoring of this type of exposure can only be done by the so called "removal techniques" (see below).
2. Skin deposition: this usually occurs when spraying the mixture
3. Contact with surfaces/crops where pesticides have been applied (re-entry workers). Depending on the type of surface (e.g. leaves, ground) different parts of the body might come into contact with the pesticide.

Several different methods are used to assess dermal exposure.

1. Surrogate skin techniques: a medium is positioned on the skin which collects the mixture and where the compound of interest is chemically analysed. The most common approach is the patch technique (WHO, 1982). Generally 10 patches are applied on the skin and/or clothing on defined areas of the following body regions: chest (1), back (1), upper (4) and lower (4) limbs. The amount of skin exposure (μ/m^2) is then extrapolated from the amount of chemical found in the patches and corrected for the skin surface actually exposed (i.e. not covered by protective equipment). Obviously this requires that the distribution of the compound is uniform across each body region where the patches are attached and in some circumstances this assumption might largely be wrong (Fenske, 1990a; Franklin *et al.*, 1981). Moreover, it is assumed that the patch captures and retains the compound in a manner similar to the skin and for most compounds this has not been validated.

Nevertheless, patch techniques might be useful to compare exposures due to different application techniques or protective equipment (Machado Neto *et al.*, 1992) or to quantify protective clothing penetration by placing patches outside and inside the clothing (Fenske, 1990b; Gold *et al.*, 1982; Nigg *et al.*, 1986, 1992).

Correlation between skin exposure and excretion of alkylphosphates (see below) was sometimes found (Weisskopf *et al.,* 1988; Aprea *et al.,* 1999). However, in several instances a better correlation was between the amount of active ingredient used and excretion of alkylphosphates (Franklin *et al.,* 1981, 1986; Fenske, 1989). Glove monitoring techniques have been used in workers re-entering the treated field because hands are mainly exposed. Limitations of this method have been highlighted (Fenske *et al.,* 1989).

2.   Chemical removal techniques: chemical deposits in selected parts of the body can be removed by washing or wiping and concentrations then measured. Washing with water/alcohol or water/surfactants are generally used to assess hand exposure (for instance after immersion exposure). The amount of compound determined in the hand wash has been found to correlate with urinary excretion of metabolites in several instances (McCurdy *et al.,* 1994; Aprea *et al.,* 1994, 1998). Wipes can be used for other skin surfaces. Removal efficiency is variable depending on the compound and on the solvent used to wash/wipe. Moreover, since the operation is usually performed after the end of exposure, some absorption may have occurred in the meantime, the extent depending on several variables including the compound, the solvents, the skin conditions. For instance, it was shown that in the case of chlorpyrifos, a one-hour delay in washing decreased the ratio, quantity removed/applied to 25% from the 50% determined immediately after end of exposure (Fenske and Lu, 1994).

3.   Fluorescent tracer techniques: fluorescent tracers are introduced into the formulation and exposed workers are subsequently observed in a dark area using longwave ultraviolet illumination. This technique allows qualitative determination of skin deposition patterns, efficiency of protective clothing and acceptability of work practices (Fenske, 1988a, 1988b; Fenske *et al.,* 1986a, 1986b, 1987; Roff, 1994; Kross *et al.,* 1996). This technique has several limitations including the requirement of introducing the tracer in the formulation, and the demonstration (still lacking) of correspondence between skin deposition or protective clothing penetration of the active ingredient and of the tracer.

Sources of exposure for fieldworkers are the crops (generally leaves and/or fruits) that have recently been treated with pesticides and the ground. The part of the residue of the pesticide on the crop which can be removed during the normal working operation is not necessarily identical to the total amount of pesticide present on and/or in the fruit/leaf. This "dislodgeable foliar residue" is then considered the critical measurement of exposure for these workers.

Specific procedures have been developed to sample and analyse foliage to determine foliar residues and their decay over time (Iwata *et al.,* 1977; Goh *et al.,* 1986; Smith, 1991; Brouwer *et al.,* 1992; Aprea *et al.,* 1994, 1997, 1999). However, the relationship between foliar residues and actual skin exposure of the worker (dermal transfer factor) cannot easily be established although a number of attempts have been reported in the literature (Popendorf and Leffingwell, 1982; Zweig *et al.,* 1985; Goh *et al.,* 1986; Stamper *et al.,* 1986; Spencer *et al.,* 1991; Krieger *et al.,* 1992; Popendorf, 1990, 1992).

16.4. Monitoring of Respiratory Exposure

Fieldworkers may be exposed to OPs as solid particulates or water-based aerosols. Concentration in air of the compound may be measured in samples collected either by a portable air sampling pump worn by the worker or by a static sampling pump. In the former case sampled air is the inhaled air. The size of the particles should also be taken into account since they may be too large, and may deposit in different parts of the airways (Hayes, 1991). The trapping system is chosen on the basis of the chemico-physical characteristics of the compound to be measured. US NIOSH, OSHA and EPA periodically publish the official/suggested methods for a number of pesticides. For risk assessment purposes, the respiratory dose is calculated from the air concentration and the estimated values for lung ventilation in adults at different degrees of physical activity. This does not take into account the bioavailability after inhalation which can be quite different among compounds and formulations.

16.5. Biological Monitoring

16.5.1. Monitoring Dose

OPs generally undergo extensive metabolism although there are instances where the compound is excreted mainly unchanged. OPs are generally hydrolysed at the P-ester bond giving the so-called "leaving group" (alcoholic moiety) and alkyl(thio)phosphates (acidic moiety). Metabolites are excreted via the urine. Therefore, OP exposures can be assessed by measuring the parent compound in plasma or urine or the metabolites in urine.

Analytical methods which allow the determination of the plasma levels exist for many OPs. These determinations are difficult or expensive for biological monitoring of occupational exposures and are less frequently used than the determination of urinary metabolites.

In workers exposed to OPs, 8 different alkylphosphates have been identified (Coye *et al.,* 1986; WHO, 1986); dimethylphosphate, dimethylthiophosphate, dimethyldithiophosphate, and dimethylphosphorothioate derive from dimethylated OPs whereas diethylphosphate, diethylthiophosphate, diethyldithiophosphate, and diethylphosphorothioate derive from diethylated OPs. Methods for the determination of urinary alkylphosphates require high resolution gas chromatography with FPD detector (Nutley and Cocker, 1993; Aprea *et al.,* 1996). Alkyphosphates are aspecific metabolites since they may derive from a large number of compounds. More specific are the "leaving groups": for instance 3,5,6-trichloropyridinol only derives from chlorpyrifos and from chlorpyrifos-methyl (Nolan *et al.,* 1984), p-nitrophenol only from parathion and parathion-methyl (Morgan *et al.,* 1977), and mono- and dicarboxylic acid from malathion exposure (Bradway and Shafik, 1977).

The interpretation of these data is difficult for the following reasons:

A. Specificity of metabolites: Alkylphosphates may derive from many different OPs which have different rates of metabolism and toxicities. For instance, certain exposures to either parathion-methyl or chlorpyrifos-methyl caused comparable excretion of dimethylphosphates and dimethylthiophosphates. However toxicological assessment of these exposures is different because the two compounds have quite a different toxicity: the rat oral LD_{50}s were 6 and >3000mg/kg, respectively (Moretto *et al.,* 1995). Also in the case of the alcoholic group, the parent compound to which the worker was exposed must be known to assess the toxicological relevance of the data. For instance, chlorpyrifos-methyl has a much lower toxicity (more than 1 order of magnitude) than the diethyl analog (Tomlin, 1997) and yet exposures to both can be measured by means of urinary excretion of 3,5,6-trichloropyridinol. On the other hand, parathion and parathion-methyl are hydrolysed to p-nitrophenol, which can be measured in urine, and have similar acute toxicity (Tomlin, 1997).

B. Relationship between urine sampling and exposure: Depending on the compound, metabolism and absorption route, the peak excretion might be reached at different times after exposure. Absorption after dermal exposure is generally slower than after ingestion or inhalation.

Certain compounds, such as chlorpyrifos (Moretto *et al.*, 1995; Aprea *et al.*, 1997; Fenske and Elkner, 1990), show a peak urinary excretion of alkylphosphates few hours after exposure. Since collection of the 24-hour post-exposure urine is not practical in the field, the timing for the collection of the spot sample must be chosen according to exposure pattern and the compound to which workers are exposed. Moreover, alkylphosphates may have different time-courses of excretion; for instance diethylphosphate peaks earlier than diethyl phosphorothioate after exposure to diazinon (Sewell *et al.*, 1999).

C. Relationship between amount found in urine and red blood cell acetylcholinesterase (AChE) inhibition:

The only established correlation between urinary metabolite excretion and effects on red blood cell (RBC) AChE (see below) is that for urinary p-nitrophenol in parathion exposed workers (Arterberry *et al.*, 1961). ACGIH set a Biological Exposure Index for workers exposed to parathion of 0.5mg p-nitrophenol/g of creatinine in urine at end of shift (ACGIH, 2000). In many instances both urinary metabolites and RBC AChE activity have been measured but in most cases no inhibition of the latter was found and therefore it could not be determined how far the concentration of urinary metabolites was from the one associated with cholinesterase inhibition (Kraus *et al.*, 1977, 1981; Popendorf *et al.*, 1979; Krieger and Thongsinthusak, 1993; Aprea *et al.*, 1998, 1999; Griffin *et al.*, 1999); less frequently minimal inhibition was observed (Spear *et al.*, 1977; Maroni *et al.*, 1990; Jauhiainen *et al.*, 1992)

In conclusion, given the high sensitivity of current techniques in analytical chemistry, the determination of plasma/urinary levels of the parent compound or its metabolite(s) is a sensitive method, more sensitive than measuring RBC AChE inhibition (see below), to monitor occupational exposures to OPs. However, it is difficult to give these data a precise toxicological significance beyond that of being a qualitative exposure index. Precise information on OP metabolism which is often lacking is necessary to estimate the administered dose from urinary levels of metabolites or parent compound. Most recently a toxicokinetic model for assessment of azinphosmethyl exposure has been developed linking the No-Observed Adverse Effect Level with urinary alkylphosphate excretion (Carrier and Brunet, 1999).

16.6. Monitoring Biochemical Effects

16.6.1. Blood Cholinesterase Inhibition

Acute toxicity of OPs is due to accumulation of AChE at nerve endings which in turn causes accumulation of acetylcholine (ACh). Excess of ACh is responsible for the clinical signs because of the ensuing overstimulaiton of parasympathetic, sympathetic, motor, and central nervous system (see relevant chapters for details). Besides in synapses, AChE is also present in the outer membrane of RBCs and to a lesser extent (about 10%) in human plasma, although its physiological function in blood is unknown.

Measurement of RBC AChE activity can be and is used to monitor occupational exposures to OPs and guidelines have been issued on methods, interpretations of results and actions to be taken (Plestina, 1984; WHO, 1986; Wilson et al., 1992).

A number of methods are available for blood cholinesterase determinations. They are not necessarily comparable and may have different accuracy and precision. Therefore, comparison between laboratories using different methods may not always be possible. USEPA reports on a workshop on cholinesterase methodologies where most of these problems were addressed (Wilson et al., 1992). A modified and simplified version of the Ellman's method (Ellman et al., 1961) has been proposed by WHO (Plestina, 1984). Under particularly difficult field conditions a kit (Tintometer method) is suggested (Plestina, 1984).

Plasma also contains pseudocholinesterases (butyrylcholinesterase), which can be inhibited by OPs. There is no known physiological substrate for these enzymes and their inhibition has no significance in terms of toxic effects (Lotti, 1995; Moretto and Lotti, 1993). The sensitivity of butyrylcholinesterase to inhibition by OPs differs from that of AChE. Table 16.1. reports a list of compounds and the enzyme they preferentially inhibit. The in vivo ratios between plasma cholinesterase and RBC AChE inhibitions also vary according to the dosage regimen (acute versus repeated) and timing of sampling after exposure. In the absence of data on RBC AChE inhibition, plasma cholinesterase activity (inhibition) is a marker of exposure rather than effect. Only if the ratio between the sensitivities to inhibition of the two enzymes is known for that particular compound, the inhibition (or the lack thereof) of RBC AChE might be extrapolated from inhibition of plasma cholinesterase.

Table 16.1. Differential sensitivity to inhibition by OPs of plasma cholinesterase and RBC AChE.

RBC AChE most inhibited Compound (reference)	Plasma cholinesterase most inhibited Compound (reference)
Dimefox (Edson, 1964)	Chlorfenvinphos (FAO/WHO, 1995)
Mevinphos (Rider *et al.*, 1975)	Chlorpyrifos (Eliason *et al.*, 1969)
Parathion (Hayes, 1963)	Demeton (Moeller and Rider, 1965)
Parathion-methyl (Rider *et al.*, 1970)	Diazinon (FAO/WHO, 1967)
	Dichlorvos (Rasmussen *et al.*, 1963)
	Ecothiophate iodide (Spiers and Juul, 1964)
	Fenitrothion (Vandekar, 1965)
	Malathion (Elliot and Barnes, 1963)
	Monocrotophos (FAO/WHO, 1996)
	Trichlorfon (Abdel-Aal *et al.*, 1970)

When interpreting RBC AChE data a number of issues should be considered: Inter-individual variability: Given the high inter-individual variability only changes of >20% on normal population average activity can be considered as not due to normal variation (Gallo and Lawryk, 1991). Moreover, there is also significant intra-individual variability. Therefore, it is suggested to compare the data with pre-exposure values and minimal differences for statistical recognition of abnormal values for both RBC AChE and plasma cholinesterase vary from 15–20% with one pre-exposure determination to 10–15% with 10 pre-exposure determinations (Gallo and Lawryk, 1991).

Ratio between RBC and nervous system AChE inhibition: It is always difficult for a given inhibitor, to know how accurately AChE inhibition in RBCs reflects that in the nervous system. Data obtained from animal studies indicate that there is a large difference among compounds in their accessibility to the nervous system. Access to RBCs is always easier than access to the nervous system but differences between the two compartments might be trivial for compounds which readily cross the blood brain barrier or relevant for those which do not. Consequently, RBC AChE data usually overestimate, though to a variable extent, nervous system inhibitions. Moreover, differences between different areas of the nervous system are conceivable and have been observed; the blood-brain barrier is generally more efficient than the nerve-brain barrier.

Reversibility of inhibition. Organophosphorylated AChE might undergo two reactions: ageing and spontaneous reactivation (see relevant chapters for details).

The rates of both reactions depend on the chemical structure of the side chain. Reversibility of inhibition must be taken into account if measurement is not performed immediately after exposure. The method used to determine the activity might also cause some reactivation of the inhibited enzyme. Rates of spontaneous reactivation vary as follows according to the side chain structure: (2-ClEtO)2>(MeO)2>(isoProO)2>(EtO)2; the presence of sulfur greatly increases the rate of reactivation of the analog compound (WHO, 1986).

Difference in the rate of reappearance of AChE activity between RBC and nervous system.

When AChE is irreversibly inhibited, the reappearance of activity depends on resynthesis of new enzyme. In RBCs it depends on new cells being produced by the bone marrow and entering the bloodstream: the rate of recovery has been calculated to be about 1% per day (Gallo and Lawryk, 1991). Animal data indicate that the half life of AChE in the nervous system is much faster (5–7 days) (Lotti, 1992).

Nevertheless, and taking into account all these issues, in most instances there is still a good correlation between levels of RBC AChE inhibition and symptoms of OP poisoning.

At least 50% AChE inhibition must be obtained in the nervous tissues to observe the first mild cholinergic signs. Severe symptoms occur at higher than 80% inhibitions and, without specific treatment, death occurs only at AChE inhibition higher than 90%. On these basis, guidelines for intervention in occupational settings have been given as described in Table 16.2. It has been suggested that workers with >30–50% RBC AChE inhibiton can return to OP exposure after AChE activity has returned to normal values (Plestina, 1984). This is not consistent with the rates resynthesis of AChE in RBC and nervous system described above. Others suggest a more flexible approach leaving the decision to the physician (HSE, 1987). California EPA requires that worker be removed from exposure when RBC AChE falls below 70% or plasma cholinesterase falls below 60% of their respective baselines. The worker can return to work when the values are >80% (Wilson *et al.*, 1997). It is not clear why plasma cholinesterase was chosen as an end-point.

16.7. Lymphocytic Neuropathy Target Esterase (NTE) inhibition

Some OPs cause a rare delayed polyneuropathy (OPIDP, see relevant chapter for details).

Commercial insecticides for which there is clear-cut evidence that they caused OPIDP in man are: chlorpyrifos, dichlorvos, methamidophos, trichlorfon, trichloronat (Lotti, 2000).

Most cases were accidental/suicidal poisonings with massive doses which caused severe cholinergic toxicity. The molecular target for OPIDP is neural neuropathy target esterase (NTE). OP pesticides are much more potent inhibitors of AChE than of NTE: based on *in vitro* data with animal and human enzymes and on in vivo data on animals, AChE is 1 or more orders of magnitude more sensitive to inhibition than NTE (Lotti, 2000). Other cases of OPIDP have been described after poisoning by tri-ortho-cresyl phophate (TOCP) (Inoue *et al.*, 1988). TOCP has very low cholinergic toxicity and, therefore, repeated intake/exposure may take place without toxic symptoms to alert the subject and for OPIDP to develop.

Table 16.2. Relationship between levels of RBC AChE inhibitions and biological/clinical effects and advised intervention measures (modified from Jeyaratnam and Maroni, 1994)

Significance	AChE inhibition	Measures required
Values indicative of or compatible with minor and reversible effects	$<30^{(1)}$	Medical surveillance needed
	$<50^{(2)}$	Working conditions to be examined to avoid exceeding such a level
Values indicative of or compatible with minor damages (initial symptoms, mild alterations of sensitive clinical indexes)	$30–60^{(1)}$ $50–70^{(2)}$	Temporary removal from exposure and analysis of working conditions needed

(1) Based on individual pre-exposure base-line.
(2) Based on normal reference values

NTE is also present in circulating lymphocytes (Bertoncin *et al.*, 1985) and its measurement has been proposed to monitor exposure to potentially neuropathic OPs (Lotti, 1987, 1989).

Scanty data so far accumulated indicate that there is a correlation between lymphocytic NTE inhibition soon after poisoning and the later development of OPIDP (Moretto and Lotti, 1998; McConnell *et al.*, 1999). When interpreting lymphocytic NTE data it should be kept in mind that: 1) available data do not allow the identification of a threshold for the NTE inhibition required to trigger the mechanism in man; 2) lymphocytic NTE activity has a large interindividual variability (Bertoncin *et al.*, 1985);

3) the possibility exists that the access of the inhibitor to the nervous system is lower than to lymphocytes; 4) reappearance of lymphocytic NTE is fast, probably faster than that in the nervous system (Moretto and Lotti, unpublished data).

Given these limitations and the characteristics of the OPs causing OPIDP, the use of this test is limited in the biomonitoring of occupational exposures and it has mainly been employed as a prognostic test for the development of OPIDP after acute OP poisoning (Moretto and Lotti, 1998).

16.8. Individual Susceptibility

In has long been known that paraoxon (the active metabolite of parathion) is hydrolysed by paraoxonase (now called PON1) and that the activity of PON1 is multimodally distributed in human populations (Ortigoza-Ferado et al., 1984). PON1 was shown to hydrolyse oxygen analogs of other OPs such as chlorpyrifos-oxon and diazinon-oxon and to play an important role in their detoxication in experimental animals since high levels of PON1 correlate with reduced sensitivity to OP poisoning (Costa et al., 1999). It has therefore been suggested that humans with low PON1 activity might be at greater risk of poisoning when exposed to certain OPs. Evidence to support this hypothesis is still lacking in humans.

16.9. Conclusions

A number of different tasks involve occupational exposures to OP insecticides. In most cases, exposure occurs mainly via the dermal route, the respiratory route being generally of minor importance. Measurement of environmental exposure or determination of urinary (or less frequently plasma) levels of the parent compound or of its metabolites is relatively easy from the analytical point of view and very sensitive.

However, data obtained from these measurements provide useful toxicological information only when compared with effects on targets of toxicity and this has been rarely done. Determination of lymphocytic NTE activity is still at an experimental stage and at the moment its use can only be recommended as a prognostic test for development of OPIDP after acute OP poisoning

References

Abdel-Al, A.M.A., El-Hawary, M.F.S., Kamel, H., *et al*. Blood cholinesterases, hepatic, renal and haemopoietic functions in children receiving repeated doses of "Dipterex". *Journal of the Egyptian Medical Association* 1970;**53**:265–71.

ACGIH. *Threshold limit values and biological exposure indices.* American Conference of Governmental Industrial Hygienist: Cincinnati, Ohio. 2000.

Aprea, C., Sciarra, G., Lunghini, L. Analytical method for the determination of urinary alkylphosphates in subjects occupationally exposed to organophosphorous insecticides and in the general population. *Journal of Analytical Toxicology* 1996;**20**:559–63.

Aprea, C., Sciarra, G., Sartorelli, P., *et al*. Biological monitoring of exposure to chlorpyrifos-methyl by assay of urinary alkylphosphates and 3,5,6-trichloro-2-pyridinol. *Journal of Toxicology and Environmental Health* 1997;**50**:581–94.

Aprea, C., Sciarra, G., Sartorelli, P., *et al*. Multi-route exposure assessment and urinary metabolites excretion of fentrothion during manual operation on treated ornamental plants in greenhouses. *Archives of Environmental Contamination and Toxicology* 1999;**36**:490–7.

Aprea, C., Sciarra, G., Sartorelli, P., *et al*. Biological monitoring of exposure to organophosphorus insecticides by urinary alkylphosphates. Protective measures during manual operations with treated plants. *International Archives of Environmental Health* 1994;**66**:333–8.

Aprea, C., Sciarra, G., Sartorelli, P., *et al*. Environmental and biological monitoring of exposure to mancozeb, ethylenethiourea and dimethoate during industrial formulation. *Journal of Toxicology and Environmental Health* 1998;**53**:263–81.

Arterberry, J.D., Durham, W.F., Elliot, J.W., *et al*. Exposure to parathion: measurement by blood cholinesterase level and urinary p-nitrophenol excretion. *Archives of Environmental Health* 1961;**3**:476–85.

Baker, E.L., Zack, M., Miles, J.W., *et al*. Epidemic malathion poisoning in Pakistan malaria workers. *Lancet* 1978;**i**:31–4.

Bertoncin, D., Russolo, A., Caroldi, S., *et al*. Neuropathy target esterase in human lymphocytes. *Archives of Environmental Health* 1985;**40**:139–44.

Bradway, D.E., Shafik, T.M. Malathion exposure studies. Determination of mono- and dicarboxylic acids and alkylphosphates in urine. *Agricultural and Food Chemistry* 1977;**25**:1342–4.

Brouwer, R., Marquart, H., De Mik, G., *et al.* Risk assessment of dermal exposure of greenhouse workers to pesticides after re-entry. *Archives of Environmental Contamination and Toxicology* 1992;**23**:273–80.

Carrier, G., Brunet, R.C. A toxicokinetic model to assess the risk of azinphosmethyl exposure in humans through measures of urinary elimination of alkylphosphates. *Toxicological Sciences* 1999;**47**:23–32.

Chester, G., Adanl, A.V., Inkmann Koch, A., *et al.* Field evaluation of protective equipment for pesticide operators in a tropical climate. *La Medicina del Lavoro* 1990;**81**:480–8.

Clarke, E.E., Levy, L.S., Spurgeon, A., *et al.* The problems associated with pesticide use by irrigation workers in Ghana. *Occupational Medicine* 1997;**47**:301–8.

Costa, L.G., Li, W.F., Richter, R.I., *et al.* The role of paraoxonase (PON1) in the detoxication of organophosphates and its human polymorphism. *Chemico-Biological Interactions* 1999;**119**–120:429–38.

Coye, M.J., Lowe, J.A., Maddy, K.J. Biological monitoring of agricultural workers exposed to pesticides: II. Monitoring of intact pesticides and their metabolites. *Journal of Occupational Medicine* 1986;**28**:628–36.

Edson, E.F. No-effect levels of three organophosphates in the rat, pig, and man. *Food and Cosmetic Toxicology* 1964;**2**:311–6.

Eliason, D.A., Cranmer, M.F., von Windeguth, D.L., *et al.* Dursban premises application and their effect on the cholinesterase levels in spraymen. *Mosquito News* 1969;**29**:591–5.

Elliot, R., Barnes, J.M. Organophosphorus insecticides for the control of mosquitos in Nigeria. *Bulletin of the World Health Organization* 1963;**28**:35–54.

Ellman, G.L., Courtney, K.K., Andres, W., Jr., *et al.* A new and rapid colorimetric determination of acetylcholinesterase activity. *Biochemical Pharmacology* 1961;**7**:88–95.

EUROPOEM The development, manteinance and dissemination of a European predicitive operator exposure model (EUROPOEM) database. A EUROPOEM database and harmonised model for predicition of operator exposure to plant protection products. A harmonised protocol for conduct of field studies of operator exposure. A tiered approach to exposure and risk assessment. AIR3 CT93–1370, Carshalton, UK. 1996.

Fenske, R.A. Correlation of fluorescent tracer measurements of dermal exposure and urinary metabolite excretion during occupational exposure to malathion. *American Industrial Hygiene Journal* 1988a;**49**:438–44.

Fenske, R.A.   Comparative assessment of protective clothing performance by measurement of dermal exposure during pesticide applications. *Applied Industrial Hygiene* 1988b;3:207–13.

Fenske, R.A. Nonuniform dermal deposition patterns during occupational exposures to pesticides. *Archives of Environmental Contamination and Toxicology* 1990a;**19**:332–7.

Fenske, R.A. Worker exposure and protective clothing performance during manual seed treatment with lindane. *Archives of Environmental Contamination and Toxicology* 1990b;**19**:190–6.

Fenske, R.A. Validation of environmental monitoring by biological monitoring. Fluorescent tracer technique and patch technique. In: *Biological Monitoring for Pesticide Exposure: Measurement, Estimation, and Risk Reduction*, ACS Symposium Series No. 382. Wang, R.G.M., Franklin, C.A., Honeycutt, R.C., Reinert, J.C. eds. The Sheridan Press; Pennsylvania, USA: 1989. p. 70–84

Fenske, R.A., Bimbaum, S.G., Methner, M.M., *et al.*   Methods for assessing fieldworker hand exposure to pesticides during peach harvesting. Bulletin of *Environmental and Contamination Toxicology* 1989;**43**:805–13.

Fenske, R.A., Elkner, K.P.   Multi-route exposure assessment and biological monitoring of urban pesticide applicators during structural control treatments with chlorpyrifos. *Toxicology and Industrial Health* 1990;**6**:349–71.

Fenske, R.A., Horstman, S.W., Bentley, R.K. Assessment of dermal exposure to chlorophenols in timber mills. *Applied Industrial Hygiene* 1987;**2**:143–7.

Fenske, R.A., Leffingwell, J.T., Spear, R.C.   A video imaging technique for assessing dermal exposure–1. Instrument design and testing. *American Industrial Hygiene Association Journal* 1986a;**47**:764–70.

Fenske, R.A., Lu, C. Determination of handwash removal efficiency: incomplete removal of the pesticide chlorpyrifos from skin by standard handwash techniques. *American Industrial Hygiene Association Journal* 1994;**55**:425–32

Fenske, R.A., Teschke, K. Study design considerations for occupational pesticide exposure assessment. In: Curry, P.B., Iyengar, S., Maloney, P.A., Maroni, M. eds. *Methods of Pesticides Exposure Assessment*. New York and London: Plenum Press; 1995. p. 51–9.

Fenske, R.A., Wong, S.M., Leffingwell, J.T. *et al.* A video imaging technique for assessing dermal exposure–II. Fluorescent tracer testing. *American Industrial Hygiene Association Journal* 1986b;**47**:771–5.

Food and Agriculture Organization/World Health Organization (FAO/WHO) (1967). Evaluations of Some Pesticide Residues in Food. Joint Meeting of the FAO Working Party and the WHO Expert Committee on Pesticide Residues. WHO/FoodAdd./667.32. WHO: Geneva. 1966.

Food and Agriculture Organization/World Health Organization (FAO/WHO) Pesticide Residues in Food, 1994. Evaluations of the Joint Meeting of the FAO panel of experts on pesticide residues in food and environment and the WHO expert group on pesticide residues. Part II Toxicological and Environmental. WHO/PCS/95.2. WHO: Geneva. 1995.

Food and Agriculture Organization/World Health Organization (FAO/WHO) Pesticide Residues in Food, 1995. Evaluations of the Joint Meeting of the FAO panel of experts on pesticide residues in food and environment and the WHO expert group on pesticide residues. Part II Toxicological and Environmental. WHO/PCS/96.48. WHO: Geneva. 1996.

Franklin, C.A., Fenske, R.A., Greenhalgh, R. *et al.* Correlation of urinary pesticide metabolite excretion with estimated dermal contact in the course of occupational exposure to guthion. *Journal of Toxicology and Environmental Health* 1981;7:715–31.

Franklin, C.A., Muir, N.I., Moody, R.P. The use of biological monitoring in the estimation of exposure during the application of pesticides. *Toxicology Letters* 1986;**33**:127–36.

Gallo, M.A., Lawryk, N.J. Organic phosphorus pesticides. In: Hays, W.J., Jr, Laws, E.R., Jr. eds. *Handbook of Pesticide Toxicology.* San Diego: Academic Press; 1991. p. 917–1123.

Goh, K.S., Edmiston, S., Maddy, K.T., *et al.* Dissipation of dislodgeable foliar residue for chlorpyrifos and dichlorvos treated lawn: implication for safe re-entry. *Bulletin Environmental Contamination and Toxicology* 1986;**37**:33–40.

Gold, R.E., Leavitt, J.R.C., Holsclav, T., *et al.* Exposure of urban applicators to carbaryl. *Archives of Environmental Contamination and Toxicology* 1982;**11**:63–7.

Griffin, P., Mason, H., Heywood, K., *et al.* Oral and dermal absorption of chlorpyrifos: a human volunteer study. *Occupational and Environmental Medicine* 1999;**56**:110–3.

Gun, R.T., Grycorcewicz, C., Estennan, A.J., *et al.* Ultralow volume application of organophosphate concentrate in grain terminals: new occupational health hazard. *British Journal of Industrial Medicine* 1988;**45**:834–7.

Hayes, W.J. Studies in humans. In: *Handbook of Pesticide Toxicology*. Volume 1. General Principles. Hayes, W.J., Jr., Laws, E.R., Jr. eds. Academic Press; San Diego: 1991. p. 215–44.

Hayes, W.J., Jr. *Clinical Handbook on Economic Poisons. Emergency Information for Treating Poisoning*, Public Health Serv. Publ. No. 476. U.S. Govt. Printing Office: Washington, D.C. 1963.

HSE. Biological monitoring of workers exposed to organo-phosphorus pesticides. Guidance note MS 17 Health and Safety Executive: London, UK. 1987.

Inoue, N., Fujishiro, K., Mori, K., *et al.* Triorthocresyl phosphate poisoning—a review of human cases. *Sangyo Ika Daigaku Zasshi* 1988;**10**:433–42.

IPCS. 1986 *Environmental Health Criteria 63*. Organophosphorus Insecticides. A General Introduction. World Health Organisation, International Programme on Chemical Safety, Geneva.

Iwata, Y., Spear, R.C., Knaak, J.B., *et al.* Worker re-entry into pesticide-treated crops. I. Procedure for the determination of dislodgeable pesticide residues on foliage. *Bulletin of Environmental Contamination and Toxicology* 1977;**18**:649–55.

Jauhiainen, A., Kangas, J., Laitinen, S., *et al.* Biological monitoring of workers exposed to mevinphos in greenhouses. *Bulletin of Environmental Contamination and Toxicology* 1992;**49**:37–43.

Jeyaratnam, J. Health problems of pesticide usage in the Third World. *British Journal of Industrial Medicine* 1985;**42**:505–6.

Jeyaratnam, J., Maroni, M. Organophosphorus compounds. *Toxicology* 1994;**91**:15–27.

Kraus, J.F., Mull, R., Kurts, P., *et al.* Epidemiological study of physiological effects in usual and volunteer citrus workers from organophosphate pesticide residues at re-entry. *Journal of Toxicology and Environmental Health* 1981;**8**:169–84.

Kraus, J.F., Richards, D.M., Borhani, N.O., *et al.* Physiological response to organophosphate residues in field workers. *Archives of Environmental Contamination and Toxicology* 1977;**5**:471–85.

Krieger, R.I. Quantitative assessment of human pesticide exposure: some defaults and assumptions. In: Curry, P.B., Iyengar, S., Maloney, P.A., Maroni, M. eds. *Methods of Pesticides Exposure Assessment*. New York and London: Plenum Press; 1995. p. 1–15.

Krieger, R.I., Ross, J.H., Thongsinthusak, T. Assessing human exposures to pesticides. In: *Methods of Pesticides Exposure Assessment*. Curry, P.B., Iyengar, S., Maloney, P.A., Maroni, M. eds. Plenum Press; New York and London: 1995. p. 129–34.

Krieger, R.I., Thongsinthusak, T.   Metabolism and excretion of dimethoate following ingestion of overtolerance peas and a bolus dose. *Food and Chemical Toxicology* 1993;**31**:177–82.

Kross, B.C., Nicholson, H.F., Ogilvie, L.K.   Methods development study for measuring pesticide exposure to golf course workers using video imaging techniques. *Applied Occupational and Environmental Hygiene* 1996;**11**:1346–50.

Lotti, M.   Central neurotoxicity and behavioral effects of anticholinesterases. In: *Clinical and Experimental Toxicology of Organophosphates and Carbamates.* Ballantyne, B., Marrs, T.C. eds. Butterworth–Heinemann; Oxford:1992. p. 75–83.

Lotti, M.   Neuropathy target esterase in blood lymphocytes. Monitoring the interaction of organophosphates with a primary target. In: *Biological Monitoring for Pesticide Exposure: Measurement, Estimation, and Risk Reduction,* ACS Symposium Series No. 382. Wang, R.G.M., Franklin, C.A., Honeycutt, R.C., Reinert, J.C. eds. The Sheridan Press: Pennsylvania, USA. 1989. p. 117–23

Lotti, M.   Organophosphate-induced delayed polyneuropathy in humans: perspectives for biomonitoring. *Trends in Pharmacological Sciences* 1987;**8**:175–6.

Lotti, M.   Organophosphorus compounds. In: *Experimental and Clinical Neurotoxicology,* 2nd Edition Spencer, P.S., Schaumburg, H.S., Ludolph, A.C. eds. Oxford University Press; New York: 2000. p. 898–925

Lotti, M.   Cholinesterase inhibition: complexities in interpretation. *Clinical Chemistry* 1995;**69**:705–11.

Machado Neto, J.G., Matuo, T., *et al.*   Dermal exposure of pesticide applicators in staked tomato (*Lycopersicon esculentum* mill) crops: efficiency of safety measure in the application equipment. *Bulletin Environmental Contamination and Toxicology* 1992;**48**:529–34.

Mackerer, C.R., Barth, M.L., Krueger, A.J., *et al.*   Comparison of neurotoxic effects and potential risks from oral administration or ingestion of tricresyl phosphate and jet engine oil containing tricresyl phosphate. *Journal of Toxicology and Environmental Health* Part A, 1999;**56**:293–328.

Maroni, M., Catenacci, G., Galli, D., *et al.*   Biological monitoring of human exposure to acephate. *Archives of Environmental Contamination and Toxicology* 1990;**19**:782–8.

McConnell, R., Delgado-Tellez, E., Cuadra, R., *et al.* Organophosphate neuropathy due to methamidophos: biochemical and neurophysiological markers. *Archives of Toxicology* 1999;**73**:296–300.

McCurdy, S.A., Hansen, M.E., Weisskopf, C.P., *et al.* Assessment of azinophosmethyl exposure in Califomia peach harvest workers. Archives of Environmental Health 1994;**49**:289–96.

Moeller, H.C., Rider, J.A. Further studies on the anticholinesterase effect of Systox and methyl parathion in humans. *Proceedings of the Federation of American Societies for Experimental Biology* 1965;**24**

Moretto, A., Capodicasa, E., Bertolazzi, M., *et al.* Biological monitoring of occupational exposures to organophosphorus insecticides. In: *Agriculture Health and Safety. Workplace, Environment, Sustainability.* McDuffie, H.H., Dosman, J.A., Semchuk, K.M., Olenchock, S.A., Senthilselvan, A. eds. CRC Press Inc., Lewis Publishers; Boca Raton, Florida: 1995. p. 217–21.

Moretto, A., Lotti, M. Poisoning by organophosphorus insecticides and sensory neuropathy. *Journal of Neurology, Neurosurgery and Psychiatry* 1998;**64**:463–8.

Moretto, A., Lotti, M. Toxicity of Pesticides. In: *Occupational Toxicology.* London: Taylor and Francis; Stacey, N.H. ed.1993. p. 177–204.

Morgan, D.P., Hetzler, H.L., Slach, E.F., *et al.* Urinary excretion of paranitrophenol and alkyl phosphates following ingestion of methyl or ethyl parathion by human subjects. *Archives of Environmental Contamination and Toxicology* 1977;**6**:159–73.

Nielsen, A., Curry, P., Leighton, T. The pesticide handlers exposure database (PHED): regulatory overview. In: *Methods of Pesticides Exposure Assessment.* Curry, P.B., Iyengar, S., Maloney, P.A., Maroni, M. eds. Plenum Press; New York and London: 1995. p. 89–94.

Nigg, N.H., Stamper, H.H., Easter, E., *et al.* Field evaluation of coverall fabrics: heat stress and pesticide penetration. *Archives of Environmental Contamination and Toxicology* 1992;**23**:281–8.

Nigg, N.H., Stamper, H.H., Queen, R.M. Dicofol exposure to florida citrus applicators: effects of protective clothing. *Archives of Environmental Contamination and Toxicology* 1986;**15**:121–34.

Nolan, R.J., Rich, D.L., Frehour, N.L., *et al.* Chlorpyrifos: pharmacokinetics in human volunteers. *Toxicology and Applied Pharmacology* 1984;**73**:8–15.

Nutley, B., Cocker, J. Biological monitoring of workers occupationally exposed to organophosphorus pesticides. *Pesticide Science* 1993;**38**:315–22.

Ortigoza-Ferado J., Richter, R.J., Homung, S., *et al.* Paraoxon hydrolysis in human serum mediated by a genetically variable arylesterase and albumin. *American Journal of Human Genetics* 1984;**36**:295–305.

Plestina, R. *Prevention, diagnosis and treatment of insecticide poisoning.* WHO/VBC/84.889 Geneva, Switzerland. 1984.

Popendorf, W. Re-entry field data and conclusions. *Reviews of Environmental Contamination and Toxicology* 1992;**128**:71–117.

Popendorf, W. Effects of organophosphate insecticide residue variability on re-entry intervals. *American Journal of Industrial Medicine* 1990;**18**:313–9.

Popendorf, W.J., Leffingwell, J.T. Regulating OP pesticides residues for farmworker protection. *Residue Reviews* 1982;**82**:125–201.

Popendorf, W.J., Spear, R.C., Leffingwell, J.T., *et al.* Harvester exposure to zolone (phosalone) residues in peach orchards. *Journal of Occupational Medicine* 1979;**21**:189–94.

Rasmussen, W.A., Jensen, J.A., Stein, W.J. *et al.* Toxicological studies of DDVP for disinfection of aircraft. *Aerospace Medicine* 1963;**34**:594–600.

Rider, J.A., Puletti, E.J., Swader, J.I. The minimal oral toxicity level for mevinphos in man. *Toxicology and Applied Pharmacology* 1975;**32**:92–100.

Rider, J.A., Swader, J.I., Puletti, E.J. Methyl parathion and guthion anticholinesterase effects in human subjects. *Proceedings of the Federation of American Societies for Experimental Biology* 1970;**29**:349.

Roff, M.W. A novel lighting system for the measurement of dermal exposure using a fluorescent dye and an image processor. *Annals of Occupational Hygiene* 1994;**38**:903–19.

Sewell, C., Pilkington, A., Buchanan, D., *et al.* Epidemiological study of the relationships between exposure to organophosphate pesticides and indices of chronic peripheral neuropathy and neuropsycholocial abnormalities in sheepfarmers and dippers. Phase 1. Development and validation of an organophosphate uptake model for sheep dippers. IOM, Institute of Occupational Medicine, Technical Memorandum Series. Edinburgh. 1999.

Smith, C.R. Dissipation of dislodgeable propargite residues on nectarine foliage. *Bulletin of Environmental Contamination Toxicology* 1991;**46**:507–11.

Soliman, S.A., Sovocool, G.W., Curley, A., *et al.* Two acute human poisoning cases resulting from exposure to diazinon transformation products in Egypt. *Archives of Environmental Health* 1982;**37**:207–12.

Spear, R.C., Popendorf, W.J., Leffingwell, J.T., *et al.* Field worker's response to weathered residues of parathion. *Journal of Occupational Medicine* 1977;**19**:406–10.

Spencer, J.R., Bissel, S.R., Sanbom, J.R., *et al.* Chlorothalonil exposure of workers on mechanical tomato harvesters. *Toxicology Letters* 1991;**55**:99–107.

Spiers, F., Juul, P. Cholinesterase activity in plasma and erythrocytes. *Acta Ophthalmologica* 1964;**42**:696–712.

Stamper, J.H., Nigg, H.N., Queen, R.M. Prediction of pesticide dermal exposure and urinary metabolite level of tree crop harvesters from field residues. *Bulletin of Environmental Contamination Toxicology* 1986;**36**:693–700.

Tinoco-Ojanguren, R., Halperin, D.C. Poverty, production, and health: inhibition of erythrocyte cholinesterase via occupational exposure to organophosphate insecticides in Chiapas, Mexico. *Archives of Environmental Health* 1998;**53**:29–53.

Tomlin, C.D.S. *The Pesticide Manual* Eleventh Edition. British Crop Protection Council: UK. 1997.

Van Hemmen, J.J., van Golstein Brouwers, Y.G.C., Brouwers, D.H. Pesticide exposure and reentry in agriculture. In: *Methods of Pesticides Exposure Assessment.* Curry, P.B., Iyengar, S., Maloney, P.A., Maroni, M. eds. Plenum Press; New York and London: 1995. p. 9–19.

Van Sittert, N.J., Dumas, E.P. Field study on exposure and health effects of an organophosphate pesticide for maintaining registration in the Philippines. *La Medicina del Lavoro* 1990;**81**:463–73.

Vandekar, M. Observations of the Toxicity of Two Organophosphorus and One Carbamate Insecticide in a Village Trial Performed by WHO Insecticide Testing Unit in Lagos During 1964, WHO Work. Doc. 65/Tox/2.64. U.S. Govt. Printing Office: Washington, D.C. 1965.

Weisskopf, C.P., Seiber, J.N., Maizlish, N., *et al.* Personnel exposure to diazinon in a supervised pest eradication program. *Archives of Environmental Contamination and Toxicology* 1988;**17**:210–12.

WHO. Field surveys of exposure to pesticides. Standard protocol. WHO/VBC/82.1 Geneva, Switzerland. 1982.

Wilson, B.W., Jaeger, B., Baetcke, K. (eds). Proceedings of the EPA Workshop on Cholinesterase methodologies. Washington, DC; Office of Pesticide Programs, USEPA. 1992

Wilson, B.W., Sanborn, J.R., O'Malley, M.A., *et al.* Monitoring the pesticide-exposed worker. *Occupational Medicine: State of the Art Reviews* 1997;**12**:347–63.

Zweig, G., Gao, R., Witt, J.M., *et al.* Exposure of strawberry harvesters to carbaryl. In: *Dermal Exposure Related to Pesticide Use.* Honeycutt, R.C., Zweig, G., Ragdsale, N.N. eds. American Chemical Society; Washington, D.C.: 1985. p. 123–38.

CHAPTER 17

The Global Picture of Organophosphate Insecticide Poisoning

Lakshman Karalliedde, Michael Eddleston and Virginia Murray

17.1. Introduction

The perceived lack of alternative practical and affordable methods for the control of vector-borne diseases and for the prevention of crop destruction by pests has resulted in the widespread use of OP insecticides. Vector-borne diseases (Curtis, 2000) and crop destruction (Gunn and Stephens, 1976) are global issues but their effects are most obviously felt in the developing world. The resulting intense but often unregulated and unsafe use of pesticides in the developing world, especially the tropics, produces the scenario for poisoning.

Pesticide poisoning results from occupational, accidental and intentional exposure. The epidemiological pattern of poisoning shows considerable variation between countries and regions, in particular between developing and industrialised countries. The starkest contrast is in the number of deaths. Developing countries use only 20% of the World's agrochemicals yet they suffer 99% of deaths from pesticide poisoning (Jeyaratnam and Chia, 1994).

The form of poisoning also differs between regions. Deliberate self-poisoning by drinking pesticides is a phenomenon that is predominantly seen in South East Asia, the Indian subcontinent, and expatriate Indian communities worldwide. In these communities, it is probably the commonest cause of poisoning requiring admission to hospital (Eddleston, 2000). In 1998, poisoning was amongst the three leading causes of hospital deaths in Sri Lanka and nearly 15,000 admissions were following OP and carbamate exposure (Health Bulletin, Ministry of Health). Over 80% of the poisonings (with OPs) in Sri Lanka result from intentional oral intake with suicidal intent (Senanayake, 1998). An earlier review of over 1000 medical records of patients with pesticide poisoning admitted to Sri Lankan hospitals showed that 73% were suicidal, 17% occupational and 8% accidental (Jeyaratnam et al., 1982).

An Ethiopian study revealed that 94% of the OP poisonings followed attempts at suicide (Abebe, 1991). In contrast, the commonest cause of pesticide poisonings in Latin America is occupational exposure.

For example, in Nicaragua, 91% of the poisonings followed such exposure (McConnell and Hruska, 1993). Approximately 25% of the poisonings in Costa Rica (Leveridge, 1998) were suicide attempts whilst 40% were due to occupational exposure and 35% due to accidental exposure. In 1996, 86,912 cases of human poisonings were reported from 67 participating Poison Control centres in the USA. This accounted for 4% of the total of poisonings and of the 20 deaths encountered, 4 were due to suicide (Litovitz et al., 1997).

Poisoning is a problem that principally affects adults more than children. Children are more commonly victims of accidental poisoning. However, since little is normally ingested in accidental poisoning, deaths are rare. However, as infant ill-health due to infectious diseases becomes less common, the contribution of poisoning to childhood morbidity and mortality is increasing, even in developing countries (Gupta et al., 1998).

Despite the enormous extent of the problem, mortality and morbidity from pesticide poisoning has received little attention. Long-term low dose occupational exposure, and its prevention have been the major priorities of health personnel in developed countries where intentional acts of pesticide poisoning are rare. To the public in industrialised/developed countries, pesticide residues in food are a major concern. These problems have low priority in the developing world. Starvation and insufficient food are major concerns of the majority of the people in developing countries. In these countries, oral intake of pesticides with suicidal intent is very common in addition to ill-health due to occupational exposure. These differences in priority have polarised research in the field of OP poisoning. As a result the necessary blend of patients, technology, and scientific manpower has yet to be harmonised to provide definitive information to the public and legislators to ensure the safe use of OP pesticides.

17.2. Estimates of Worldwide Pesticide Poisonings

In 1972, the WHO collected statistics from 19 countries and concluded that "there were as many as 500,000 cases of pesticide poisonings per year". It considered the problem to be unacceptably large and called for work to be put into both substantiating this estimate and controlling the problem (WHO, 1973). In 1977, using notifications from several governments and surveys of nine countries, WHO estimated the number of deaths globally to be about 20,640 a year.

In 1981, OXFAM, updated the WHO figures and considered pesticide-related poisonings worldwide to number around 750,000 each year. Later in the decade, the Economic and Social Commission of Asia and the Pacific (ESCAP) suggested that pesticide poisoning incidents might amount to two million a year, with as many as 40,000 fatalities (Foo, 1985).

A nationwide study of acute pesticide poisonings admitted to Sri Lankan hospitals in 1979 (Jeyaratnam et al., 1982) revealed 10,000 admissions and almost 1000 deaths in a country of 12 million population. The public health implication of this finding was emphasised by the number of deaths, which was almost twice the total number of deaths caused by malaria, poliomyelitis, whooping cough, diphtheria and tetanus; the traditional public health problems of developing countries.

In 1985, the WHO estimated that one million cases of unintentional pesticide poisoning resulted in 20,000 deaths (Levine, 1986), a figure similar to that reported by Jeyaratnam (1985).

Henao and colleagues in 1993, concluded after analysing the results of various studies on pesticide poisoning in Latin America, that in the smallest countries in that region there were at the very least 1000–2000 poisonings a year and that 10–20% of poisoned patients were under 18 years old. The groups of pesticides involved in the majority of acute poisonings were the OPs, carbamates and paraquat.

Studies of occupational intoxication in Asia (Jeyaratnam et al., 1987) showed that about 3.2% of pesticide users considered themselves to have suffered ill-effects from the use of pesticides. On this basis there would be 26.5 million cases of pesticide intoxications in agricultural workers in a year in developing countries. The WHO claim that between 2–3% of agricultural workers in developing countries suffer from some form of intoxication and that 10–12% of those cases are fatal (WHO, 1990).

Recent annual estimates of the global incidence of unintentional pesticide poisonings range from 2.9 million acute poisonings and 220,000 associated deaths (Jeyaratnam, 1990) to 2–5 million poisonings and 40,000 fatalities (WHO, 1990; Fernando, 1995; McConnell and Hruska, 1993).

17.3. Problems with these Estimates of Worldwide Incidence

These estimates of the global incidence of pesticide poisoning in general and OP poisoning in particular have been predictably contentious as comprehensive epidemiological studies are not available.

The numbers are derived from hospital data or are extrapolated from a few studies looking at certain aspects of pesticide poisoning such as those associated with occupational exposure (Jeyaratnam *et al.*, 1987). There are many problems in this approach.

17.3.1. *Problems Associated with Health Facilities*

The incidence of pesticide or toxic chemical-related deaths is likely to be grossly underestimated, not only because of the lack of proper records but also because attending physicians and health practitioners fail to recognize symptoms of pesticide poisoning (Forget, 1991). In a study from East Africa, Mbakaya *et al.*, (1994) reported that more than 40% of the health care professionals interviewed could not recognise pesticide poisoning cases.

Richter and Safi, (1997) suggested that pesticide poisoning among Israeli agricultural workers and their families is under-reported because in many cases the association between illness and toxic exposures is not recognised by primary care physicians or nurses. Many deaths from acute poisoning in the Indian subcontinent and quite probably in most other developing countries occur prior to the patient reaching hospital (Senanayake and Pieris, 1996). Therefore, in order to obtain realistic numbers of poisoning, it is necessary to study the records of coroners, police surgeons, institutions offering private medical care, and institutions offering care in traditional medicine e.g. Ayuruvedha, Unani, or Chinese medicine (Karalliedde, 2000).

17.3.2. *Problems Associated with Health Care Seeking Behaviour*

The number of those affected and actually going to hospital and being recorded varies markedly. Health care-seeking behaviour following pesticide exposure varies from country to country, district to district, and even community to community dependent at least partly upon facilities available for treatment.

Studies have found 70% presenting to hospital in Indonesia and Malaysia and 83% in Sri Lanka, but only 8.4% presenting to hospital in Thailand (Jeyaratnam *et al.*, 1987).

A recent study of Indonesian pesticide sprayers revealed that less than 1% sought care at health centres with symptoms related to spraying as most accepted a certain degree of illness as an integral part of their agricultural work (Kishi *et al.*, 1995). In Paraguay, around 10% of those with symptoms related to pesticide exposure treated themselves and frequently used analgesics (Dinham, 1993).

17.3.3. Problems Associated with Record Keeping and Reporting

There could be great variation in the official records of those who sought hospital treatment. In Thailand, the Epidemiological Surveillance Report recorded 2094 cases of pesticide poisoning in 1985 with no deaths while the National Environmental Board reported 4046 cases with 289 deaths (Jeyaratnam, 1992). In many countries like Ecuador (Dinham, 1993), there is gross under-reporting of hospital admissions due to a lack of a system for collecting information.

Dr Flavio Zambroni of the Poison Control Centre in Campinas, Sao Paulo, Brazil, estimated that for each case of poisoning recorded in the hospitals or clinics, there could be as many as 250 unreported victims—mainly due to a lack of doctors with toxicological knowledge (Dinham, 1993).

A further reason for under-reporting of cases of occupational poisoning is the desire of farmers not to have to pay compensation. Labourers are sometimes coerced into not reporting their illness by their employer. McConnell and Hruska (1993), Keifer *et al.* (1996) estimated that two-thirds of poisonings go unrecorded in Nicaragua,

In South Africa, Poison Centres around the country consistently report consultations for possible pesticide poisoning far in excess of national notifications (London and Myers, 1993). A study of fatalities seen at Cape Town mortuary in 1979 suggested that only 5% of cases of fatal pesticide poisonings had been notified (Coetzee, 1981). More recent surveys of hospital admissions suggested that approximately 20% of cases (fatal and non fatal) were being notified in South Africa (Emanuel, 1992; London and Myers, 1993). Among the stated causes for underreporting were failure of health personnel to notify and misdiagnosis of milder forms of poisoning. Even in the UK, barriers to reporting ill-health following OP exposure have been identified by the Working Group on Organophosphates of the Committee on Toxicity of Chemicals in Food, Consumer Products and Environment (Department of Health, 1999).

These include consequences for employment, the large numbers in self-employment and a culture of stoicism among agricultural workers.

Further, there were no means of gauging the overlap between the different official reporting data systems.

In the US, farm operators report adverse health effects more frequently than the reported incidence of occupational pesticide poisonings (Lichtenberg and Zimmerman, 1999).

17.3.4. The Medico-Legal Structures

In countries like India attempted suicide is an offence and notification to the police is required. As a result, many subjects or their families seek medical attention in institutions where record keeping and notification procedures are not as rigid as in governmental institutions (Karalliedde, 2000).

17.4. Factors Influencing the Incidence of Serious Poisoning

Multiple factors affect the incidence of serious poisoning in the developing world, from the availability of highly toxic substances to their unsafe manufacture, storage and use. Countries of the industrialised world have effective legislation related to pesticides but unfortunately, effective legislation is the exception rather than the rule throughout the developing world and its absence in great part explains the heavy load of deaths due to pesticide poisoning in the World's poorer regions.

17.4.1. Legislation

The ultimate responsibility for controlling the use of pesticides and minimising health hazards rests with national governments. Enacted legislation generally controls the registration, manufacture, import, storage, transport and sale of pesticides, usually involving systems of prior approval or licensing.

Registration of pesticides is the core issue since it determines whether a pesticide can be used legally in a country and the conditions for its use. Nearly all countries have developed comprehensive and well-structured legislation, but there is considerable variation in the degree of enforcement.

Model legislation has often been passed without either the political will or the financial resources to implement it—even the process of registration may impose a strain on the technical and financial resources of developing countries.

Separation of politics from the revenue implications of pesticides is also very difficult in the developing world.   This is a major factor contributing to the production, import and use of pesticides classified as hazardous by the WHO (1993) in developing countries.   Many of the pesticides manufactured in India are known to be hazardous and are no longer produced elsewhere (Dinham, 1993).   Governments tend to be cognisant of revenue and foreign exchange expenditure and allow sales to continue for extended periods after implementing local bans.

Table 17.1. lists the most commonly used OP pesticides in Asia, Central America, and East Africa and their classification by hazard according to WHO recommendations (LD_{50} mg/kg). Ia, Extremely hazardous; Ib, Highly hazardous; II, Moderately hazardous; III, Slightly hazardous. The classification is based primarily on the acute oral and dermal toxicity to the rat (IPCS WHO/PCS/98.21)

Even where the production and importation of certain hazardous pesticides is banned, smuggled supplies can often still be found.   Paraguay offers an example. In 1990, total reported imports of pesticides to Paraguay amounted to $US 22.94 million, based on customs records.   However, Dr Carlos Cawette, Head of the Pollution Control Department of the Environmental Health Services (SENASA) believes that as little as 20% of pesticides used are brought in to the country legally. Pesticides available on the market have frequently being acquired illegally or have been locally reformulated or re-mixed. Often they are without labels.   A similar situation appears to exist in Ecuador and Venezuela (Dinham, 1993).   An investigation by Greenpeace showed that over 50% of the pesticides available on the Greek market were included in the UN list of substances that have been banned or 'restricted' in other countries.

This interpretation needs to be cautious as the term 'restricted' in approval systems indicates the restriction of a pesticide to a particular crop for which specific approval has been given.   Although the machinery to vet the importation of pesticides has been put in place in Kenya, Tanzania and Uganda, these appear to be ineffective since pesticides banned in the developed countries can easily be purchased and used in any three of these countries.   No official regulations exist which govern the distribution of pesticides (African Newsletter on Occupational Health and Safety, 1999; Ngowi, 1997; Ngowi et al., 1994).

Table 17.1. The most commonly used OP pesticides in Asia, Central America, and East Africa and their classification by hazard according to WHO

Region and agent	Classification by hazard	LD 50- mg/kg
Asia		
Malathion	III	100
Parathion-methyl	Ia	14
Diazinon	II	422
Monocrotophos	Ib	14
Central America		
(Nicaragua, Guatemala, Honduras, El Salvador, Panama)		
Parathion-methyl	Ia	14
Methamidophos	Ib	30
Chlorpyrifos	II	135
Diazinon	II	422
Fenitrothion	II	503
Malathion	III	2100
Terbufos	Ia	wide range reported
East Africa		
(Tanzania, Kenya, Uganda)		
Chlorpyrifos	II	135
Diazinon	II	422
Dichlorvos	Ib	56
Dimethoate	II	150
Fenitrothion	II	503
Malathion	III	2100

adapted from Wesseling *et al.*, 1997; Mbakaya *et al.*, 1994

Current pesticide safety legislation and administration in many countries may be characterised by extensive duplication, overlap and poor co-ordination among a range of state departments. Because of the multiple administrative bureaucracies, the potential for gaps exist in the legislative framework (London and Myers, 1995).

17.4.2. Manufacture of Pesticides

In 1953, Bidstrup and colleagues reported neuropathy in 3 workers engaged in laboratory production of mipafox in the UK.

This was probably the first report of toxicity during the manufacturing processes. The situation has changed greatly since this time in the industrialised world where strict regulations ensure worker protection during the manufacturing processes. However, the level of monitoring of both workplace conditions and workers' health in manufacturing plants in developing countries varies greatly. There is a growing perception that industry does not welcome the monitoring of workers' health by the medical profession, particularly in rapidly industrialising countries in Asia (personal communication Surjit Singh, 2000).

On the whole, reports regarding ill-health amongst workers in such manufacturing plants are scarce in the medical literature. For example in Costa Rica where formulating plants are on the increase, 54 cases of poisonings of workers in formulation plants were registered at the National Insurance Institute in 1986 (Dinham, 1993). However, other pesticide factory workers involved in the manufacture of EPN, leptophos, methamidophos, trichlorfon, diazinon, dimethoate, phenthoate and malathion complained of a number of symptoms which could be associated with exposure to these OPs. Symptoms included numbness in legs and hands, pain in both legs, memory difficulty, tiredness and abdominal discomfort (Otto et al., 1990).

A cross-sectional study of pesticide applicators and formulators from 2 Egyptian plants where a wide range of pesticides including OPs were manufactured was carried out by Amr et al. (1997). Significantly higher frequencies of psychiatric disorders were found in formulators who had been directly exposed to the chemicals for at least 40 hours per week for 9 months or longer, during at least two consecutive years.

17.4.3. Storage and Sale Outlets

Haynes (1985) studied storage conditions in four African nations, six South-East Asian countries, and Fiji. Undesirable situations such as pesticides being stored next to fertilisers, seeds, food or drink, a general lack of record keeping, the absence of provision for spills, a lack of labels, corroded and leaking containers, and improper repackaging were common. The study indicated that most of the problems encountered might have been reduced if training had been given to shopkeepers/storage facility handlers before they were supplied with these agents.

Unsafe storage and sale is widespread. Almost every rural grocery store in Sri Lanka has shelves full of many brands of pesticides in bottles of various sizes and shapes (Berger, 1988). Pesticides and foodstuffs are often stored together in the supermarkets in Venezuela (Dinham, 1993) with obvious problems for mistakes and contamination. Pesticides are frequently decanted in these shops from large containers into small bottles for sale to smallholders, resulting in spills. There is widespread sale of pesticides in bottles also used for domestic products, with no labels.

In Kenya, a wide range of pesticides are sold at small open markets (kiosks), grocery stores and supermarkets. The vendors purchase these chemicals in bulk containers, repackage them in to small containers of various sizes which are unlabelled. The customers rely on the traders' verbal instructions (as there are no labels) as regards their use and handling (Mwanthi and Kimani, 1990).

The conditions of sale are also of concern. A survey of 20 shops selling pesticides in Costa Rica was carried out by the PPUNA (Programa de Plaguicidas: Desarrollo, Salud y Ambiente) between April and June 1991. They found that all shops lacked ventilation and that the smell of pesticides was strong in many shops and in warehouses. No protective clothing or equipment was used by the employees who handle pesticides (Dinham, 1993). In an audit of farm pesticide stores in Western Cape (South Africa), more than half were found to be unlocked at the time of inspection and a number of farms had no secure locking facility. In addition, almost half of the farms had excess residual stocks of pesticides including chemicals no longer registered for use and about a third of the farms were unable to dispose of empty containers because of prohibitive costs (London, 1992a; 1992b).

Unsuitable storage can produce problems in the field. This is primarily due to the production of toxic transformation products secondary to either the nature of the container or the climatic conditions in which storage takes place. Two spray men working in public health occupations in Alexandria, Egypt, experienced acute toxicity with cholinesterase levels being depressed for 18 days following exposure due to improper storage of diazinon in tin-plated sheet steel containers, resulting in the production of sulfotep and mono-thio-TEPP; two degradation products that are more toxic than diazinon (Soliman et al., 1982). The emulsifiable concentrate (60%) was not in compliance with the WHO's standard specifications regarding emulsion stability. A similar occurrence in Pakistan due to conversion of malathion to isomalalthion caused widespread ill health amongst sprayers in Public Health Programmes (Baker et al., 1978; Shihab, 1976)

17.4.4. Labelling

Eighty percent of South African farm workers cannot read or write (Dinham, 1993). In addition, at least 20 languages are spoken in South Africa suggesting that labels used on pesticide containers which are normally written in one language, often English would be ineffective. Similar situations exist in much of the developing world where the multitude of local languages makes the provision of labels appropriate to the specific locality prohibitive, even if workers are able to read them.

In Kenya, labelling in both English and Kiswahili was legislated in 1982. However, as most users were women whose literacy rate was approximately half that of the males, the impact was minimal (Kimani and Mawantha, 1995).

Results of a survey in English-speaking Saint Lucia (Caribbean) showed that half of the 130 pesticide users surveyed had received more than 'introductory' training in safe use of pesticides and most said they always found labels or directions affixed to pesticide containers. However, about half said they never or only sometimes understood the labels, and many of those who said they understood, did not always follow the instructions (McDougall *et al.*, 1993).

Labelling is a desirable and necessary procedure. However, the information provided to the workers of the developing countries needs to relate to their specific environment. It would be more helpful if other effective forms of health education and communication were also developed. A further complication is the practical value of instructions in case of exposure such as "contact a doctor" or "wash immediately with water" in an environment where health facilities are scarce, telephones beyond the reach of the vast majority, and clean water unavailable.

17.4.5. Work Conditions

The developing world constitutes three quarters of the World's population occupying three quarters of the earth's land mass. Approximately 830 million workers are involved in agriculture in these countries (Jeyaratnam and Chia, 1994). However, the effects of climate, poverty and illiteracy put basic precautions beyond the reach of most agricultural workers in developing countries. The majority of people using pesticides are small scale farmers working on their own plot of land without pooled resources with which to buy safety equipment.

Workers known to be at highest risk of exposure in agriculture include applicators and mixers (Moses, 1983; Coyle and Fenske, 1988).

Less than 20% of farm workers in high exposure jobs received safety training in handling pesticides in the 1970's in South Africa (Emanuel, 1983; London, 1992b). However, recent legislation in South Africa (Department of Manpower, 1993) makes mandatory the training of safety representatives and workers who are in contact with potential toxins.

Following a study in rural agricultural community (Githungiri) in Kenya, Kimani and Mawantha (1995) found that more women than men were at risk of agrochemical exposure. Approximately 70% of the farm personnel who handled these chemicals all year around were women and girls. A substantial number of women were also involved in the retail trade of pesticides. These women repackaged pesticides into plastic and brown paper bags for sale at open-air markets. Often, the pesticides were placed next to farm produce such as fruit, vegetable, potatoes and cereal. Chee (1990) observed that 80% of the chemical sprayers of palm oil and rubber plantations in Malaysia were women.

The inequitable economic, social, educational and sometimes racial relationship between farmers and labourers in many countries create semi-feudal societies where farm-workers are frequently exploited. Many do not question their employers, as employment is difficult to find. Workers may be compelled to use the equipment and pesticides provided by the farm owners. Workers are paid by the acreage sprayed and the frequency with which spraying is carried out. Thus, irrespective of ill-health or weather conditions, poverty drives the labourers to work long hours, spray frequently and hurriedly, without recourse to recommended exposure-free periods and potentially with total disregard to other safety instructions.

17.4.6. Protective Clothing, and Guidelines for Safe Use

The Control of Substances Hazardous to Health Regulations (COSHH), in the UK, presents detailed guidance to reduce the risk of exposure to all chemicals including pesticides. The industry has provided guidelines for their safe use. They provide the precautions to be taken regarding weather, wind, and protective clothing, and also procedures to follow after dangerous exposure. The enforcement or acceptance of these and similar recommendations have considerably reduced the incidence of pesticide poisoning in developed countries with temperate climates.

Personal Protective Equipment (PPE) has to be both suitable to allow the job in hand to be carried out and adequate for protection from exposure, according to EC directives.

Many workers and their employers in developing countries cannot afford PPE and also find them unbearable for work in hot humid conditions.

Even in the UK, full compliance with PPE recommendations is poor. A Health and Safety Executive (HSE) pilot technical development survey that measured exposure of 11 orchard sprayers in 1996 and 32 sprayers in 1997 found only 2 out of 11 operators in un-cabbed tractors complying fully with PPE recommendations (Pesticide News, 1998). Although water-proof trousers were worn by 90% of users and water-proof footwear by 88%, only 23% wore gloves, 7% wore face coverings and 3% used head coverings.

Many sheep farmers consider PPE to be impractical to wear, and argue that dipping sheep while wearing PPE is simply not practicable (Pesticide News, 1998).

The situation in the developing world is far worse. Only about 5% of Ecuadorian agricultural workers use protective clothing when working with hazardous pesticides (Dinham, 1993) and a study in Ethiopia (Lakew and Mekkonnen, 1998) revealed that there was virtually no use of any protective equipment even if available.

17.4.7. Improper Disposal of Containers

In South Africa, despite the Hazardous Substances Act 1973 which states that empty pesticide containers must be disposed of in a responsible manner—either punctured and flattened, or buried—drums are generally left in the fields or orchards. In a study of 27 farms in the Hex River valley of Western Cape, 51% of farmers claimed that they had a problem with the disposal of empty containers and unwanted chemicals. Approximately 18% had unwanted chemicals which they could not dispose of and 70% had empty containers lying around. Only 7% of the farmers knew of companies that could dispose of chemical waste. As a result, pesticide containers are often not discarded correctly and were then reused by workers ignorant of the danger. For example, in April 1989, 50 Transkei migrants employed on a potato farm in the Orange Free State were poisoned after drinking water from a disused drum which had contained monocrotophos. A three-year-old child died and 8 people became critically ill (Dinham, 1993).

Philip Masia of the South African Farmworker Education Project commented that "you are talking about people who earn so little that they cannot even afford a bucket...so they use whatever container will hold water..." (Dinham, 1993).

In Kenya, empty chemical containers are used by women to store edibles such as sugar, salt and for carrying drinking water or milk (Kimani and Mwanthi, 1995).

This type of problem is present worldwide. Over 10 million containers per year are disposed of inadequately in Parana, Brazil, often being dumped in rivers, on plantations, or by roadsides. They are frequently re-used for transport of food and water or burnt without adequate controls (Dinham, 1993)

17.5. Occupational Exposure

Ill-health associated with exposure to OP pesticides during manufacture, mixing and preparation of formulations and application is of growing concern. It may be the result of the increasing intensity with which these agents are used in agriculture, public health and gardening. The places of their manufacture are expanding to regions in the world with wide variations in climate, conditions of work, supervision and legislation related to workers safety and environmental pollution. Multinational companies, under the pressure of strict occupational and environmental health legislation in developed countries, have now relocated their plants to developing countries (Hernberg, 1992).

Occupational exposure differs in developed and developing countries. In developing countries

- Most industrial activity takes place in small shops or is located in houses or backyards. Parasitic and infectious diseases, malnutrition, poor housing, a tropical climate and the mindset imposed by poverty, have effects on the working population. Expensive gloves, aprons and face shields recommended for use in temperate climates are considered cumbersome and restrictive in the tropics (Dinham, 1993; Jeyaratnam, and Chia, 1994).

- The widespread use of child labour. Despite labour laws prohibiting the employment of young people in dangerous occupations, many of the sprayers poisoned in the province of Theqar in Iraq, during a malaria eradication programme, were those between 14 and 17 years old (Shihab, 1976). In Nicaragua, during the 1980s, involvement of the young work force in the war necessitated the application of pesticides by children. This resulted in an increase of poisoning in children from 12.7% in 1984 to 17.1% in 1987 (McConnel and Hruska, 1993). Harari *et al.* (1997) reported on the 'unacceptable occupational exposure to toxic agents among children in Ecuador'.

The biochemical confirmation of exposure to lead, OPs and mercury among children employed in different occupations highlighted the need to control or prevent such exposures.

- Haphazard use. In one Indonesian study (Kishi *et al.*, 1995), the majority of workers mixed several pesticides at full strength in a container, often a narrow mouthed bottle, without any gloves. In nearly half of spray operations, the equipment was faulty, and there was considerable wetting of bare skin and clothes with little or no wash-down immediately available. No farmer wore industry-recommended protective clothing and the little clothing that they did wear did not cover the skin and was, for the most part, permeable cotton.

- Working habits: pesticides are normally applied by workers using their own sprayers for which only a few basic designs exist. Small landholders usually use a lever-operated knapsack sprayer (LOK). Assessment of the LOK sprayers used in the Muda irrigation scheme in Malaysia (Anas *et al.*, 1987) found that 20% of them had serious faults or were badly damaged. The study also revealed that the farmers lacked knowledge about operating the sprayers and maintaining them. Another study revealed that farmers chose a particular brand of sprayer mainly for its weight, size, ease or comfort rather than for safety factors including the ease of repair, and availability of spare parts (Jusoh *et al.*, 1987).

The working habits of a group of adults living on potato farms in Montufar canton in northern Ecuador were reported by Cole *et al.*, 1997, 1998. Of the pesticides used, methamidophos (OP), carbofuran (carbamate) and mancozeb (dithiocarbamate) were the commonest (80% of pesticide usage) and application was almost always by means of a back pack. These workers were noted to mix pesticides with their bare hands or a stick. Leaking back-sprays, the non-use of protective clothing other than rubber boots (38 out of 40 workers) and storage of pesticides in the farm-houses and unsafe pesticide disposal practice were all noticed. Farm residents were found to have lower neuropsychological scores and more peripheral neuropathy symptoms than non-farm controls.

Non-toxic model pesticides and tracer dyes were applied to rice, vegetable, mango, cotton and coffee crops in the Philippines, Thailand, Tanzania and Malawi, using knapsack and ULV spinning disc sprayers. Tracer dye falling on the operator during application was measured for each type of crop sprayed. Mean gross dermal deposits of dye were : rice 97mg/h ; mango 257 mg/h; vegetables 103 mg/h; cotton 220 mg/h; coffee 95 mg/h (Ambridge *et al.*, 1990).

In a study of the effect of OP insecticides in 81 pest control workers from the Northern Omo State farm in Ethiopia, it was found that the mean plasma and red cell cholinesterase levels were 50 % lower than pre-exposure levels in 16% and 40% respectively (Lakew and Mekonnen, 1998). This study revealed that the workers were ignorant about toxicity of pesticides and risk of pesticides exposure. There was near total absence of personal protective devices and what was available was improperly used.

The following extracts from the literature illustrates some aspects relevant to occupational exposure particularly in the developing countries (Dinham 1993).

"...with no protective gear, no gloves and with feet exposed, the applicator walks straight into the area that has just being sprayed...In fact as he sprays for the next three to four hours, some of the spray falls on his bare feet and legs and his cotton overall is heavily soaked in spray..."

"...worker in charge of the pump and pesticide tank mixes the pesticide in the tank and then pumps it to applicators with hose pipes...wearing a cotton overall that is drenched in dichlorvos...regular clothes are under this overall and are drenched as well. He has rubber gloves which are wet with pesticide. He wears a respirator but not for long, because he complains that it is uncomfortable in the hot and humid weather...He will remain in his soaked clothes in this small pump house for 8–10 hours. He is also wearing gumboots, so some pesticide drips in to the boots from the clothes. The hose pipe leaks under pressure within the pump house..."

"...on a large flower farm, workers spray a cocktail of pesticides from their knapsacks, while others weed close by...the workers who are weeding are directly exposed to spray mist for long hours...they have cotton overalls which get drenched in the pesticides, but they have to wear these clothes the whole day..."

"...farmers are required to provide employees, whether seasonal, migrant or full time with safety equipment for spraying such as chemical-resistant clothing...A survey conducted (Farm workers Research and Resource Project 1989/90) revealed that only 4 of 39 workers were supplied with sufficient protective gear... the rest were given nothing or overalls... and only one of the interviewed workers knew the name of the chemical used...."

"...sprayers usually mix pesticides with their hands and sometimes even taste it to ensure the right consistency before spraying..."

"...sprayers wear only shorts and do not wear any other cloth round their mouth, hands or legs... Even if men wish to do so, they cannot wear full clothes as landlords do not like their labour well dressed, seeing this as a mark of power and disrespect....."

"...young girls between 10–15 years old are employed on a daily basis to pick worms after the field is sprayed... they pick with their bare hands and are paid .20 paise for a small basket of worms.... There is no bar on entering recently sprayed fields..."

"...workers do not have access to clean water to wash off pesticides which have contaminated their skin...they cannot leave the field to change clothes...they resume work after a drink or smoke..."

Poisoning was common during malaria eradication campaigns (Baker *et al.*, 1978; Shihab, 1976) during the early periods of OP application. This was largely due to poor working practices: e.g. the wearing of clothes wet with pesticides for several days without washing; extensive skin contact during filling and pressurisation of spray tanks; mixing of malathion mixtures with bare hands; blowing through clogged spray nozzles to clear the obstruction (Baker *et al.*, 1978).

A group of expatriate workers from developing countries (predominantly ethnic Asians) employed for at least two years in farming in the United Arab Emirates and exposed to OPs were studied by Gomes *et al.* (1998). Exposure status was determined using acetylcholinesterase activity (acetylcholinesterase activity was reduced by a mean of 16% in the exposed group compared with controls). Irritated conjunctiva, watery eyes, blurred vision, runny nose, wheeze, chest tightness in the last month were all reported significantly more frequently in established farm workers. These workers also reported dizziness, headache, restlessness, sleeplessness, muscular pain, abdominal pain or weakness often or sometimes.

Indian workers who sprayed fenthion for 5–6 hours daily without using any protective clothing (spraying 1500–2000 litres of fenthion per month) for a mean duration of 8.5 years reported a number of minor symptoms like headache, giddiness, ocular symptoms and parasthesiae after spraying.

After a three-week withdrawal period, there were improvements in motor function and disappearance of abnormal EMG findings, which were detected the day after exposure (Misra *et al.* 1988).

17.5.1. Occupational Exposure in Developed Countries

17.5.1.1. Usage of pesticides

The developed world uses a great deal of pesticides including OPs. For example, UK farmers treated over one million hectares with 395 tonnes of OP insecticides in 1994, representing almost a third of all insecticide applications. Between 1992 and 1994, usage of dimethoate increased by 89% and that of chlorpyrifos almost 8 fold (Pesticide News 34, 1996). Houses and lawns in the United States receive a total of approximately 20 million annual chlorpyrifos treatments and 82% of US adults have detectable levels of a chlorpyrifos metabolite (3,5,6-trichloro-2-pyridinol) in the urine (Steenland *et al.,* 2000). Nearly all families studied in Missouri from June 1989 to March 1990 used pesticides at least one time per year and two thirds used pesticides more than five times per year (Davis *et al.,* 1992).

17.5.1.2. Effects

Although effective legislation limits human exposure to the pesticides in the developed countries, some studies have found detrimental effects of pesticides in agricultural workers. Gadoun (1996) studying the New York Pesticide Poisoning Registry from 1990 to 1993 found that 28 subjects satisfied the criteria for suspected or confirmed poisoning among lawn care and tree service applicators. The most common class of pesticides applied were OPs (71%). Twenty of the reported workers were symptomatic. Personal Protective Equipment was used routinely by 22 of the 27 applicators from whom information was available.

Stokes and colleagues (1995) found a loss of vibration sense in 68 male pesticide applicators licenced in New York State to spray apple orchards. The mean vibration threshold scores (which estimate the somato-sensory function of the peripheral nervous system) were significantly higher for the dominant and non-dominant hands among pesticide applicators.

The pesticide used by 86% of the sprayers was an OP and each worker had sprayed for a mean of 20 years. This work supported the findings of Svendsgaard *et al.* (1998), and of McConnell *et al.*, (1994), in production workers in Egypt and Nicaragua.

In contrast Danielle *et al.*, (1992) studying pesticide applicators (Washington State, USA) who were exposed mainly to azinphos-methyl (57% of the 57 applicators spent 10 days or more directly involved in spraying activities during study period) found no evidence of clinically significant adverse changes in neuropsychological tests using the Neurobehavioural Evaluation System. Another study from Washington stated that employees working on apple farms exposed to azinphos-methyl and possibly to phosmet or parathion-methyl via foliar OP residues did not show any abnormalities in peripheral neurophysiological function after working for 80 hours or more in the season during which the study took place (Engel *et al.*, 1998)

Californian State employees who loaded diazinon in to spreading equipment and applied granules wearing appropriate protective clothing (disposable coveralls, rubber boots and gloves, face shields, full face respirators) for a mean duration of 39 days did not reveal any significant differences on neuropsychological screening compared with a control group (Maizlish *et al.*, 1987).

Holmes and Goan (1956) studied the ground and flying crews of airplane insecticide spraying companies based in Colorado. Thirty of 44 men had values below normal for blood cholinesterase but all denied symptoms at time the blood samples were taken. Two of the men who had very low values were admitted to hospital in the subsequent two days. A later study from Israel (Richter *et al.*, 1992) of ground crews and pilots occupied in aerial spraying as well as field workers exposed to OPs showed an association between exposure and illness, even though no individuals with acute poisoning were found. Cantor and Silberman (1999) studying mortality among aerial pesticide applicators and flight instructors found that aircraft accidents were a major cause of mortality for both groups. Compared with flight instructors, aerial applicator pilots were at significantly elevated risk for all major causes of death.

Weinbaum *et al.* (1995) examined the OP related illness-data reported to the Workers Health and Safety Branch at the California Department of Food and Agriculture in the years 1984–1988. There were 878 cases with systemic illness and 199 cases of skin disease or eye injury. They observed that mixer/loader applicators had more severe illnesses as did those exposed to residue on crops and commodities. There was a strong association of diethyl OPs with severity of systemic illness.

The largest number of safety violations occurred in the summer. In 1987, 26% of the reported pesticide related illnesses in California were associated with disability and 2–3% of the reported cases were hospitalised.

Ames *et al.* (1995) studied agricultural workers in an attempt to investigate whether exposure to OPs sufficient to produce acetylcholinesterase inhibition but no evidence of frank toxicity was associated with chronic neurological sequelae. Though the study sample was relatively small, there was no demonstrable difference from controls except in a single test from the neuropsychological battery. This study suggested at most, a low incidence of long-term sequelae following exposures sufficient to depress cholinesterase activities (COT Report, Department of Health, 1999).

Symptoms related to OP or carbamate exposure were reported by tree planters in British Columbia and significant inhibition of RBC AChE was observed in nearly 16% of individuals (Robinson *et al.*, 1993). A study (Pickett *et al.*, 1998) did not provide strong support to the hypothesis that pesticide exposure was an important risk factor for suicide amongst farmers in Canada. Another study from Canada surveyed malathion exposure among elevator and dock workers who handle grain (Dimich- Ward *et al.*, 1996).

Schnitzer and Shannon (1999) reported the growth of the Occupational Pesticide Poisoning Surveillance program at Texas from 1987 to 1996. The evolution from a passive system to an active surveillance program expanded the number of reported cases (from 9 workers in 1987 to 99 workers in 1996) and strengthened inter-agency collaborations.

Ward *et al.* (2000) reported a method for identifying personnel potentially exposed to agricultural pesticides using a remote sensing and a Geographic Information system.

17.5.2. Sheep Dip

There are approximately 95,000 sheep farms in the UK. Because of ecto-parasites, sheep need to be dipped in insecticidal solutions. These are classified as veterinary pharmaceuticals and not as pesticides and are regulated as such. Dipping involves roughly 300,000 people. Health effects of sheep dips have been the subject of many reports (Forbat and Skehan, 1992; Sims and Cook, 1992; Murray *et al.*, 1992).

A study of data from reports of the Appraisal Panel for Suspected Adverse Reactions to Veterinary Medicines revealed that 651 reports of suspected adverse reactions due to OP sheep dips were received since 1985. Prior to 1991 the reports received each year were relatively few (ranging from 5–19 each year); greater numbers were reported in 1991, 1992 and 1993 (127, 129 and 180 reports respectively) but reports fell to 17 in 1998 (Veterinary Medicines Directorate, 1999).

In 1995, Stephens et al., studied 146 sheep farmers and observed abnormalities in tests of sustained attention and speed of information processing. These neuropsychological defects caused controversy and debate in the medical and lay literature. The study had an extremely poor response rate, the reasons for which were not clear and there were a number of confounding variables (Watts, 1995; O'Brien et al., 1995; Davies, 1995; Pesticide B Network, Pesticide Action News). Rees (1996) concluded that sheep dipping was strenuous and dirty work and that sheep farmers found it difficult to wear personal protective equipment and avoid skin contamination in the dip. In this limited study, farmers did not appear to have significant OP toxicity despite inadequate handling precautions. Niven et al. (1996) showed that UK sheep dippers using OPs had only relatively low levels of urinary metabolites. Nevertheless, The Pesticide Trust estimates that at least 1000 sheep farmers suffer from some adverse effect of OP sheep dips (Pesticide News). Controversies associated with these issues have not been resolved to date.

17.5.3. Greenhouse Workers

Intensive growing under hotter and more humid conditions in southern Europe poses differing problems from those encountered in northern Europe.

Bazylewicz-Walczak et al. (1999) observed that female workers exposed to OPs in greenhouses had longer reaction times and reduced motor steadiness. Such women also complained of increased tension, depression and fatigue. Intense exposure to pesticides was also considered to encourage acts of self-harm amongst workers. El Poniente, the eastern area of Almeria Province (Southern Spain) has the highest density of greenhouses in the world and 73% of the workforce is employed in agriculture. At least 79% of all pesticide fatalities reported to the central reference hospital at Almeria Province were due to suicides.

The suicide rate in El Poniente was 15–25 per 100,000 and pesticides were used by 40–47% to commit suicide. Parron *et al.* (1996) considered that there was increased risk of suicide associated with exposure to pesticides in intensive agricultural areas. However, the possibility of confounders makes the assumption of a causal relationship unwise.

17.6. Accidental Poisonings

Most of the poisonings involving groups of people have been accidental. An estimated 3000–5000 cases of accidental poisonings occur annually in the US according to the Environmental Protection Agency (EPA, 1995). Zweiner and Ginsburg (1988) reported from Dallas that virtually all pesticide poisonings in children were accidental and occurred in the home and 70% were due to ingestion of an improperly stored compound.

Among 148 outbreaks (excluding Bhopal and three probable epidemics of pesticide-related suicide) reported between 1951–90, the known number of cases was 24,731 with 1065 deaths (4.3% case fatality); these are probably massively underestimated. Among the known outbreaks the most commonly identified toxins were OPs (58), carbamates (23), chlorinated hydrocarbons (23) and organic mercurials (11). Food was the most common vehicle of exposure in these epidemics (83) followed by skin contact (26), multiple types of exposure (22) and respiratory exposure (16) (Levine and Doull, 1992).

17.7. Contamination of Food During Transport, Storage and Preparation

Foodstuffs that are contaminated and confused with pesticides are usually powders and crystals, such as flour and sugar that are held in sacks. These occur at sites of food manipulation such as canteens, hospitals, restaurants, cafeterias.

Contamination of foodstuff during transport or storage is common (e.g. parathion stored in a bottle thought to be cooking oil poisoned 25 people at a wedding). Accidental use of pesticide in food preparation, due to their similarity to food products is another common cause of poisoning.

Populations affected may be large since these foods are often distributed widely either on their own or in products such as bread and commonly affects several members of a family near a source of distribution e.g. bakery, food store.

Latency is usually short and evolution of outbreak rapid. Mass or multiple poisonings have been reported from USA, India, China, Canada, Egypt, Peru, Colombia, Sri Lanka, Pakistan, Iraq, Guyana, Morocco, Yugoslavia, Malaysia, Jamaica, Mexico, Costa Rica, Switzerland, Iran, Senegal, Turkey, Venezuela and South Africa (Ferrer and Cabral, 1991; Jeyaratnam and Chia, 1994; Perold and Bezuidenhout, 1980; Bhalla and Jajoo, 1999). However, many such occurrences are probably not reported or recorded.

The scenarios that give rise to the high risk of accidental poisoning in the homes of workers in developing countries is illustrated by the following report.

Indonesia: A visit to the homes of farmers and agricultural workers revealed that 84% stored agricultural chemicals at home and 75% were stored within the living or kitchen area. 82% of pesticides were within easy reach of children. Twenty-two percent of the containers were partially or completely unsealed and 50% were leaking their contents. Over one half of those surveyed stated that they used agricultural pesticides in much higher concentrations than those licensed by the Department of Health for home and garden use. In 76% of the households, the wife or children washed the farmers field clothing, mixed in with family laundry in nearly two-fifths of the households (Kishi *et al.,* 1995).

This report from **Peru**: Mass poisoning reported 1999, highlights the situation in many developing countries.

"27 children (aged 3–14 years) died in a remote Andean village (Tauccamarca) after eating a government–donated breakfast contaminated with parathion on 22nd October 1998. Another 20 children were poisoned and required medical treatment. The graphic description of a village woman according to Media Sources of the incident is possibly worthy of quote. 'The kids were screaming, vomiting and grabbing their bellies. Some were dead, others were writhing on the grass and still more were on the school patio. We had no idea what to do'. The children collapsed outside the school, on the dirt roads leading to their homes, and in the doorways of their parent's houses. The conditions prevalent in rural developing communities where OP poisonings occur are illustrated by other extracts from the report. Healthy children attempted to lead sick children to their homes but many died along the way. Some villagers were able to carry their children to the town of Huasac, a 1.5 hour walk from Tauccamarca, where they could be evacuated to a hospital in the city of Cusco, several hours away. Parents of the victims said that if there were a road to their village, or if they had medical services there, some of the children might have been saved".

17.7.1. Contamination of Water Supplies, Water, Vegetables and Fruit

Accidental poisoning from low-dose chronic exposure is a risk in many countries where OP pesticides have been detected in food at higher than recommended safety limits. However, these findings have come from small percentages of produce and a generalisation can be made that over 90% of the produce from plantations that use pesticides do not contain dangerous levels of insecticides, particularly when the recommendations for safe use of insecticides and for harvesting are followed.

While the risk appears to be low in industrialised countries, the US Environment Working Group (EWG) claims that each day one million children under 5 consume unsafe levels of OP insecticide residues (parathion-methyl, dimethoate, chlorpyrifos, pirimiphos-methyl and azinphos-methyl) in the US (Pesticide News, 1998). The UK's Ministry of Agriculture, Fisheries and Foods figures for 1995 show that 1–2% of carrots contain OP residues up to 25 times higher than expected. However, less than 2% of all foods tested contained levels of insecticide above safe approved limits. The OPs implicated include chlorfenviphos, quinalphos and triazophos. It has been suggested that vegetarians and people on weight reducing diets which necessitate a diet rich in fruits and vegetables may be at increased risk (Ratner *et al.*, 1983).

Potential for contamination is greater in the developing world. For example, continuous aerial spraying of cotton in Egypt pollutes the special canal irrigation system that is used for growing other crops for consumption (Dinham, 1993). Chang Yen *et al.* (1995) studied the residual levels of organophosphate pesticides in vegetables in Trinidad, West Indies. A market basket survey of produce conducted between October 1996 and May 1997 showed that 10% of produce exceeded the internationally acceptable maximum residue limits (MRLs) for the respective pesticides. Approximately 83% of celery samples exceeded MRLs and among the OPs associated were methamidophos, diazinon, triazophos, dimethoate. They observed that the application rates that had been used exceeded the manufacturer's recommendations and that there was disregard for recommended pre-harvest intervals after pesticide application. From Hong Kong, Lau (1990) reported vegetable-borne pesticide poisoning, and in 1993 Ting *et al.* observed acute methamidophos poisoning caused by contaminated green leafy vegetables.

17.7.2. Exposure after Household Pest Extermination and Head Lice Treatment

There have been occasions, fortunately rare, of accidental OP poisoning following its use to exterminate pests in households (Richter et al., 1992). In India, 60 men succumbed to food poisoning after eating a lunch cooked in a community kitchen. On the morning of the outbreak, the kitchen had been sprayed with malathion for household pests whilst the raw materials for the cooking were stored in open jute bags (Chaudhry et al., 1998). Health effects due to improper use of chlorpyrifos and other insecticides in a kindergarten to destroy cockroaches was reported by Fischer and Eikmann (1996). The airborne concentrations of diazinon, chlorpyrifos and bendiocarb after application in offices peaked 4 hours after spraying and surface concentrations were higher at 24 and 48 hours when compared to 1 hour after spraying (Currie et al., 1990). Entry in to unventilated rooms after spraying within 24 hours can cause ill-health.

Following the use of OP agents in homes, symptoms could develop within 36 h in about 25% of children (Zweiner and Ginsburg, 1988). These intoxications in children probably follow skin absorption from contaminated skin, contaminated carpets and linen. These are rare events and involve small numbers compared to occupational and intentional poisonings. However, such occurrences need to be documented in order to ensure adherence to safety protocols.

In children, treatments of head lice may occasionally cause toxicity (Opawoye and Haque, 2000).

Another potential source of accidental poisoning is from No-pest strips (dichlorvos) and flea collars. Davis et al. (1992) observed that families in Missouri failed to recognise and reduce insidious exposures from such sources. Pest strips containing dichlorvos may lead to chronic exposure as a study in an experimental room (chamber) revealed indoor air concentration values exceeding accepted daily intake (Weis et al., 1998)

17.8. Intentional Poisoning

Intentional ingestion of OPs for the purpose of self-harm is essentially a developing world phenomenon (Eddleston *et al.,* 1998; Eddleston, 2000). It is particularly concerning because the incidence is rising and many deaths involve OP agents considered as hazardous by the WHO and restricted in the West. Deliberate self-poisoning occurs predominantly in young age groups (16–30 yrs) (Senanayake, 1998; Karalliedde and Senanayake, 1986) although there appears to be increasing numbers in all age groups over the age of 14. The widespread availability of OP agents, the lack of safe storage facilities, and the publicity given to deaths associated with OP ingestion are important aetiological factors.

Studies of self-harm with pesticides have been numerous, in particular from Asia and especially from Sri Lanka (reviewed in Eddleston, 2000). Case series have been reported from all parts of the tropics. OPs have become the self-harm poison of choice in multiple regions—from Guyana in the 1960s (Nalin, 1973) to Japan in the 1990s (Eddleston, unpublished observations). In some parts of the world, for example Sri Lanka, an increase in incidence of self-harm with OP pesticides has coincided with an increase in deaths from self-harm.

A study during 1995 and 1996 recorded 2559 adults admitted with acute poisoning to Anuradhapura General Hospital, Sri Lanka—a secondary referral centre for 900,000 people. Of these patients, 325 (12.7%) died; OPs and carbamates were responsible for 914 admissions and 199 deaths. They placed a heavy burden on the hospital's ITU, OP poisoned patients occupied 41% of the medical intensive care beds during this period. While the mean case fatality rate for OPs was 22%, it reached 60% during some months (Eddleston *et al..,* 1998). Review of hospital records and those of the National Health Statistics Office revealed a 4-fold increase in case number between 1984 and 1995 (Eddleston *et al.,* 1998; 1999).

In a study of cause of death from 37,125 death certificates issued in the district of Kandy, (population 1,048,317 in the 1981 census) Sri Lanka over 20 years showed that 77% of the deaths due to poisoning were due to pesticides. Nearly 50% of the deaths occurred outside the city limits, at homes or in small rural hospitals. Mortality due to pesticide poisoning showed an increasing trend during the 20 years from 11.8 deaths/1000 deaths to 43 deaths/1000 deaths. This trend was most obvious in the rural areas in the district where deaths due to pesticides rose from 8/1000 to 70/1000 (Senanayake and Peiris, 1995).

There are many socio-cultural aspects associated with oral intake of OP agents with suicidal intent. While ease of access is important, there appear to be other cultural factors that determine which poison will be used. In a study of immigrant workers in Saudi Arabia and Kuwait, it was the Asian workers who most frequently ingested OPs. Similarly, in the multiethnic communities of Fiji and Africa, it was Asians who most often chose OPs for suicide (Mahgoub *et al.*, 1990; Mowbray, 1986).

17.9. Homicidal Poisonings

Globally, homicidal OP poisoning is unusual. However, in certain districts of Bangladesh, these pesticides appear to have become a common method for homicide. OP poisoning was reported to be more often due to homicide than to self-harm in these communities (Khan *et al.*, 1985; Begum *et al.*, 1989).

The most recent report of homicidal use was from Iceland (Bjornsdottir and Smith, 1999) where a South African religious leader reported ill-health probably after OP intoxication.

17.10. Concluding Remarks

Although the exact numbers remain contentious, it is clear that pesticide related ill-health in general, and OP associated ill-health in particular present an international public health problem. Its global epidemiology raises several issues. The international organisations such as the FAO and WHO, together with the pesticide industry, have been actively attempting to improve the safety of pesticide use in the developing world.

In 1982, the FAO started writing an International Code of Conduct on the Distribution and Use of Pesticides - this was adopted formally in 1985. The code is voluntary and aims "to increase international confidence in the availability, regulation, marketing and use of pesticides". This work by the FAO and industry coincided with great public disquiet about pesticide use in the tropics after the publication of 'A growing problem: pesticides and the third world poor' by David Bull. In particular this code stated that "pesticides whose handling and application require the use of uncomfortable and expensive protective clothing and equipment should be avoided, especially in the case of small scale users in tropical climates".

Each country has its own unique pattern of legislation, registration schemes and enforcement. The FAO has been supported by the pesticide industry (through its trade association GCPF—formerly GIFAP) and the WHO to develop a scheme for harmonisation of requirements for registration. Again with the WHO, the FAO is also working to harmonise schemes for approval, classification and labelling of pesticides and to develop values for Accepted Daily Intake (ADI). The FAO's Plant Production and Protection Division has established a programme to help developing countries safely dispose of obsolete pesticide stocks.

The World Health Organization through its Office of Occupational Health recommends global strategies and programmes for occupational health in various sectors, including agriculture. The Environmental Health Programme and the International Programme on Chemical Safety (IPCS-WHO/ILO/UNEP) publish detailed safety and health information about aspects of environment and chemicals. The IPCS has over the years developed programmes and protocols for harmonised collection of data on poisoning. Further, IPCS has conducted workshops and seminars in developing countries for teaching and training of trainers in the prevention and management of poisoning. The Council of Europe and the European Union are active in developing and enforcing legislation associated with the registration and use of pesticides. The Codex Committee on Pesticide Residues is active in developing guidelines for residue limits of pesticides on foodstuffs. The industry itself has set up Safe Use Projects in Kenya, Thailand, and Guatemala to improve pesticide use and safety (Ellis, 1998).

Thus there is no apparent lack of effort and enthusiasm to minimise the health hazards of pesticides. However, even though these efforts have been going on for 20 years in some cases, their effectiveness has been limited. More and more people are dying from OP pesticide poisoning each year.

In northern districts of Sri Lanka for example, a country that has recently passed legislation aiming to improve pesticide safety, cases admitted to hospital continue to rise markedly (4-fold between 1985 and 1995) (Eddleston *et al.*, 1999).

It is clearly necessary to re-examine past and present strategies for prevention and find improved ways with which to not only prevent further increases in poisoning incidence but also drastically reduce the current unacceptable level of morbidity and mortality.

The following strategies are worthy of consideration:

1. Epidemiological studies to facilitate audit: OP poisoning is prevalent in diverse cultures, socio-economic groups and climates. Several countries where the incidence is high do not have the structure or the resources for accurate record keeping. There is an urgent need for better epidemiological studies, at least to provide realistic assessments of the magnitude of the problem. It could be argued that it is known to be a major health problem and such studies would be a waste of resources. However, good epidemiological studies are necessary to make accurate assessments of benefits or changes, particularly following the implementation of programmes for prevention or control.

2. Training of junior medical staff: The junior medical officers who offer the first line of care in many countries do not receive any training in the management of poisoning and there are no programmes of continuing medical education in toxicology. Most junior doctors rely on their meagre exposure to toxicology during the undergraduate curriculum and to outdated medical texts to manage patients (Karalliedde, 2000). It has been recognised that a major problem is the failure or delay in associating symptoms and signs with pesticide poisoning by medical personnel (Richter and Safi, 1997; Mbakaye et al., 1994; Forget, 1991). Toxicology is not a recognised speciality in several of these countries. Continuing education in the form of seminars and conferences organised by international organisations are often unavailable to these young doctors. Texts and journals or any form of current literature is not affordable by nearly all junior doctors of developing countries. It is necessary to focus training and teaching to the medical personnel who actively manage the patients.

3. Provision of equipment and essential medications to peripheral hospitals: The lack of facilities for mechanical ventilation and of essential medications necessitate the movement of very sick patients on arduous journeys to institutions where such facilities exist.

The economies of developing countries are stretched by provision of care for diseases like malaria, tuberculosis, gastro-intestinal disorders and often cannot cope with the additional demands made by poisoning. For example, Nepal, a country with a population of 22 million has a national supply of less than 25 functioning mechanical ventilators for all patients (Karalliedde, 2000). International organisations should focus their attention on peripheral or rural hospitals with a view to equipping such institutions with the essentials for management of poisoning. Pesticide poisoning is essentially a rural phenomenon.

4. Health education: Strategies for health education should take into consideration the dialects, social and cultural attitudes and the literacy rates of the communities targeted. There do not appear to be any universal formulae. The medical officers require information regarding the pesticides that are used in a particular region. In most instances, the pesticide to which exposure has taken place is not known with certainty which causes delays and on occasions inappropriate treatment. All products available with information facilitating their identification should be available to all medical personnel.

5. Safety precautions and training of workers: Accidental and occupational poisonings could be realistically minimised or eliminated even in developing countries. This could be achieved by appropriate health education and training strategies modulated to suit particular communities. Posters, news papers, radio broadcasts or television programmes provide choices from which selection should be practical and strategic. Aspects such as labelling, use of personal protective equipment, guidelines for safe use etc would prove effective if appropriate for the community.

6. Guide lines for treatment: Nationally or regionally agreed guidelines for management should be available to all medical and nursing staff. The situation is not eased by the controversies that exist in OP poisoning management amongst those with expertise in the field. For example, controversy still exists as to the efficacy, timing and dosage of oxime therapy. However, broad principles of management can be agreed upon and circulated in preference to protocols developed by individuals which may not receive widespread acceptance.

7. Industry supplying OP pesticides should develop and expand systems for providing suitable educational programmes to communities where their products are used.

8. National Governments or State Administrators need to coordinate and streamline its regulatory and administrative functions in order to create a coherent framework for promotion of chemical safety in agriculture (London and Myers, 1995).
9. International agreement is necessary, urgently, to ban the manufacture of at least the pesticides classified as Extremely Hazardous by the IPCS/WHO.

Acknowledgement

We wish to acknowledge the work of Gráinne Cullen, whose literature searches and initial work helped immensely in the preparation of this chapter.

References

Abebe, M. Organophosphate pesticide poisoning in 50 Ethiopian patients. *Ethiopian Medical Journal* 1991;**29**:109–18.

African Newsletter on Occupational Health and Safety 1999:9:FIOH, Helsinki, Finland

Ames, R.G., Steenland, K, Jenkins, B., *et al.* Chronic neurologic sequelae to cholinesterase inhibition among agricultural pesticide applicators. *Archives of Environmental Health* 1995;**50**:440–4.

Ambridge, E.M., Haines, I.H., Lambert, M.R. Operator contamination during pesticide application to tropical crops. *Medicina del Lavoro* 1990;**81**:457–62.

Amr, M.M., Halim, Z.S. and Moussa, S.S. Psychiatric disorders among Egyptian pesticide applicators and formulators. *Environmental Research* 1997;**73**:193–9.

Anas, A.N., Jusoh, M.M., Heong, K.L., *et al.* A field observation of lever operated knapsack sprayers owned by the rice farmers in the Muda irrigation scheme. In *Proc. International Conference on Pesticides in Tropical Agriculture*, Kuala Lumpur, Malaysian Plant Protection Society 1987.

Baker, E.L., Warren, M., Zack, M., *et al.* Epidemic malathion poisoning in Pakistan Malaria workers. *Lancet* 1978;**i**:31–4.

Bazylewicz-Walczak, B., Majczakowa, W., Szymczak, M. Behavioural effects of occupational exposure to organophosphorus pesticides in female greenhouse planting workers. *Neurotoxicology* 1999;**20**:819–26.

Begum, J.A., Choudhury, M.M. and Ara, G. A study of poisoning cases in four hospitals of Bangladesh. *Bangladesh Medical Journal* 1989;**18**:60–4.

Berger, L.R. Suicides and pesticides in Sri Lanka. *American Journal of Public Health* 1988;**78**:826–8.

Bhalla, A., Jajoo, U. Food poisoning due to organophosphorus compounds. *National Medical Journal of India* 1999;**12**:90.

Bidstrup, P.L., Bonnell, J.A., Beckett, A.G. Paralysis following poisoning by new organic phosphorus insecticide (mipafox). *British Medical Journal* 1953;**1**:1068.

Bjornsdottir, U.S., Smith, D. South African religious leader with hyperventilation, hypophosphataemia and respiratory arrest. *Lancet* 1999;**354**:2130.

Cantor, K.P., Silberman, W. Mortality among aerial pesticide applicators and flight instructors: follow up from 1965–1988. *American Journal of Industrial Medicine* 1999;**36**:239–47.

Chang Yen, I., Bekele, I., Kalloo, C. Use patterns and residual levels of organophosphate pesticides on vegetables in Trinidad, West Indies. *Journal of AOAC International* 1999;**82**:991–5.

Chaudhry, R., Lall, S.B., Mishra, B., *et al.* A foodborne outbreak of organophosphate poisoning. *British Medical Journal* 1998;**317**:268–9.

Chee, Y.L. Poisoning women workers. Ecoforum: A publication of the *Environmental Liaison Centre International*, Global Coalition for Environment and Development 1990;**14**:5.

Choudhry, A.W. Health hazards of pesticide use in Africa. In: Lehitnen S, Kurppa K, Korhonew E, Saarinen eds. Proceedings of the East Africa Regional symposium on Chemical accidents and Occupational Health. Institute of Occupational Health, Helsinki, 1989. p. 70–4.

Coetzee, G.J. *The epidemiology of pesticide mortality in the Western Cap'.* Cape Town: Department of Community Health, University of Cape Town 1981.

Cole, D.C., Carpio, F., Julian, J., *et al.* Assessment of peripheral nerve function in an Ecuadorial rural population exposed to pesticides. *Journal of Toxicology Environmental Health* Part A 1998;**55**:77–91.

Cole, D.C., Carpio, F., Julian, J., *et al.* Neurobehavioural outcomes among farm and non farm rural Ecuadorians. *Neurotoxicology and Teratology* 1997;**19**:277–86.

COTT Report: Committee on Toxicity of Chemicals in Food, Consumer products and the Environment. Organophosphates. Department of Health UK 1999.

Cook, R.R. Health effects of organophosphate sheep dips. *British Medical Journal* 1992;**305**:1502–3.

Coyle, M.J., Fenske, R. Agricultural workers. In: Levy, B.S. (ed). *Critical choices for South Africa—An agenda for the 1990s*. Cape Town: Oxford University Press 1988.

Curtis, C. Personal communication 2000.

Currie, K.L., McDonald, E.C., Chung, L.T., *et al.* Concentrations of diazinon, chlorpyrifos and bendiocarb after application in offices. *American Industrial Hygiene Association Journal* 1990:51:23-7.

Daniell, W., Barnhart, S., Demers, P., *et al.* Neuropsychological performance among agricultural pesticide applicators. *Environmental Research* 1992;**59**:217–28.

Davies, D.R. Neuropsychological effects of exposure to sheep dip. Letter. *Lancet* 1995;**345**:1632.

Department of Manpower. Occupational Health and Safety Act. Government Gazette 337; No 14918. Pretoria. Government Printers 1993.

Dimich-Ward, H., Dittrick, M., Graf, P. Survey of malathion exposure among elevator and dock workers who handle grain. *Canadian Journal of Public Health* 1996;**87**:141–2.

Dinham, B. The Pesticide Hazard. The Pesticide Trust. Zed Books, London. 1993 with the country reports from **Brazil**: Reinaldo Onofre Skalisz : State Council for Defence of the Environment, Gert Roland Fischer (PAN Brazil), Onaur Ruano. **Costa Rica**: Luisa .E.Castillo and Catharina Wesseling (Programa de Plaguicidas:Desarrollo, Salud y Ambiente (PPUNA), Universidad Nacional, Heredia, Costa Rica. **Ecuador**: Ing. Agr. Mercedes Bollandos (Fundacion Natura) **Paraguay**: Jorge Abbate (Alter Vida) **Venezuela**: Porfiria Mendonza de Linares(CIDELO, Lara) **Egypt**: Dr El Sebae, Professor AA Abdel-Gawaad South Africa: Kate Emanuel (Environment and Development Agency and Group for Environmental Monitoring, Johannesburg). **India**: Dr Daisy Dhamaraj (PREPARE, Madras), Dr A.T.Dudani, Sanjoy Sengupta (Voluntary Health Association, India) **Malaysia**: Pesticide Action Network (PAN) Asia and Pacific.

Eddleston, M. Patterns and problems of deliberate self-poisoning in the developing world. *Quarterly Journal of Medicine* 2000; in press.

Eddleston, M., Ariaratnam, C.A., Meyer, W.P., *et al.* Epidemic of self-poisoning with seeds of the yellow oleander tree (*Thevetia peruviana*) in northern Sri Lanka. *Tropical Medicine and International Health* 1999;**4**:266–73.

Eddleston, M., Sheriff, M.H., Hawton, K. Deliberate self-harm in Sri Lanka—an overlooked tragedy in the developing world. *British Medical Journal* 1998;**317**:133–5.

Ellis, W.W. Private-public sector co-operation to improve pesticide safety standards in developing countries. *Medicina del Lavoro* 1998;**89**:S112–S122.

Emanuel, K. *'Poisoned Pay: Farmworkers and the South African Pesticide Industry'*. Johannesburg: Group for Environmental Monitoring and the Pesticide Trust. 1992.

Engel, L.S., Keifer, M.C., Checkoway, H. *et al.* Neurophysiological function in farm workers exposed to organophosphate pesticides. *Archives of Environmental Health* 1998;**53**:7–14.

Fernando R. Pesticide poisoning in Asia-Pacific region and the role of a regional information network. *Journal of Toxicology Clinical Toxicology* 1995:3:677-82.

Ferrer, A., Cabral, R. Toxic epidemics caused by alimentary exposure to pesticides: a review. *Food Additives and Contaminants* 1991;**8**:755–75.

Fischer, A.B., Eikmann, T. Improper use of an insecticide at a kindergarten. *Toxicology Letters* 1996;**88**:359–64.

Foo, G.S. The pesticide poisoning report: A survey of some Asian countries. Malaysia: International Organization of Consumers Unions. 1985.

Food and Agriculture Organisation of the United Nations. International Code of Conduct on the Distribution and Use of Pesticides. *Rome: Food and Agriculture Organisation of the United Nations*. 1990.

Forbat, J.N., Skehan, J.D. Health effects of organophosphate sheep dips. *British Medical Journal* 1992;**305**:1503.

Forget, G. Pesticides and the third world. *Journal of Toxicology and Environmental Health* 1991;**32**:11–31.

Gadon, M. Pesticide poisonings in the lawn care and tree service industries. A review of cases in the New York State Pesticide Poisoning Registry. *Journal of Occupational and Environmental Medicine* 1996:38:794-9.

Gomes, J., Lloyd, O.L., Revitt, D.M. The influence of personal protection, environmental hygiene and exposure to pesticides on the health of immigrant farm workers in a desert country. *International Archives of Occupational and Environmental Health* 1999;**72**:40–5.

Greenaway, C. and Orr, P. A foodborne outbreak causing a cholinergic syndrome. *Journal of Emergency Medicine* 1996;**14**:339–44.

Gunn, D.L., Stevens, J.G.R. *Pesticides and human welfare*. Oxford University Press 1976.

Gupta, S., Govil, Y.C., Misra, P.K., *et al.* Trends in poisoning in children: Experience at a large referral teaching Hospital. *National Medical Journal of India* 1998;**11**:166–8.

Harari, R, Forastiere, F., Axelson, O. Unacceptable " occupational" exposure to toxic agents among children in Ecuador. *American Journal of Industrial Medicine* 1997:**32**:185-9.

Haynes, I.H. Problems of pesticide storage in developing countries. *Chemistry and Industry* 1985;**16**:621-3.

Health Bulletin, Department of Health, Sri Lanka 1999.

Henao, S., Finkelman, J., Albert, L., *et al.* De plaguicidas y salud en las Americas. Mexico, DF, *Centro Panamericano de Ecologia Humana y Salud*: 1993.

Hernberg S. Foreward. In: *Occupational Health in Developing Countries*. Jeyaratnam, J. ed. Oxford Medical Publications 1992.

Holmes, J.H., Gaon, M.D. Observations on acute and multiple exposure to anticholinesterase agents. *Trans American Clinical Association* 1956;**68**:86-101

IPCS, International Programme on Chemical safety. Multilevel course on the safe use of pesticides and on the diagnosis, treatment of pesticide poisoning. WHO/IPCS/94.3. Geneva: *World Health Organization,* 1994.

Jeyaratnam, J. Acute pesticide poisoning: a major global health problem. *World Health Statistics Quarterly* 1990;**43**:139-44.

Jeyaratnam, J. Acute poisonings caused by chemicals. In: *Proceedings of the International Symposium on Health and Environment in Developing Countries*, Haikko, Finland, 1986. Institute of Occupational Health, Helsinki. 1986. p. 39-44.

Jeyaratnam, J., Chia, K.S. *Occupational Health in National Development*. World Scientific. Singapore. 1994.

Jeyaratnam, J. Health problems of pesticide usage in the Third World. *British Journal of Industrial Medicine* 1985;**42**:505-6.

Jeyaratnam, J. *Occupational Health in Developing Countries. Oxford Medical Publications*. Oxford University Press. 1992.

Jeyaratnam, J., De Alwis Senewiratne, R.S., Copplestone, J.F. Survey of pesticide poisoning in Sri Lanka. *Bulletin of the World Health Organisation* 1982;**60**:615-9.

Jeyaratnam, J., Lun, K.C., Phoon, W.O. Survey of acute pesticide poisoning among agricultural workers in four Asian countries. *Bulletin of the World Health Organisation* 1987;**65**:521-7.

Jusoh, M., Anas, A.N., Heong, K.L., *et al.* Features of lever operated knapsack sprayer considered important by the Muda rice farmers in deciding which sprayer to buy. In Proceedings of International Conference on Pesticides in Tropical Agriculture, Kuala Lumpur, Malaysian Plant Protection Society 1987.

Karalliedde, L. Report to WHO SEARO, IPCS and Guys and St Thomas Hospital Trust. Retrospective Survey 1999–2000.

Karalliedde L, Senanayake N. Acute organophosphorus insecticide poisoning: a review. *Ceylon Medical Journal* 1986;**31**:93–100.

Kasilo, O.J., Hobane, T., Nhachi, F.B. Organophosphate poisoning in urban Zimbabwe. *Journal of Applied Toxicology* 1991;**11**:269–72.

Keifer, M., McConnell, B., Pacheco, A.F., *et al.* Estimating underreported pesticide poisoning in Nicaragua. *American Journal of Industrial Medicine* 1996:**30**:195–201.

Khan, N.I., Sen, N. and Al-Haque, N. Poisoning in a medical unit of Dhaka Medical College Hospital in 1983. *Bangladesh Medical Journal* 1985;**14**:9–12.

Kimani, V.N. Mwanthi, M.A. Agrochemicals exposure and health implications in Githunguri location, Kenya. *East African Medical Journal* 1995:**72**:531-5.

Kishi, M., Hirschhorn, N., Djajadisastra, M *et al.*. Relationship of pesticide spraying to signs and symptoms in Indonesian farmers. *Scandinavian Journal of Work and Environmental Health* 1995;**21**:124–33.

Lakew, K., Mekonnen, Y. The health status of northern Omo State Farm workers exposed to chlorpyrifos and profenofos. *Ethiopian Medical Journal* 1998;**36**:175–84.

Lau, F.L. Vegetable-borne pesticide poisoning. *Hong Kong Practitioner* 1990;**12**:1193-7.

Leveridge Y., R. Pesticide poisoning in Costa Rica during 1996. *Veterinary and Human Toxicology* 1998;**40**:42–4.

Levine, R. S. Assessment of mortality and morbidity due to unintentional pesticide poisonings. Unpublished Doc WHO/VBC 186–929. Quoted by Levine and Doull (1992).

Levine, R.S., Doull, J. Global estimates of acute pesticide morbidity and mortality. *Review Environment Contamination and Toxicology* 1992;**129**:29–50.

Lichtenberg, E., Zimmerman, R. Adverse health experiences, environmental attitudes, and pesticide usage behavior of farm operators. *Risk Analysis* 1999;**19**:283–94.

Litovitz, T.L., Smilkstein, M., Felberg, L., *et al.* 1996 Annual report of the American Association of Poison Control Centers Toxic Exposure Surveillance System. *American Journal of Emergency Medicine* 1997;**15**:447–500.

London, L. Agrichemical hazards in the South African farming sector. *South African Medical Journal* 1992a;**81**:560–4.

London, L. Pesticide safety on farms in the Stellenbosch area. Report to the Health Department, Stellenbosch Division of the Western Cape Regional Services Council. Cape Town: Department of Community Health, University of Cape Town 1992b.

London, L., Myers, J.E. Agrichemical hazards and the work process in agriculture in the Western Cape. Occupational Health Research Unit report No 1. Cape Town: Department of Community Health, University of Cape Town, Rondesbosch 1993.

London, L., Myers, J.E. Critical issues for Agrichemical safety in South Africa. *American Journal of Industrial Medicine* 1995;**27**:1–14.

Mahgoub, O.M., Al-Freihi, H.M., Al-Mohaya, A.M., *et al.* Deliberate self-harm in the migrant population in the Eastern Province of Saudi Arabia. *Saudi Medical Journal* 1990;**11**:473–7.

Maizlish, N., Schenker, M., Weisskopf, C., *et al.* A behavioural evaluation of pest control workers with short-term, low-level exposure to the organophosphate diazinon. *American Journal of Industrial Medicine* 1987;**12**:153–72.

Mbakaya, C.F.L., Ohayo-Mitoko, G.J.A., Ngowi, V.A.F., *et al.* The status of pesticide usage in East Africa. *African Journal of Health Sciences* 1994;**1**:37–41.

McConnell, R., Hruska, A.J. An Epidemic of Pesticide Poisoning in Nicaragua: Implications for Prevention in Developing Countries. *American Journal of Public Health* 1993;**83**:1559–62.

McConnell, R., Keifer, M., Rosenstock, L. Elevated quantitative vibrotactile threshold among workers previously poisoned with methamidophos and other organophosphate pesticides. *American Journal of Industrial Medicine* 1994;**25**:325–34.

McDougall, L., Magloire, L., Hospedales, C.J., *et al.* Attitudes and practices of pesticide users in Saint Lucia, West Indies. *Bulletin Pan American Health Organisation* 1993;**27**:43-51.

Misra, U.K., Nag, D.,Khan, W.A., *et al.* A study of nerve conduction velocity, late responses and neuromuscular synapse functions in organophosphate workers in India. *Archives of Toxicology* 1988;**61**:496–500.

Moses, M. Pesticides. In: *Environmental and Occupational Medicine.* Rom, W.R. ed. Boston: Little Brown and Company. 1983. p. 547–71.

Mowbray, D.L. Pesticide poisoning in Papua New Guinea and the South Pacific. *Papua New Guinea Medical Journal* 1986;**29**:131–41.

Murray, V.S., Wiseman, H.M., Dawling, S., *et al*. Health effects of organophosphate sheep dips. *British Medical Journal* 1992;**305**:1090.

Mwanthi, M.A., Kimani, V.N. Health hazards of pesticides. *World Health Forum* 1990:**11**:430.

Nalin, D.R. Epidemic of suicide by malathion poisoning in Guyana. Report of 264 cases. *Tropical and Geographical Medicine* 1973;**25**:8–14.

Niven, K.J.M, Robertson, A., Waclowski, E.R., *et al*. Occupational hygiene assessment of exposure to insecticides and effectiveness of protective clothing during sheep dipping operations (Report TM/94/04). Edinburgh, UK, *Institute of Occupational Medicine* 1994 (revised 1996).

Ngowi, A.V.F. The evaluation of the effects of pesticides on farm workers in the coffee growing areas of Tanzania. MSc. Thesis. *University of Manchester, UK*, 1997.

Ngowi, A.V.F., Maeda, D.N., Stephens, J. East Africa Pesticide network project. EAPN-Tanzania. Technical Report. September, 1989–June 1994. *Tropical Pesticides Research Institute*, Arusha, Tanzania 1994.

O'Brien, S.J., Cambell, D.M., Morris, G.P. Neuropsychological effects of exposure to sheep dip. Letter. *Lancet* 1995;**345**:1632.

OECD. Guidance Document for the Conduct of Studies of Occupational Exposure to Pesticides During Agricultural Application. OECD Environmental and Safety Publications, Series on Testing and Assessment, No 9. Paris: Environmental directorate, *Organisation for Economic Co-operation and Development* 1997.

Ohayo-Mitoko, G.J.A., Heederik, D.J.J., Kromhout, H., *et al*. Acetylcholinesterase inhibition as an indicator of organophosphate and carbamate poisoning in Kenyan Agricultural workers. *International Journal of Occupational and Environmental Health* 1997;**3**:210–20.

Opawoye, A.D. and Haque, T. Insecticide/organophosphorus compound poisoning in children.http:/www.kfshrc.edu.sa/annals/182/97-225.html.

Organizacion Internacional del Trabajo. Los asalariados agricolas: condiciones de empleo y de trabajo. Oficina Internacional del grabajo, programa de Activadades Sectoriales, Ginebra, Suiza, TMAWW:1996.

Otto, D.A., Sollman, S., Svendagaard, D., *et al*. Neurobehavioural assessment of workers exposed to organophosphorus pesticides. In: Advances in Neurobehavioural Toxicology: Applications in Environmental and Occupational Health. Johnson, B.L., Anger, W.K., Durao, A., Xintaras, C. eds Lewis Publishers; Michigan, 1990. p. 306–22.

Parron, T., Hernandez, A.F., Villanueva, E. Increased risk of suicide with exposure to pesticides in an intensive agricultural area. A 12 year retrospective study. *Forensic Science International* 1996;**79**:53–63.

Perold, J.G., Bezuidenhout, D.J.J. Chronic organophosphate poisoning. *South African Medical Journal* 1980;**57**:7–9.

Pesticide News, 1996, 1998.

Pickett, W., King, W.D., Lees, R.E., *et al.* Suicide mortality and pesticide use among Canadian farmers. *American Journal Industrial Medicine* 1998;**34**:364–72.

Ratner, D., Oren, B., Vigder, K. Chronic dietary anticholinesterase poisoning. *Israel Journal of Medical Sciences* 1983;**19**:810–4.

Rees, H. Exposure to sheep dip and the incidence of acute symptoms in a group of Welsh sheep farmers. *Occupational and Environmental Medicine* 1996;**53**:258–63.

Richter, E.D., Safi, J. Pesticide use, exposure and risk: A joint Israeli-Palestinian Perspective. *Environmental Research* 1997;**73**:211–8.

Richter, E.D., Chuwers, P., Levy, Y., *et al.* Health effects from exposure to organophosphate pesticides in workers and residents in Israel. *Israel Journal of Medical Sciences* 1992;**28**:584–98.

Richter, E.D., Kowalski, M., Leventhal, A., *et al.* Illness and excretion of organophosphate metabolites four months after household pest extermination. *Archives of Environmental Health* 1992;**47**:135–8.

Senanayake, N., Peiris, H. Mortality due to poisoning in a developing agricultural country: trends over 20 years. *Human and Experimental Toxicology* 1995;**14**:808–11.

Senanayake, N. Organophopshorus insecticide poisoning. *Ceylon Medical Journal* 1998;**43**:22–9.

Shihab, K. Malathion poisoning among spray-men. *Bulletin Endemic Diseases* 1976;**17**:69–74

Sims, P. Health effects of organophosphate sheep dips. *British Medical Journal* 1992;**305**:1502–3.

Singh Surjit. Personal Communication 2000.

Soliman, S.A., Sovocool, G.W., Curley, A., *et al.* Two acute human poisoning cases resulting from exposure to diazinon transformation products in Egypt. *Archives of Environmental Health* 1982;**37**:207–12.

Steenland, K., Dick R.B., Howell, R.J., *et al.* Neurologic function among termiticide applicators exposed to chlorpyrifos. *Environmental Health Perspectives* 2000;**108**:293–300.

Stephens, R., Spurgeon, A., Calvert, I., *et al.* Neuropsychological effects of long-term exposure to organophosphates in sheep dip. *Lancet* 1995;**345**:1135–9

Stokes, L., Stark, A., Marshall, E., *et al.* Neurotoxicity among pesticide applicators exposed to organophosphates. *Journal of Occupational and Environmental Medicine* 1995;**52**:648–653.

Svendsgaard, D., Soliman, S., Otto, D., *et al.* Assessment of neurotoxicity in workers occupationally exposed to organophosphorus pesticides. Research Triangle Park. NC.US Environmental Protection Agency 1988 (EPA document CR-811178).

Ting, S.M., Chan, T.Y.K., Wong, W.K.K., *et al.* Acute methamidophos poisoning caused by contaminated green leafy vegetables. *Southeast Asian Journal of Tropical Medicine Public Health* 1993;**24**:402–3.

Veterinary Medicines Directorate. Suspected Adverse Reaction Surveillance Scheme. Report to the Veterinary Products Committee of Suspected Adverse Reactions received 1985-1998 and the Findings of the appraisal panel for Human Suspected Adverse Reactions from meetings in 1998. 1999. Addlestone.

Ward, M.H., Nuckols, J.R., Weigel, S.J., *et al.* Identifying populations potentially exposed to agricultural pesticides using remote sensing and a Geographic Information system. *Environmental Health Perspectives* 2000;**108**:5–12.

Watt, A.H. Letter. Neuropsychological effects of exposure to sheep dip. *Lancet* 1995;**345**:1631.

Weinbaum, Z., Schenker, M.B., O'Malley, M.A., *et al.* Determinants of disability in illness-related to agricultural use of organophosphates (OPs) in California. *American Journal of Industrial Medicine* 1995;**28**:257–74.

Weis, N., Stolz, P., Kroos, J., *et al.* Dichlorvos insect strips indoors: pollution and risk assessment. *Gesundheitwesen* 1998;**60**:445–9.

Wesseling, C., McConnell, R., Partanen, T., *et al.* Agricultural pesticide use in developing countries: Health effects and research needs. *International Journal of Health Services* 1997;**27**:273–308.

WHO (World Health Organization). Safe use of pesticides. Twentieth report of the WHO expert committee on insecticides. WHO Technical Report Series, No 513. World Health Organization, Geneva. 1973.

WHO. Informal consultation on planning strategy for the prevention of pesticide poisoning. WHO/VBC/86.296. World Health Organization, Geneva 1986.

Working Group on Organophosphates of the Committee on Toxicity of Chemicals in Food, Consumer Products and Environment (Department of Health UK 1999).

World Health Organization. IPCS, Chemical Safety, Fundamentals of Applied Toxicology, Training Module 1, Appendix 2. World Health Organisation, Geneva 1992.

World Health Organization. Public health impact of pesticides used in agriculture. Geneva: World Health Organization, 1990.

World Health Organization. WHO Recommended Classification of Pesticides by Hazard and Guidelines to Classification 1992. World Health Organisation, Geneva 1993.

Zwiener, R.J., Ginsburg, M. Organophosphate and carbamate poisoning in infants and children. *Pediatrics* 1988;**81**:121–6.

INDEX